Practical Atlas of Ruminant and Camelid Reproductive Ultrasonography

Practical Atlas of Ruminant and Camelid Reproductive Ultrasonography

Editor-in-chief

Luc DesCôteaux, D.M.V., M.Sc., Dipl. ABVP (Dairy)
Professor
Ambulatory clinic of ruminant health management
Faculté de médecine vétérinaire
Université de Montréal
St-Hyacinthe (Québec)
CANADA

Associate Editors

Giovanni Gnemmi, D.V.M., Dipl. ECBHM
BovineVet
Premosello Chiovenda
ITALY

Jill Colloton, D.V.M.
Bovine Services, LLC
Wisconsin
USA

WILEY-BLACKWELL
A John Wiley & Sons, Inc., Publication

Edition first published 2010

Blackwell Publishing was acquired by John Wiley & Sons in February 2007. Blackwell's publishing program has been merged with Wiley's global Scientific, Technical, and Medical business to form Wiley-Blackwell.

Editorial Office
2121 State Avenue, Ames, Iowa 50014-8300, USA

For details of our global editorial offices, for customer services, and for information about how to apply for permission to reuse the copyright material in this book, please see our website at www.wiley.com/wiley-blackwell.

Library of Congress Cataloging-in-Publication Data

Practical atlas of ruminant and camelid reproductive ultrasonography / editor-in-chief, Luc DesCôteaux ; associate editors, Giovanni Gnemmi, Jill Colloton.
p. ; cm.
Includes bibliographical references and index.
ISBN-13: 978-0-8138-1551-0 (alk. paper)
ISBN-10: 0-8138-1551-7 (alk. paper)
1. Veterinary obstetrics–Atlases. 2. Ruminants–Generative organs–Ultrasonic imaging–Atlases. 3. Camels–Generative organs–Ultrasonic imaging–Atlases. I. DesCôteaux, Luc. II. Gnemmi, Giovanni. III. Colloton, Jill.
[DNLM: 1. Genital Diseases, Female–veterinary–Atlases. 2. Pregnancy, Animal–Atlases. 3. Reproductive Techniques, Assisted–veterinary–Atlases. 4. Ruminants–Atlases. 5. Ultrasonography–veterinary–Atlases. SF 887 P895 2010]
SF887.P67 2010
636.2'0898047543–dc22

2009015928

A catalog record for this book is available from the U.S. Library of Congress.

Set in 10/12.5pt Palatino by SNP Best-set Typesetter Ltd., Hong Kong

Drawings by Caroline DesCôteaux

TABLE OF CONTENTS

PREFACE

Ultrasound enables us to see what we cannot hear. If a picture is worth 1,000 words, a live, three-dimensional, ultrasonographic image can tell an even more compelling and accurate story. Ultrasonography has added a new dimension to the traditional physical examination, including transrectal palpation, of the reproductive tract.

Ultrasonographic technology has made major strides during the last quarter of a century. However, mastering the skill and art of ultrasonography requires patience, diligence, and persistence, which generally means a slow learning curve. *Practical Atlas of Ruminant and Camelid Reproductive Ultrasonography* was conceived and developed to facilitate the learning process. The three primary authors assembled an international team of 25 experienced collaborators from 11 different countries to produce a comprehensive treatise on the use of ultrasonography in the management of reproduction in cattle, sheep, goats, water buffalo, zebu, and camelids. Cattle are the reference model for reproductive technology as it has been for all species in the areas of artificial insemination, embryo transfer, in vitro fertilization, nucleus transfer, and cloning. It is nice to see that economic species beyond *Bos taurus* are included.

Chapters 1 and 2 guide practitioners and researchers through the basic principles and guidelines of ultrasonography and scanning techniques. Anatomy of the bovine reproductive tract, with special emphasis on the ovary and the uterus, is reviewed in Chapters 3, 4, and 5. Thus the stage is set to focus on pregnancy diagnosis and detection of twins (Chapter 6), evaluation of fetal viability and fetal gender determination (Chapter 7), and advanced reproductive technology (ET, IVF, cloning) (Chapter 8). Chapter 9 addresses the breeding soundness evaluation (BSE) of the bull, and Chapters 10, 11, and 12 highlight the water buffalo, small ruminants, and camelidae, respectively. The detailed information and perspective of more than 450 illustrations (ultrasound images, photographs, and drawings) throughout the *Atlas* reflect the collective knowledge and expertise of the coauthors of the respective chapters. A helpful didactic feature is the inclusion of a summary of practical aspects to remember at the end of each chapter.

In the 21st century, owners expect and demand more from their veterinarians with respect to technology and procedures concerning specific assessment of the reproductive status of their animals, i.e., early pregnancy diagnosis, fetal viability, and ovarian activity. An exciting aspect is that the readily available equipment can be taken to the farm. The benefits of an accurate diagnosis justify the expense of the equipment and the expertise, while the sonographer reaps the benefits of satisfaction and motivation to be on the cutting edge of technology.

The *Atlas* also provides glimpses of new or alternative methods when it discusses the use of color Doppler ultrasonography to study angiogenesis and its role in fetal development, and the use of a small curvilinear probe. *Practical Atlas of Ruminant and Camelid Reproductive Ultrasonography* is a valuable global educational resource because it fine-tunes reproductive programs. Visual learning is superior to verbal learning, and the knowledge acquired by visual learning is retained better. The *Atlas* abounds with more than 400 authentic images.

Congratulations to the editor-in-chief, Dr. Luc DesCôteaux, associate editors Dr. Giovanni Gnemmi and Dr. Jill Colloton, and their coauthors, whose diligent work has resulted in a premier publication.

Maarten Drost D.V.M., Dipl. ACT
Theriogenologist
University of Florida
www.drostproject.vetmed.ufl.edu

Acknowledgments

To my wife Michèle and our children, Caroline, Anick, and Francis, who supported me and showed immense patience while this very long project was brought to fruition.

To my employer, the Université de Montréal, which allowed me a sabbatical in order to concentrate on this book project and improve my network of contacts in the field of ruminant reproductive ultrasonography.

To Jill and Giovanni, my friends and associate editors, for their open-minded attitude, ideas, experience, generosity, and encouragement.

To the authors of each chapter, who were willing to share their knowledge and expertise to offer this practical guide for use in all fields of ruminant reproduction.

To the École Nationale Vétérinaire de Toulouse, where I spent my sabbatical and received all necessary assistance. I will treasure my memories of this hospitable, sunny, and windswept corner of France, whose hills and valleys provide the ideal environment for a long-distance triathlon devotee.

To Anick, Caroline, and Andréanne, for their help in processing countless illustrations.

To all future readers for your commitment to furthering your understanding and expertise in ultrasonography in order to sharpen your decision-making abilities in an increasingly competitive practice environment.

And to all whom I might have forgotten to mention and yet who provided their precious assistance and encouragement, I extend my most sincere thanks.

Luc DesCôteaux

Introduction

Four years ago, my two associate editors and I came up with the idea of creating a practical guide to ultrasound imaging in ruminant and camelid reproduction. Our goal was straightforward: to assemble a practical, concise, and well-illustrated reference document for veterinary practitioners and teachers who want to use ultrasound technology, currently the most efficient and least invasive diagnostic tool, with the ultimate goal of improving reproductive performance in ruminants.

Practical Atlas of Ruminant and Camelid Reproductive Ultrasonography is a unique aid to learning and covers reproduction in all small and large ruminants: domestic, companion, and exotic (buffalo and zebu); male and female; and camelids. It is the fruit of efforts in international teamwork, combining the expertise of 25 authors, all specialists in related fields.

Whether it is read on a per subject basis or used as a reference for special situations in practice, this book contains many useful features. There are tables of ultrasound markers that can be used as guides during the reproductive examination, and the *Atlas* can be placed beside the imaging unit for handy reference. The important practical aspects to remember are presented at the end of each chapter, and several multiple-choice questions provide readers with the opportunity to evaluate their comprehension.

This guide provides valuable assistance in setting up a diagnostic imaging service in your everyday practice to take the most appropriate and responsible approaches to treatment, offer new and specialized services to your clients, and open doors to a new clientele.

Luc DesCôteaux, D.M.V., M.Sc., Dipl. ABVP (Dairy)
Editor-in-chief

From the Associate Editors

Ultrasonography in production animal reproduction has progressed over the years from a technique used by a small group of elite farmers and veterinarians to an opportunity accessible to everyone anywhere in the world. The cosmopolitan origin of the coauthors of *Practical Atlas of Ruminant and Camelid Reproductive Ultrasonography* is proof of this. Furthermore, the *Atlas* is an ideal bridge between the world of research and the world of practice. One cannot exist without the other.

Only through real cooperation and deep intellectual discussion is it possible to build the foundation for constructive growth. This is the spirit that led us to produce this work. The editor-in-chief, associate editors, and coauthors have varying opinions, which sometimes led to difficult debates, but always we remained loyal to the goal and open to each other's ideas.

Today I cannot think of any production animal reproduction management system that does not benefit from ultrasonography. Veterinarians, producers, and researchers must keep this in mind as we learn how to maximize the value of ultrasound in production animal reproduction.

Change requires a huge effort, mostly intellectual. The *Atlas* is an apologia to skeptics who think it is possible to function adequately without ultrasonography.

My sincere thanks go to all our coauthors, who are pioneers in this art and extraordinary experts in their fields.

Luc DesCôteaux has been an indefatigable orchestra director. Without his patience and especially his tenacity this work would still be only an idea. Jill Colloton is a great practitioner whose daily work in the field develops into extraordinary ideas for research. She is not afraid to debate with those of different opinions or to alter her thinking when they produce logical arguments.

It has been an honor to take part in producing this book. It has enabled me to grow through interaction with my colleagues. Even more importantly, it has allowed me to share with our readers my extraordinary enthusiasm for this remarkable technique. Thanks to all of you.

Giovanni Gnemmi, D.V.M., Dipl. ECBHM
Associate Editor

As a "plain vanilla" D.V.M. it has been a terrific honor for me to be involved with *Practical Atlas of Ruminant and Camelid Reproductive Ultrasonography*. It says much about our profession that the finest minds in practice, research, and academia are not only willing but quite eager to converse with their colleagues in the field. I encourage every reader of the *Atlas* to communicate with the editors, coauthors, and authors listed in the References section at the end of each chapter. Bovine reproductive ultrasound has advanced greatly since its inception, but the field is still in relative infancy. Input from practitioners and producers will drive research to the most productive path.

I am proud to be part of a profession that values field veterinarians, producers, university academicians, and corporate researchers equally. I am also proud to be associated with people who dedicate their precious time with little recompense to advance our profession. Luc DesCôteaux devoted an entire sabbatical year to organizing, editing, writing, and promoting this book. Giovanni Gnemmi found time beyond his busy practice, teaching, and travels to write, research, and contact potential coauthors. These coauthors contributed their time and expertise without ever asking "What's in it for me?" Thank you all for a job well done!

Jill Colloton, D.V.M.
Associate Editor

Contributors

Dr. Gregg ADAMS, professor
Veterinary Biomedical Sciences, Western College of Veterinary Medicine, University of Saskatchewan, Saskatoon, Saskatchewan, Canada

Dr. Heinrich BOLLWEIN, professor
Clinic of Cattle, University of Veterinary Medicine, Hannover, Germany

Dr. Sébastien BUCZINSKI, professor
Département de sciences cliniques, Faculté de médecine vétérinaire, Université de Montréal, Québec, Canada

Dr. Paul D. CARRIÈRE, professor
Département de biomédecine, Faculté de médecine vétérinaire, Université de Montréal, Québec, Canada

Dr. Sylvie CHASTANT-MAILLARD, professor
Unité de Reproduction, École Nationale Vétérinaire d'Alfort, Maisons-Alfort, France

Dr. Jill COLLOTON
Bovine Services, LLC, Wisconsin, USA

Dr. Heraldo Marcus Rosi CRUVINEL
Instituto Federal de Educação Ciência e Tecnologia do Triangulo Mineiro—Campus Paracatu, Paracatu—State of Minas Gerais, Brazil

Dr. Sandra CURRAN
Ultrascan, Inc., Madison, Wisconsin, USA

Dr. Luc DESCÔTEAUX, professor
Département de sciences cliniques, Faculté de médecine vétérinaire, Université de Montréal, Québec, Canada

Dr. Jean DUROCHER
Dairy herd health coordinator, Valacta (Québec DHI), St-Hyacinthe, Québec, Canada

Dr. Véronique GAYRARD, professor
Physiologie et Thérapeutique, École Nationale Vétérinaire de Toulouse, Toulouse, France

Dr. Giovanni GNEMMI
BovineVet, Premosello Chiovenda, Italy

Dr. Antonio GONZALEZ-BULNES
Departamento de Reproduccion Animal, Instituto Nacional de Investigacion y Tecnologia Agraria y Alimentaria, Madrid, Spain

Dr. Réjean C. LEFEBVRE, professor
Département de sciences cliniques, Faculté de médecine vétérinaire, Université de Montréal, Québec, Canada

Dr. Graeme B. MARTIN, professor
Institute of Agriculture, The University of Western Australia, Crawley, Australia

Dr. Motozumi MATSUI, professor
Department of Clinical Veterinary Medicine, Obihiro University of Agriculture and Veterinary Medicine, Obihiro, Japan

Dr. Akio MIYAMOTO, professor
Graduate School of Animal and Food Hygiene, Obihiro University of Agriculture and Veterinary Medicine, Obihiro, Japan

Dr. Víctor H. PARRAGUEZ, professor
Departamento Ciecias Biologicas Animales, Facultad de Ciencias Veterinarias, Universidad de Chile, Santiago, Chile

Dr. Nicole PICARD-HAGEN, professor
Pathologie de la reproduction, École Nationale Vétérinaire de Toulouse, Toulouse, France

Dr. Luis A. RAGGI, professor
Departamento Ciecias Biologicas Animales, Facultad de Ciencias Veterinarias, Universidad de Chile, Santiago, Chile

Dr. Marcelo RATTO, professor
Department of Animal Science, Faculty of Veterinary Sciences, Universidad Austral de Chile, Valdivia, Chile

Dr. Sebastiano SALE
Medico Veterinario, Dorgali (NU), Italy

Dr. Francisco SALES ZLATAR
Instituto de Investigaciones Agropecuarias (INIA), Centro Regional de Investigacion Kampenaike, Punta Arenas, Chile

Dr. Brad STROUD
Stroud Veterinary Embryo Services, Weatherford, Texas, USA

Dr. Carolina VIÑOLES-GIL
Programa de carne y lana, Instituto Nacional de Investigacion Agropecuaria, Tacuarembo, Uruguay

Practical Atlas of Ruminant and Camelid Reproductive Ultrasonography

CHAPTER ONE

Principles and Recommendations, Essential Concepts, and Common Artifacts in Ultrasound Imaging

Véronique Gayrard, Paul D. Carrière, and Luc DesCôteaux

Introduction

This chapter outlines the principles of ultrasound imaging using recommendations and fundamental concepts that are the basis of ultrasound use in theriogenology. The first part describes the different characteristics of ultrasound equipment with regard to image quality and the different uses of ultrasound in female reproduction in ruminants. The second part expands on the general principles of ultrasound imaging; these concepts are essential to understanding how image quality and diagnostic value can be improved according to the characteristics and imaging modes of the different types of ultrasound equipment. The third part presents the principal artifacts encountered when inspecting the genital organs. Understanding these artifacts is essential in forming a rational interpretation of an ultrasound examination and improving diagnostic accuracy.

Description and Practical Recommendations in the Choice of Ultrasound Equipment with a View to Image Quality

The ultrasound apparatus consists of a probe that is connected by a cable to a console. The console includes an electronic case, a command keyboard, and a monitor with an imaging screen (Figure 1.1). A

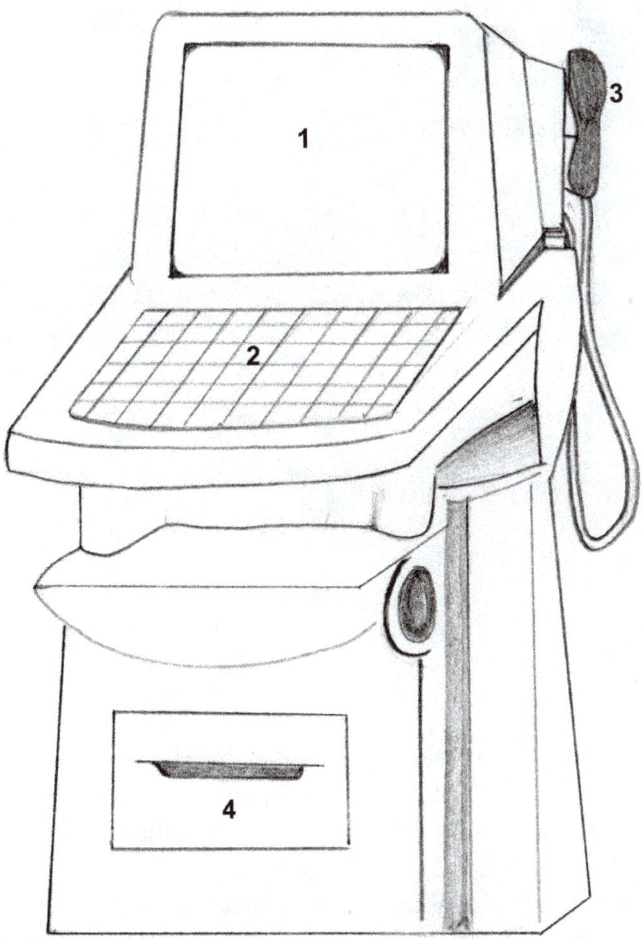

Figure 1.1. Principal components of the ultrasound apparatus. 1: Monitor; 2: Command keyboard; 3: Probe; 4: Printer.

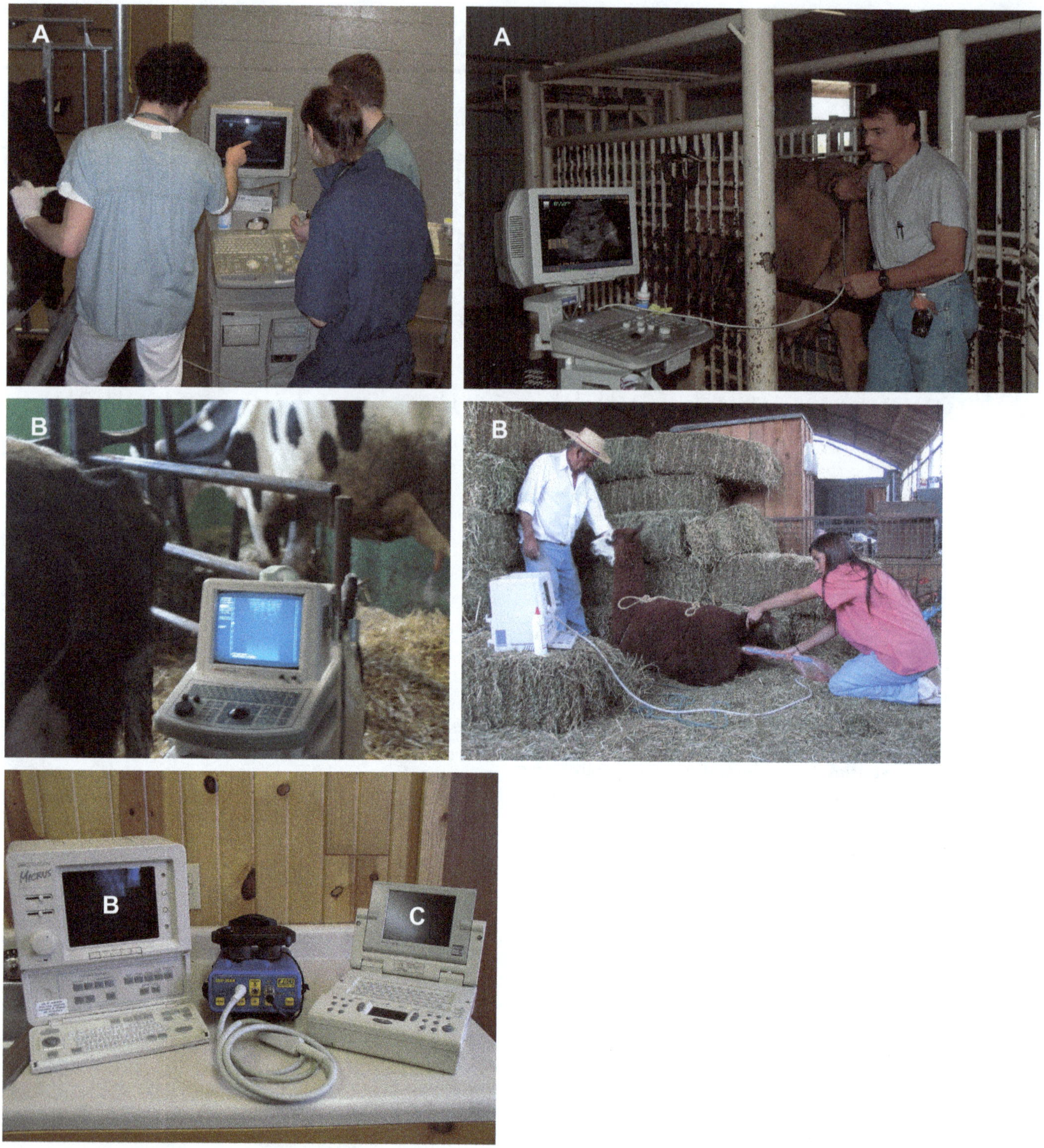

Figure 1.2. The different types of ultrasound units. A: Nontransportable hospital grade ultrasound unit; B: Transportable hospital grade ultrasound unit; C: Portable ultrasound unit.

voltage regulator located between the electric cable and the apparatus prevents damage to the electronic system caused by fluctuations in electric potential, particularly during electric storms. Three overall categories of equipment are used in female ruminant reproduction: nontransportable hospital grade ultrasound units, transportable hospital grade ultrasound units that can be used on farms, and portable ultra-

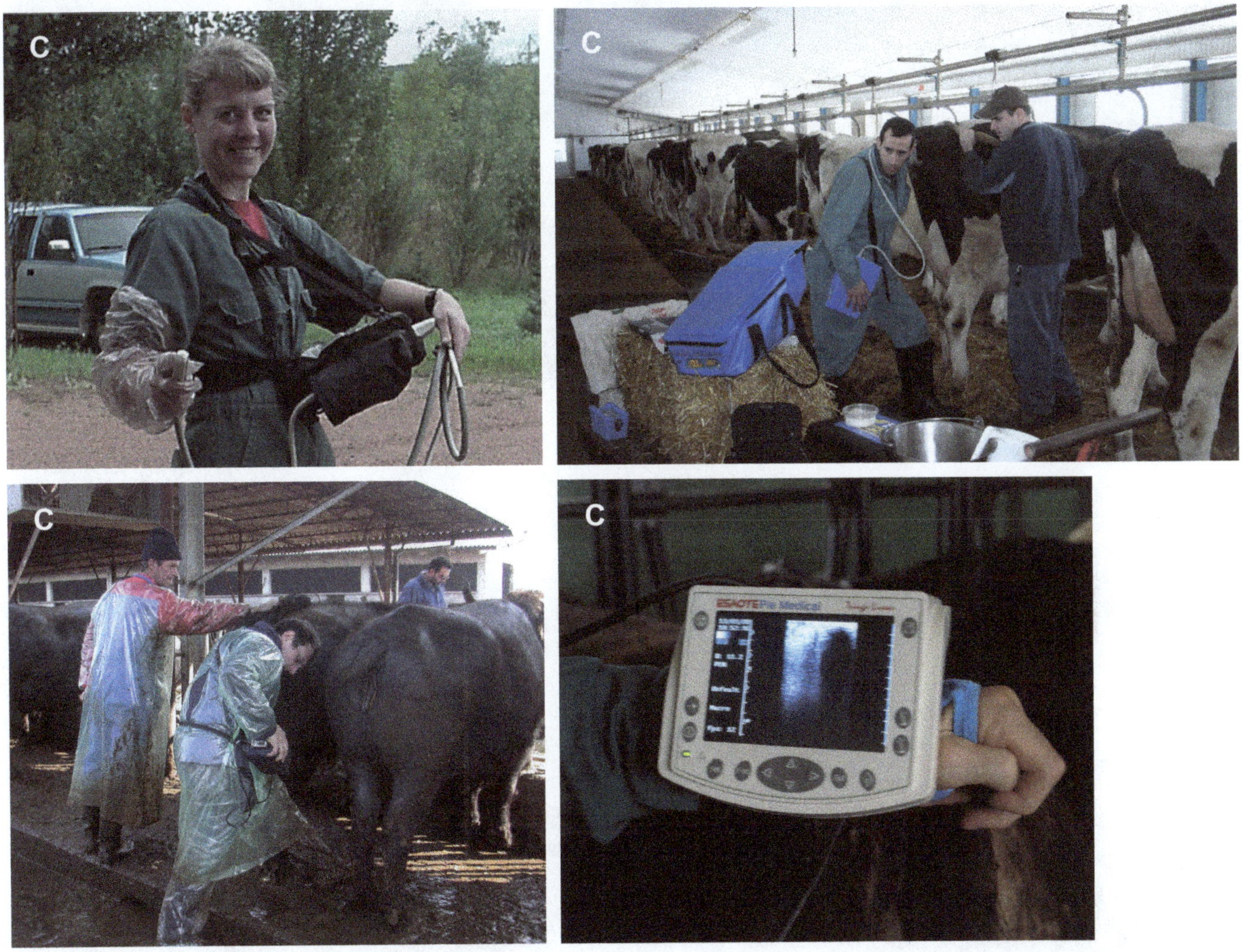

Figure 1.2. *Continued*

sound units (Figure 1.2). The quality of the ultrasound images depends essentially on the characteristics of the probe and the way the ultrasound image is processed.

Choosing a probe

The probe is made of crystals with piezoelectric properties (quartz, certain ceramics). The crystals dilate and contract when electrical impulses are applied, with a frequency in the order of magnitude of their own resonance frequency, which produces an ultrasound wave.

Probe types

Probes are classified according to whether they provide a linear or sector scan of the tissue section with the ultrasound beam[1,4,7,10] (Figures 1.3, 1.4). Linear scan probes contain a large number of crystals (128–256) aligned along the longitudinal axis of the probe over a length of 5 to 15 cm. The section is scanned electronically by sequential ignition of the crystals along the probe. Linear scan probes generate a rectangular-shaped image of constant and sufficient width to cover the region being examined. A larger zone can be viewed if the crystals are placed on a convex surface. This is the case with a convex or curved linear probe that generates an image which could be as large as the one produced by a linear probe at the surface, but which expands with the depth of the image.

Mechanical sector probes contain a small number of rotating crystals, a single crystal with an oscillating mirror, or a single oscillating crystal. Sector probes produce a fan-shaped image that is very narrow at the surface and which expands with depth (Figure 1.4).

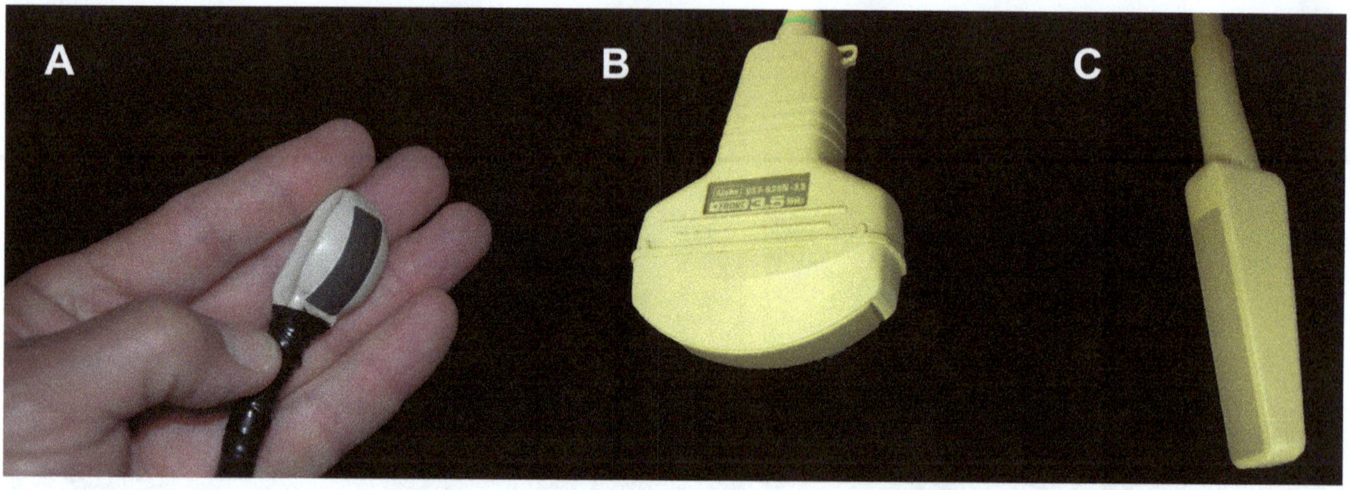

Figure 1.3. The different types of probes. A: Convex or curved linear probe; B: Sector probe; C: Linear probe.

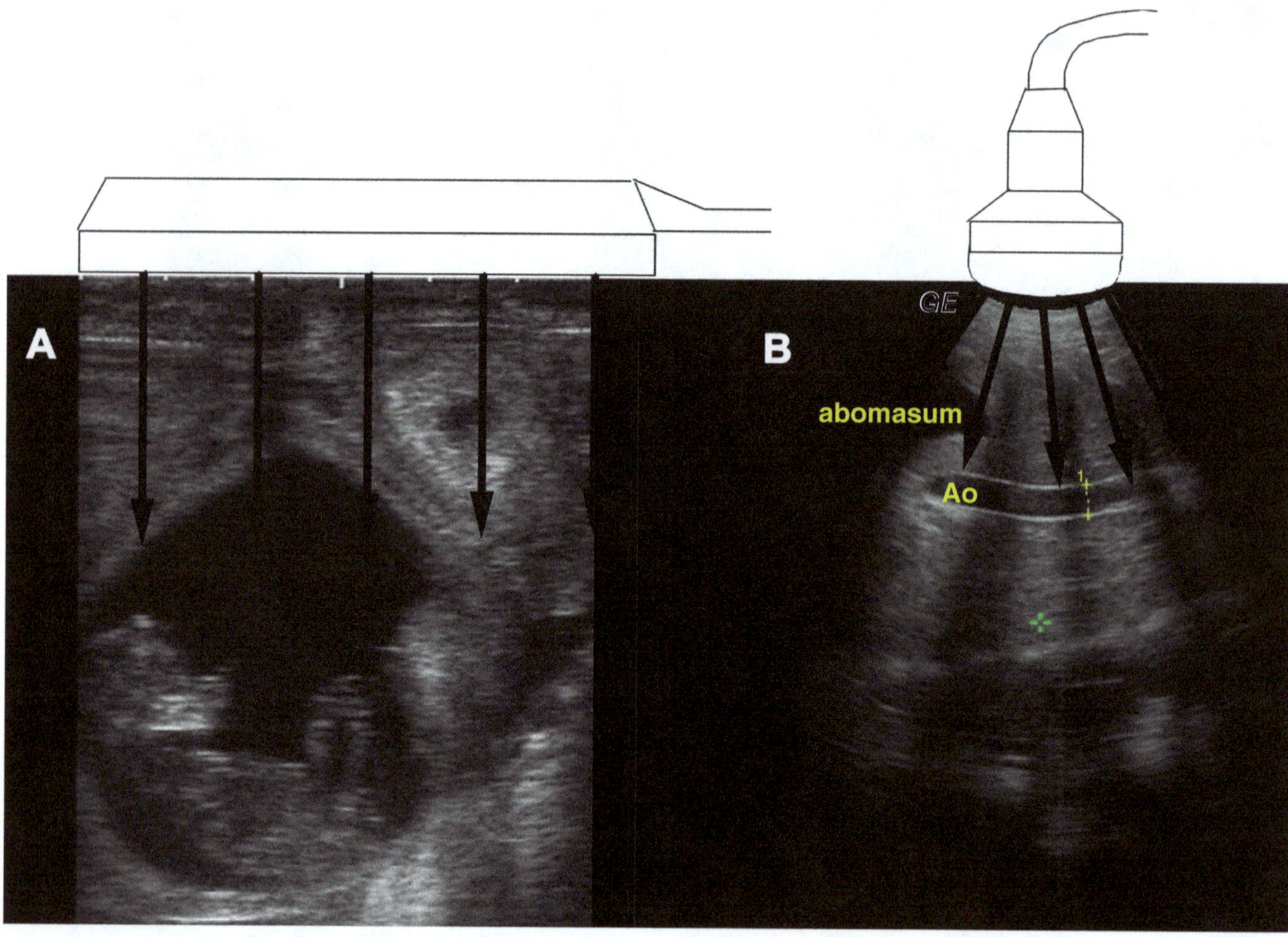

Figure 1.4. The different probe types and their scanning surface. A: Linear probe; B: Sector probe.

Table 1.1.
Advantages, disadvantages, and principal use of the different probe types in theriogenology

Probe Types	Sector Probe	Linear Probe	Convex or Curved Linear Probe
Advantages	Small surface of contact in the near field	High resolution in the near field	High resolution in the near field
Disadvantages	Weaker resolution in the near field	Greater surface of contact	Good surface of contact but smaller than the linear probe Divergence in the far field
Use	Intravaginal probe in small ruminants Transvaginal folliculocentesis in cattle for in vitro fertilization Abdominal examination in small ruminants Evaluation of fetal health in advanced gestation of cattle	Rectal probe for most large ruminants (males and females) Examination of the testicles	Evaluation of the ovaries in superovulation Preferred by some practitioners for transrectal examination of the reproductive system

This allows the veterinarian to view large structures located deep in the body and to produce images through narrow acoustic windows, such as between two ribs. With electronic sector probes the crystals are aligned but the resulting image is identical to the one obtained with a convex or curved linear probe. Sector scans are obtained by a phase difference in the signals transmitted and received by the crystals. The linear scan probes are preferred for transrectal ultrasound examinations of bovine reproductive organs because their shape permits safer manipulation in the rectum. Most linear probes have grooves or indicators that facilitate manipulation in terms of properly orienting the probe. Table 1.1 presents the advantages, disadvantages, and main uses of the different types of probes in theriogenology.

Frequency and power of resolution

The frequency represents the number of crystal oscillations per second (number of hertz, Hz) and depends on the crystal's characteristics (type and thickness of the matter). The frequencies used in medical imaging are between 2 and 10 megahertz (MHz), where 1 MHz is 1 million cycles per second, 50 times greater than the maximum frequency of audible sound by the human ear—hence the name *ultrasound*. The high bandwidth probes with a broad-spectrum frequency (from 4 to 8 MHz) emit different frequencies depending on the electrical impulse applied. These probes, like multifrequency probes with crystals of different resonant frequencies, allow variations in frequency without having to change probes.

Axial resolution

Frequency has a major influence on image quality because it controls the axial resolution, the equipment's ability to discriminate between two structures located close together on the ultrasound propagation axis[4,5] (Figure 1.5). To obtain good axial resolution a high frequency is required, but because penetration is inversely proportional to frequency it is the depth of examination that guides the choice of the probe frequency[2] (Table 1.2).

Lateral resolution

Lateral resolution is the equipment's ability to distinguish between two adjacent structures that are located at the same depth. Lateral resolution depends on the diameter of the ultrasound beam, which varies according to the probe's frequency and the depth of observation. To improve lateral resolution the ultrasound beam diameter is decreased by focalization[3] (Figure 1.6). The best lateral resolution is obtained in the focal zone, a short distance (a few cm) on each side of the focal point, which corresponds to the center of the narrowest part of the focalized ultrasound beam. The focal distances of the probes used in transrectal ultrasound are 7.0, 3.5, and 2.0 cm deep for the respective frequencies of 3.5, 5.0, and 7.5 MHz[4]. In the first approach good quality images can be obtained at up to twice the focal distance. The number and depth of the focalization points can be set at or below the depth of the objects to be viewed. It should be noted that setting multiple focal points decreases frame rate.

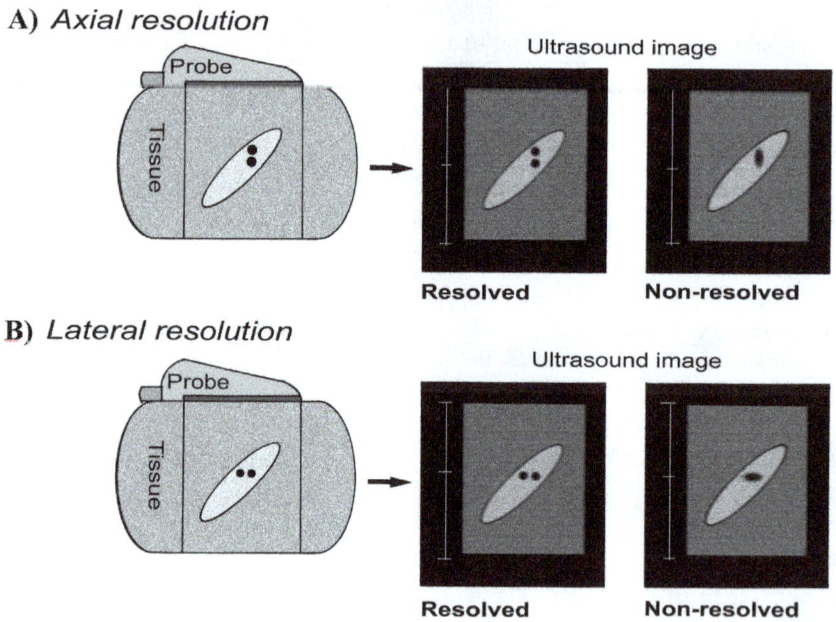

Université de Montréal

Figure 1.5. Ultrasound image resolution (illustration by Dr. Guy Beauregard). A: Axial resolution—capacity to distinguish between two nearby structures that are located along the ultrasound wavelength propagation axis; B: Lateral resolution—capacity to distinguish between two nearby structures located at the same depth.

Table 1.2.
Characteristics and indications of probes with different frequencies used in theriogenology

3 MHz	5 MHz	7.5 MHz
Best field depth (0–20 cm)	Intermediate field depth (0–12 cm)	Reduced field depth (0–7 cm)
Lower resolution	Good resolution	Higher resolution
Advanced gestation Postpartum uterus	Routine pregnancy diagnosis Determining fetal sex	Follicles and corpus luteum Early pregnancy diagnosis Determining fetal sex

Table 1.2 recapitulates the characteristics and the indications for the different frequencies used in theriogenology[2].

Image processing

The ultrasound beam emitted by the probe penetrates the tissues of the body where it undergoes numerous reflections. The reflected waves, or echoes, are captured by the probe and the ultrasound information is converted into electronic signals. The analog electronic signals are immediately amplified and then digitalized via an analog-digital converter and sent to the monitor to provide a "live" image in gray scale with 16, 64, or 256 shades of gray (Figure 1.7).

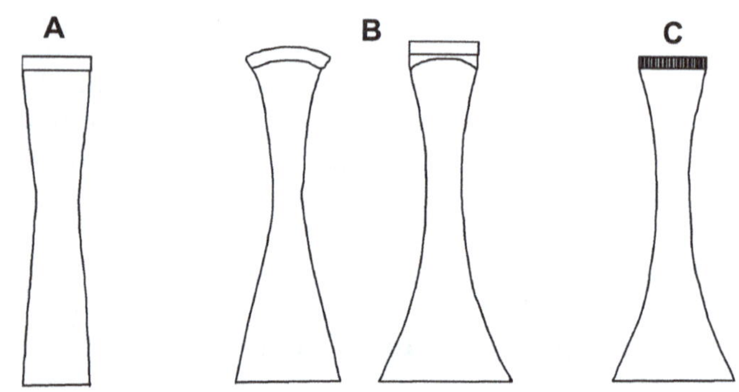

Figure 1.6. Focalization of the ultrasound beam (according to Fishetti and Scott 2007). A: The beam is nonfocalized and expands in the distant field; B: Mechanical focalization obtained by the curve of the crystals or with an acoustic lens; C: Electronic focalization obtained by playing off the delays in the excitation of the crystals.

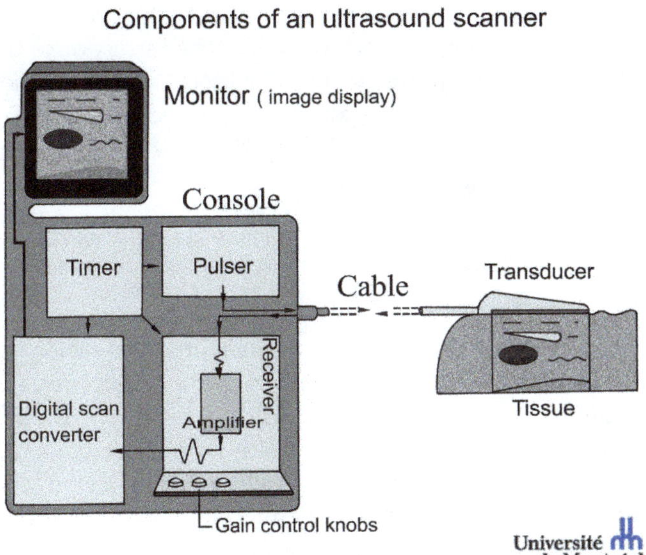

Université de Montréal

Figure 1.7. Ultrasound image processing (illustration by Dr. Guy Beauregard). The ultrasound beam emitted by the piezoelectric crystals from the probe penetrates body tissues where it undergoes numerous reflections. The reflected waves, or echoes, are captured by the probe and the ultrasound information is converted into electronic signals. The analog electronic signals are immediately amplified and then digitalized via an analog-digital converter; then they are sent to the monitor to provide a "live" image in gray scale with 16, 64, or 256 shades of gray. The gain settings that control the level of amplification of the echoes are adjusted by the operator.

The main objective of image processing is to produce images with uniform brightness. The returning echo is a weak signal that needs to be amplified. In particular, the echoes from deeper structures are weaker than those from tissues closer to the surface. Signal amplification increases the amplitude of the echoes to adjust the brightness of the image. Adjustment by the operator is carried out manually by looking at the image. Three gains must be adjusted:

- One gain for the overall image that has the same effect on all echoes (general gain)
- One gain for the near field
- One gain for the distant (deeper) field

An onscreen marker helps highlight the point(s) of focalization. The entire depth or only a part of the image can be viewed with the *zoom* control that magnifies the image. To study an image more carefully, it can be set using the *freeze* control. An image can also be split in two, allowing the user to identify and preserve an image onscreen while continuing the ultrasound examination. The digital images can also be printed, saved, and pulled up to complete patients' medical files.

General Principles and Essential Concepts to Improve Image Quality

Physical properties of ultrasound

A sound wave can be described by its various properties: velocity (v), intensity, length, and frequency. Wave velocity is the speed of pressure variation in the medium; it depends solely on the characteristics of the medium (elasticity, density). In body tissues the average speed of propagation is approximately 1540 m/s, with the exception of bone tissue (4080 m/s) and lung tissue (600 m/s because of the presence of air)[4]. This means that an ultrasound wave is propagated in tissues over a distance of 1.5 mm in 10^{-6} s.

Wave amplitude, which corresponds to the amplitude of particle movement, determines the intensity of the wave. Intensity is the quantity of energy that crosses the unit of surface area per unit of time and is expressed in watts per cm^2 (W/cm^2).

Frequency expresses the number of vibrations of the ultrasound source per unit of time. Frequency is therefore identical to the number of waves that pass through a given point in the medium per second and to the number of times that the particle vibrates per second. The unit of frequency measurement is the hertz (Hz). Ultrasound is defined as being any sound wave with a frequency above 20,000 Hz.

The wavelength (λ), which is characterized by both the wave and the medium through which it passes, measures the spatial extent of one vibration cycle. It is related to frequency (f) and to velocity by the equation $\lambda = v/f$. Therefore, the length of a wave in a water medium (velocity = 1540 m/s) at a frequency of 5 million Hz (5 MHz) is 0.3 mm. The wavelength has a major significance for diagnosis because it determines the axial and lateral resolutions that are respectively in the order of 2 to 4 times and 3 to 10 times the length of the wave[6]. Therefore, at a frequency of 5 MHz the axial and lateral resolutions are respectively included between 0.6 and 1.2 mm, and 0.9 and 3 mm depending on the quality of the apparatus. The greater the frequency the shorter the wavelength, resulting in better axial and lateral resolutions.

How echoes are formed

Ultrasound waves interact with the tissues they penetrate. Reflection produces the echoes that result in the echographic image. Reflection occurs when the ultrasound wave meets an acoustic interface, which is the interface between two media with different acoustic impedances (Figure 1.8). The acoustic impedance (z) of a tissue is the product of the density of the medium (ρ) and the velocity (v):

$$z = \rho \times v \tag{1.1}$$

The acoustic impedance describes the greatest or least resistance of a given medium to the penetration of ultrasound waves. It is weak in air and very high in bone tissue. The relative importance of the intensity of the echo compared to that of the incident wave, i.e., the wave that meets the interface, depends on the value of the interface, which is the difference in acoustic impedance of the media of the interface. Therefore, most of the energy is transmitted through the weaker interfaces and explores the tissues located deeper in the body. Hence, the transmitted wave is less intense than the incident wave. Air and bone impedances are very different from that of soft tissue. In particular, the acoustic impedance of air is much less than soft tissue. Therefore at the soft tissue/air interface, more than 99% of the energy is reflected. For this reason, clipping the hair and using an appropriate gel to minimize air pockets is recommended prior to transabdominal ultrasound examinations.

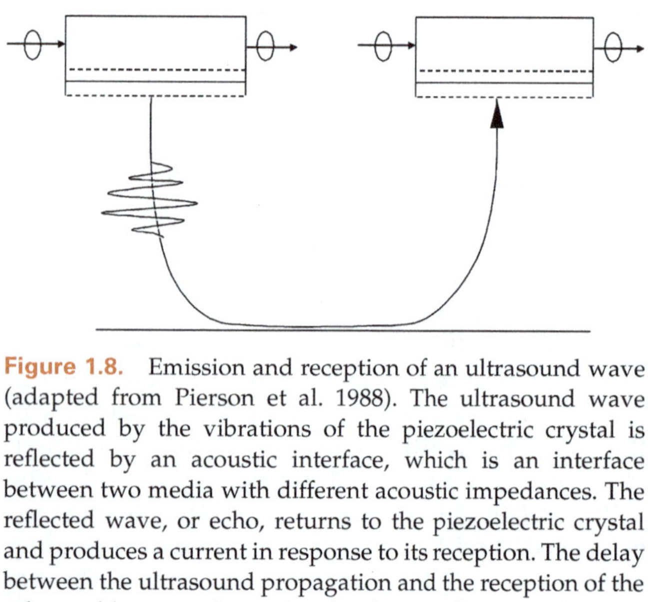

Figure 1.8. Emission and reception of an ultrasound wave (adapted from Pierson et al. 1988). The ultrasound wave produced by the vibrations of the piezoelectric crystal is reflected by an acoustic interface, which is an interface between two media with different acoustic impedances. The reflected wave, or echo, returns to the piezoelectric crystal and produces a current in response to its reception. The delay between the ultrasound propagation and the reception of the echo enables us to determine the distance between the crystals and the interface.

The reflected wave or echo returns to the piezoelectric crystal where it produces a current in response to the perception of the echo. The delay between the ultrasound wave propagation and the reception of the echo enables us to determine the distance between the crystals and the interface.

Attenuation

The energy of the wave is attenuated during its propagation through the tissues. Attenuation corresponds to the decrease in intensity of the wave as it progresses through the tissues, which limits the depth of the tissues that can be explored. Attenuating mechanisms are the interactions during which energy is removed from the incident beam to be either reemitted in different directions (reflection, refraction, diffusion) or absorbed (absorption) by the tissues and transformed into heat (Figure 1.9).

Refraction

Refraction is the deviation of the transmitted ultrasound wave as it is propagated through a medium with a different velocity (soft tissue/liquid interface). Refraction occurs only if the interface is not perpendicular to the wave. The wave reflected at an angle equal to the angle of incidence does not return toward the source of the emission and the transmitted wave is deviated with regard to the incident wave (Figure 1.9C). This phenomenon occurs frequently during examinations of the reproductive system because of the various spherical liquid structures encountered (follicles, embryonic vesicle, ovarian cysts, etc.) The deviation of the transmitted wave by refraction is the source of a visual artifact known as a *shadow cone*, which will be described later.

Diffusion

Diffusion is the reflection of a small fraction of the energy of the ultrasound wave in several directions by targets that are smaller than the wavelength (Figure 1.9B). Diffusion is also observed when the wave hits an irregular surface that effectively decreases the size of the continuous interface.

Absorption

Absorption is the transformation of energy into heat when the wave is propagated in a homogenous medium. Therefore, the ultrasound wave intensity

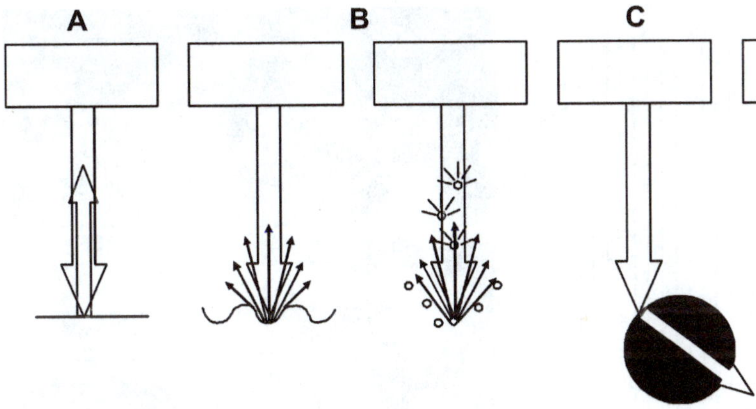

Figure 1.9. The attenuation mechanisms of the ultrasound wave (according to Ginther 1995). A: Reflection is the return of part of the wave (and its energy) in the form of an echo; B: Diffusion is a reemission of the ultrasound energy in all directions due to reflections by small interfaces or a rough surface; C: Refraction is the deviation of the ultrasound wave; D: Absorption is the transformation of ultrasound energy into heat.

decreases exponentially with the depth of penetration in the tissue. Absorption depends on the tissue type: It is very low in liquids and very high in bone and air. The coefficient of attenuation of soft tissue that takes into account both absorption and diffusion is proportional to the frequency and has an average value of 0.5 dB per MHz and per cm[6,7]. Therefore, at equal attenuation levels, the penetration distance of ultrasound is weaker when the frequency is high. Consequently, an increase in frequency reduces the penetrating distance of the ultrasound waves.

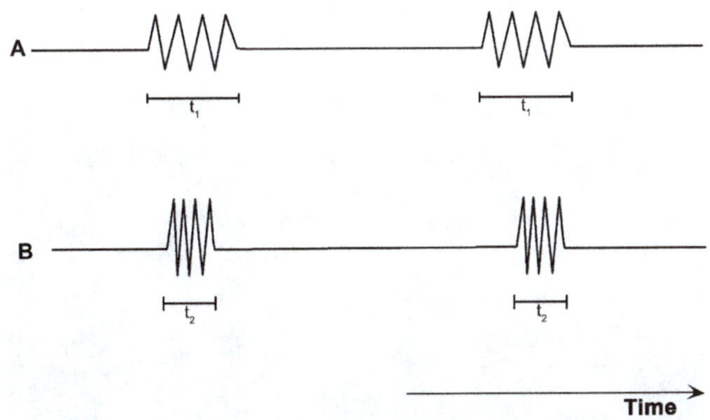

Figure 1.10. Diagram of the ultrasound burst as a function of frequency. The frequency is lower in A than in B. The result is that the duration occupied by the burst t_1 is greater than t_2, the time occupied by a burst emitted with a higher frequency probe. This is due to the fact that a burst is formed by the same number of cycles (3 or 4). We also observe long silences, or time intervals without emission, between two bursts. During these periods of silence the echoes are captured by the probe.

Image formation

The crystal undergoes a series of short electrical impulses that causes a short series of vibrations called a *burst* (Figure 1.10). Intervals of quiescence allow the echoes to be captured by the same crystals. One thousand bursts can be emitted per second, in spite of the pauses between each pulsation. The number of vibrations in a burst is the same (3 to 4) at any frequency. As a consequence, an increase in frequency translates into a decrease in the duration of the burst, thus improving axial resolution. The burst is propagated in the underlying tissues and the volume explored by the burst is called the *sonic beam*.

B-mode (brightness mode) ultrasound refers to the section of the image obtained by automatic, rapid, and sequential scanning of the plane of the section as established by the orientation of the probe[10] (Figure 1.11). In this mode we can produce images of tissue sections that are similar to histological sections of the plane scanned by the ultrasound beam (Figure 1.4). By slowly moving the probe over the area of interest (ovary, fetus, etc.), the veterinarian is able to create a mental and spatial image of the information. This compilation of image sections resulting in a three-dimensional mental image assumes its true importance in determining the sex of the fetus (Chapter 7).

The ultrasound beam will encounter different interfaces and produce detectable echoes. These echoes are

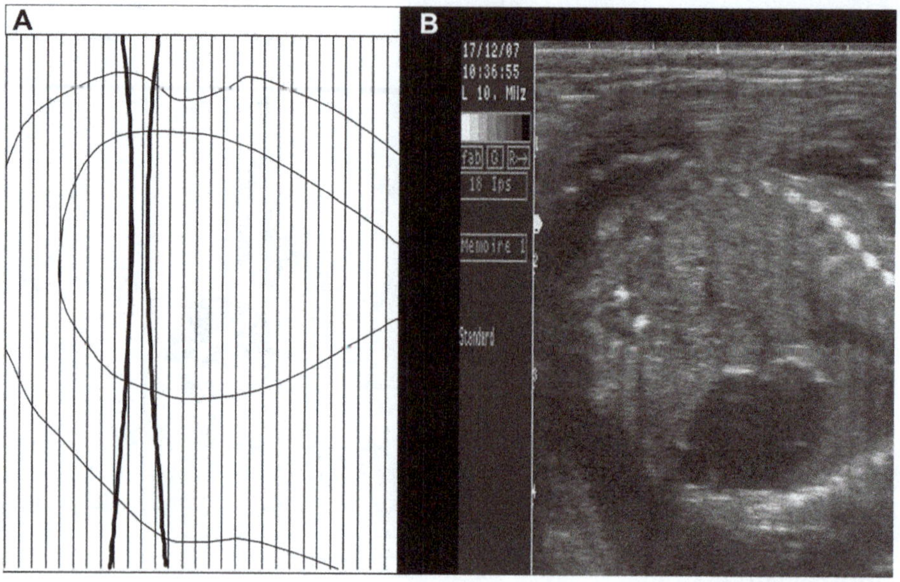

Figure 1.11. Image formation in B-mode or two-dimensional ultrasound (adapted from Whittingham 2007). A: The ultrasound beam moves laterally along the plane of the section with the sequential ignition of a group of crystals. B: Thoracic cage of a fetus (10.0 MHz probe; depth of 5 cm). The information from a beam creates a vertical line on the screen and the image is produced from the echoes coming from the different scan lines that form the plane of the section.

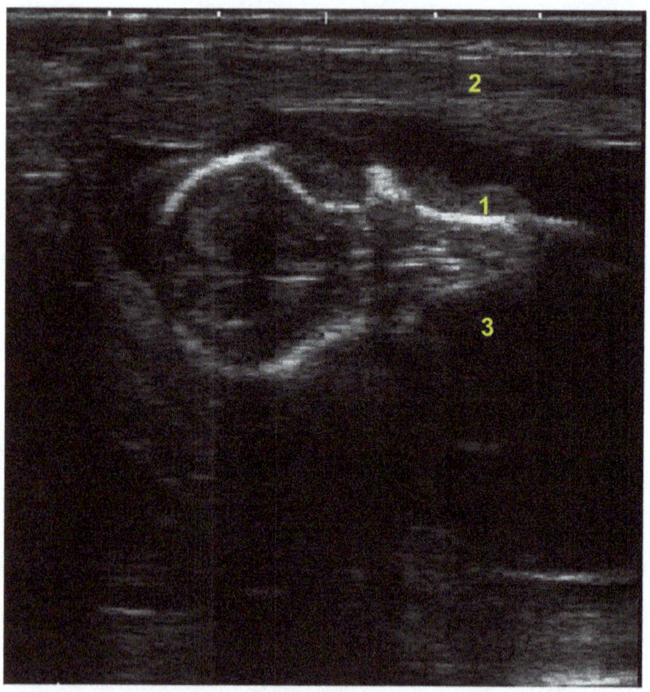

Figure 1.12. Representation of the amplitude of the echo on the head of a 70-day-old fetus, using the gray scale (10.0 MHz probe; depth of 4 cm). 1: Very dense tissue reflector: pixels are bright (white); 2: Intermediately dense tissue reflector: pixels are gray; 3: No reflector: pixels are black. The highly echogenic areas (skull of the fetus) are shown in white on the screen, whereas the nonechogenic structures (amniotic liquid) are shown in black. The structures with intermediate echogenicity (uterine wall) are shown in shades of gray. Each point (pixel) shown on the screen has a brightness that varies somewhere between total (white) and null (black).

processed to produce the ultrasound image, each element of which is called a *pixel*. The image appears on the screen with a depth that is determined by the latency of the return of the echo. The information from a beam produces a vertical line on the screen and the image is formed from the echoes coming from different scan lines that compose the plane of the section (Figure 1.11).

The brightness of the different parts of the image varies according to the intensity of the echo: anechogenic structures (follicle liquid, amniotic and allantoic fluid, urine) appear black, and highly echogenic structures (bone, gas) appear white. The structures with intermediate echogenicity are represented in shades of gray (Figure 1.12). The speed of image formation is typically between 20 to 30 images per second. Therefore the ultrasound images produced in real time change when the structures move (e.g., heartbeats) or when the probe is moved[9].

Common Artifacts

Artifacts are often observed in the ultrasound examination of reproductive organs because of the many pockets of air or liquid. Understanding the different types of artifacts is essential in improving the diagnostic value of ultrasound images[4,7,8].

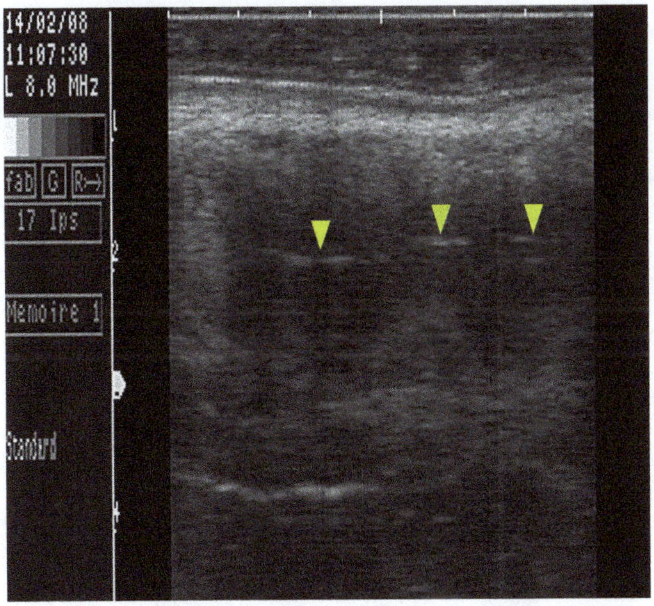

Figure 1.13. Specular reflections in the folds in the bovine cervix (8 MHz probe; depth of 4.5 cm). The cervix is shown in its longitudinal axis in a nonpregnant cow. In the cervical canal the specular reflections (arrows) are caused by the reflection of the ultrasound beam off the surface of the folds in the cervical wall. This occurs because the cervical wall is a smooth surface, larger than the beam, and parallel to the probe.

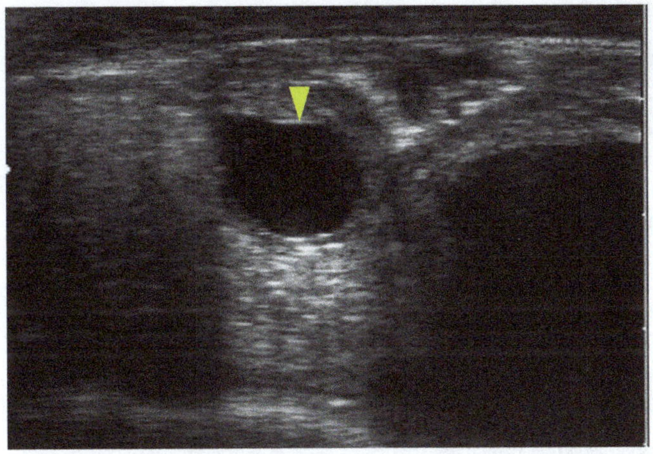

Figure 1.14. Specular reflections in an ovarian follicle in a cow (10.0 MHz probe; depth of 4 cm). In this image a specular reflection (arrow) is created by the reflection of the ultrasound beam off the dorsal part of the follicle. The adjacent areas do not give a specular reflection because the echoes are reflected at a different angle than the angle of impact. If the probe is moved to the surface where the beam hits at a perpendicular angle the specular zone moves as well. The majority of the beam that provides the specular reflection penetrates deeper into the tissues and also hits the ventral part of the follicle perpendicularly, resulting in a second specular reflection.

Specular reflection

Specular reflection occurs when the beam falls on a smooth surface that is larger than the beam and parallel to the probe. Only one impulse that hits a specular reflector at a perpendicular angle will be registered as an echo on the screen. An impulse that hits an interface at a nonperpendicular angle will be reflected at the same angle, and the interface will not be detected. This means that the amplitude of the echo will depend not only on the difference in acoustic impedance between the two tissues of the interface, but also on the angle of impact.

Specular reflections occur frequently in the reproductive system due to the many folds in the wall of the cervix (Figure 1.13) and the surface of ovarian follicles (Figure 1.14), all of which cause specular reflections.

Nonspecular reflections

Nonspecular reflections (diffuse reflections) result from the reflections off rough surfaces or surfaces that are narrower than the beam. Contrary to specular reflections, the amplitude of the echo from nonspecular reflectors does not depend on the incident angle of the beam. The ultrasound impulse is about 2–3 mm wide in the focal zone; therefore, interfaces that are less than 2–3 mm in size provide nonspecular images. As well, when the beam hits a rough surface the effective interface is narrower than the beam width. In diffusion a very small fraction of the reflected energy returns to the probe (1/1000 of the amplitude of a specular echo). With the different shades of gray, these diffused echoes allow the user to recognize tissues. Because the amplitude is independent of the incident angle the gray shades of these structures remain relatively constant no matter how the probe is oriented. Diffusion provides most of the echoes that identify the structures. The corpus luteum is a source of nonspecular echoes (Figure 1.15).

Shadow artifacts

With a normal image, a black zone corresponds to the absence of a reflector, such as occurs with a fluid-filled

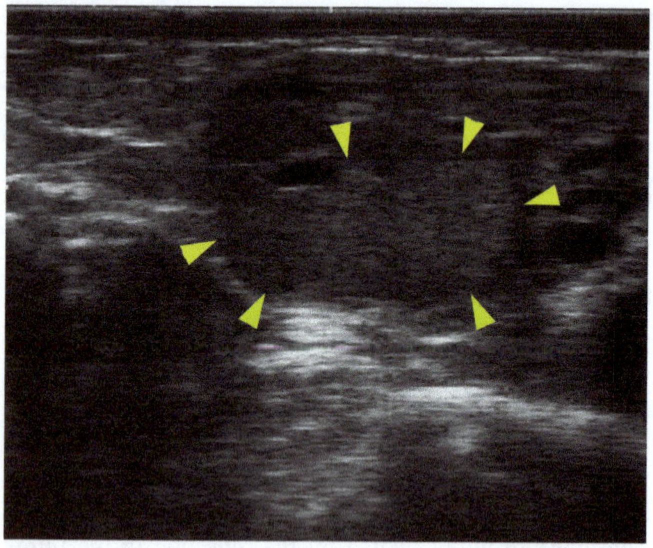

Figure 1.15. Nonspecular images: corpus luteum (8.0 MHz probe; depth of 4 cm). The corpus luteum is a source of nonspecular echoes. The echostructure of the corpus luteum is due to the echoes diffused by the many small heterogeneous structures such as capillaries and connective tissue. The gray tone is relatively constant no matter how the probe is oriented.

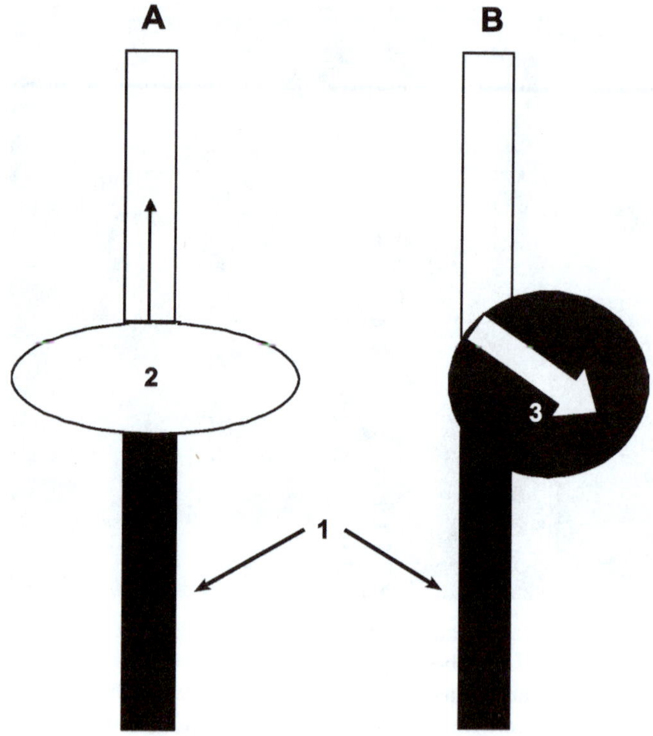

Figure 1.16. Source of shadow artifacts (adapted from Ginther, 1995). Shadowed areas (1: appearing black on the screen) can sometimes be artifacts. Normally, a black image on the screen corresponds to a tissue, such as follicular liquid, that does not emit an echo because it does not contain a reflector. A: Black hole artifacts can appear because the beam is blocked by a very dense reflector (e.g., bone (2), air/tissue interface) that reflects the entire echo. The underlying area will not be seen, even though it contains reflectors. B: The deviation of the beam transmitted by refraction on a smooth, curved structure will create a shadowed area because these areas are not hit by the beam. This occurs especially in the presence of pockets of liquid (3: follicles, ovarian cysts, etc.).

structure. However, the areas that appear black on the screen can also be artifacts. Figure 1.16 shows the possible sources of these shadow artifacts. One shadow is caused by a blocked or deviated beam. The black area on the ultrasound image corresponds to the area of tissue from which the ultrasound wave is not retransmitted back to the probe.

A shadow can result from a beam that is blocked by a very dense reflector such as the pelvic bones (Figure 1.17) or the refraction of the beam from beside a liquid-filled cavity (follicles, amnion, etc.). The ultrasound beams that hit the cavity tangentially will result in a shadow cone (Figure 1.18).

Enhancement artifacts

Enhancement artifacts occur frequently due to the presence of liquid-filled cavities. When crossing a cavity the beam is not attenuated, and its amplitude for a given depth is greater when it crosses a liquid structure. This type of increase indicates the presence of liquid and helps identify a liquid structure such as a follicle (Figure 1.19).

Reverberation artifacts

Reverberation refers to the production of "illegitimate" echoes due to two or more reflectors located on the trajectory of the ultrasound wave. The first reflector is generally the skin/probe interface or rectal wall/probe interface. The second reflector can be an air pocket or bone tissue. Reverberation is due to the repeating rebound of the echo between the two reflectors until the extinction of the echo by attenuation. This gives rise to a pileup of echoes on the screen. The first is legitimate, whereas the others are reverberations that become progressively weaker and move toward the

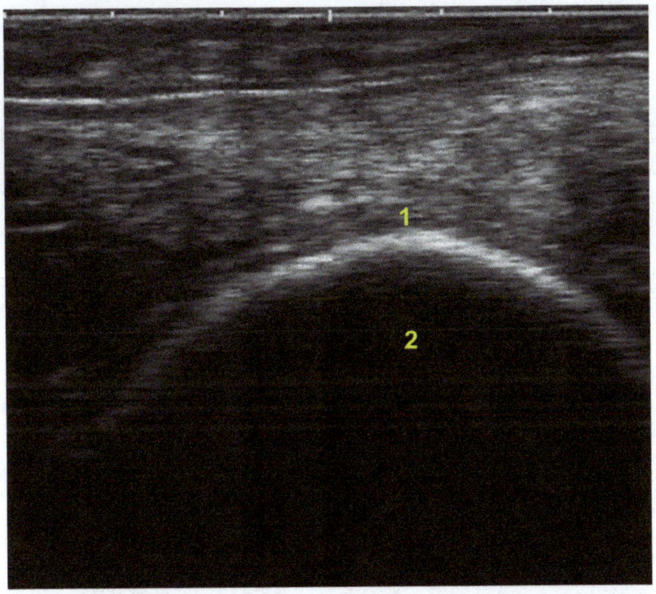

Figure 1.17. Example of shadow artifacts (8.0 MHz probe; depth of 5 cm). 1: Pelvic bones; 2: Shadow artifacts resulting from a high level of reflection off the pelvic surface.

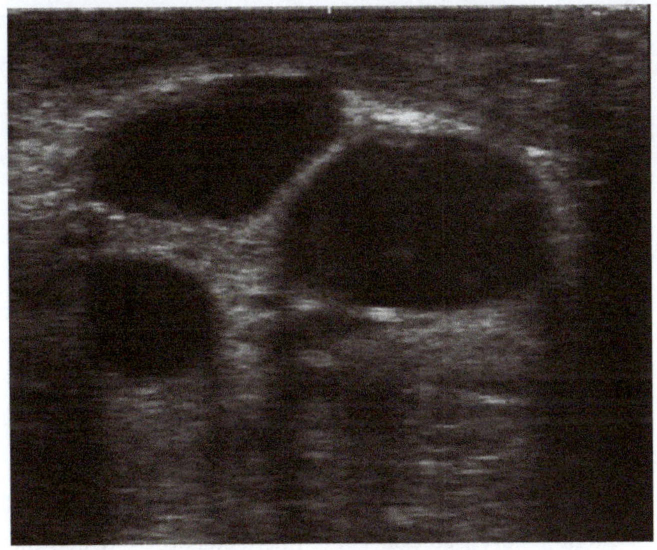

Figure 1.18. Shadow cone (8.0 MHz probe; depth of 5 cm). The beams that hit the follicles tangentially will result in shadow cones.

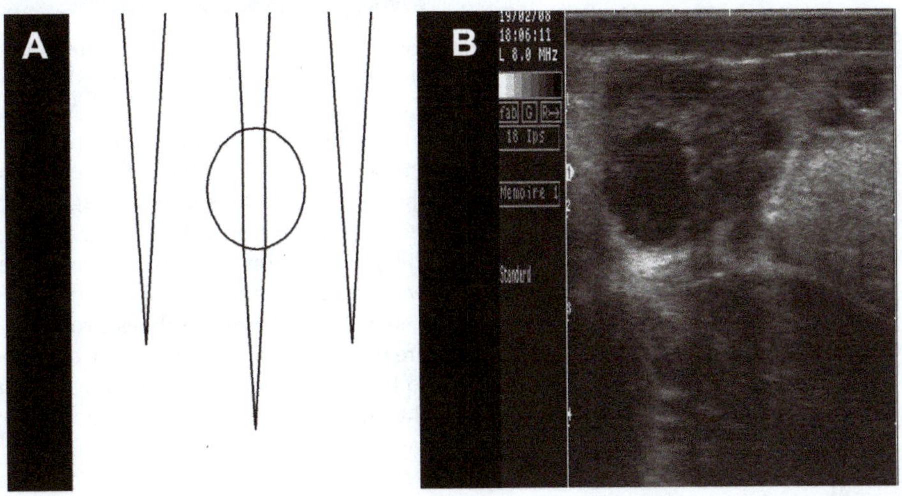

Figure 1.19. Enhancement artifact (adapted from Ginther 1995). A: The amplitude of an echo depends on all the attenuations it undergoes before being reflected. When the beam crosses a liquid area (in the middle of the illustration) it is not attenuated and its amplitude is relatively greater than that of the beam that was attenuated by the adjacent tissues; this causes a column of brighter echoes underneath the liquid structure. B: A typical enhancement artifact is shown in the image that appears right before a follicle, which appears clearly whiter than the adjacent areas, even though the tissue structures are the same for this depth over the entire width of the ultrasound image (8.0 MHz probe; depth of 4.5 cm).

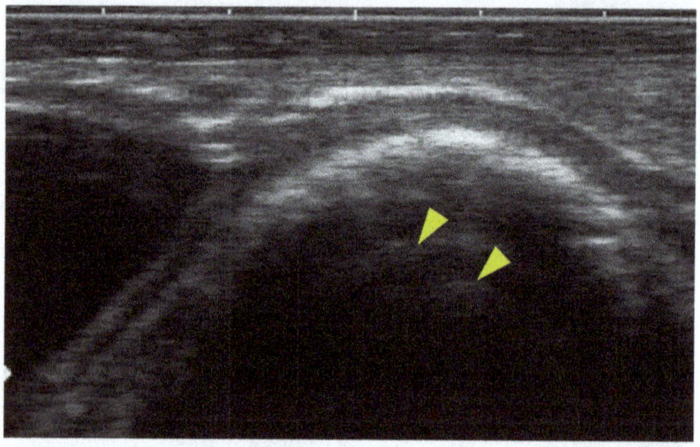

Figure 1.20. A reverberation artifact (8.0 MHz probe; depth of 3.5 cm). Reverberation is the phenomenon by which the echo rebounds one or many times between two interfaces with high acoustic impedance until the echo is extinguished by attenuation. The figure shows the example of reverberation due to the rebound of waves between the soft tissue/bony pelvis interface and the interface of the probe placed on the rectal wall with high acoustic impedance (no gel). The beam will go back and forth three times between the two interfaces. The first back-and-forth pass results in a legitimate echo on the screen. The second and third passes result in reverberations (arrows), which are images that do not correspond to echogenic structures located outside the first image. This is due to the fact that the first echo will rebound off the probe/rectal wall interface and then go toward the pelvis. The second echo takes more time to be produced, and is "seen" lower on the image, in a shadowy area. In light of attenuation, the echoes will be increasingly difficult to distinguish.

bottom of the screen. Given the decreasing strength of the reverberated echoes, these can also be called *comet-tail artifacts* (Figure 1.20).

Mirror image artifact

A mirror image artifact occurs with a very reflective interface. A second image of a structure (mirror image) is obtained beyond the highly reflective interface (Figure 1.21). This artifact is explained by the reflected wave being returned toward the structure at the surface of the pelvis. The echoes produced by the structure are reflected again to the surface of the pelvis and return to the probe with a time lag that causes the erroneous position of the second image of the structure.

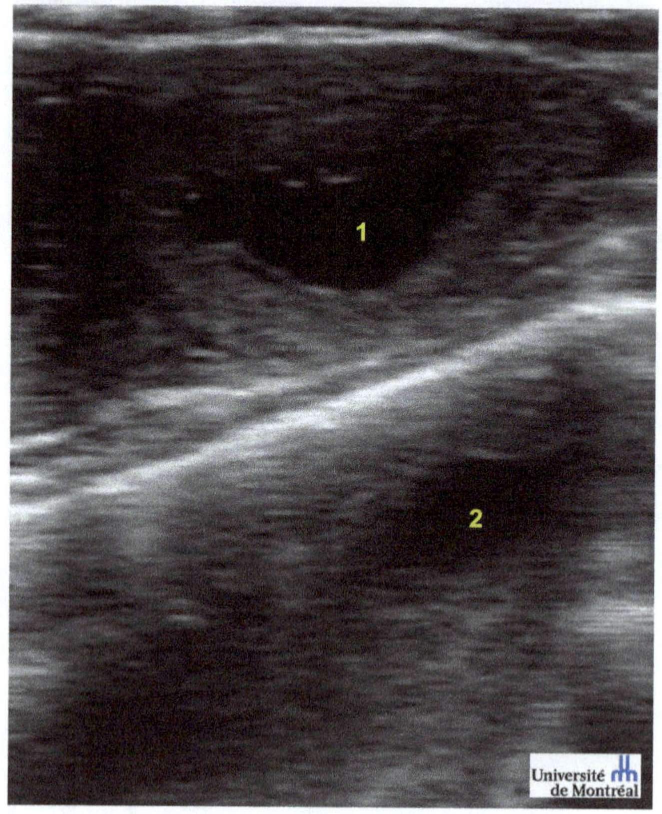

Figure 1.21. Example of a mirror image during early pregnancy diagnosis in a cow (5 MHz probe; depth of 7 cm). Courtesy of the Université de Montréal. 1: A section of a uterine horn containing embryonic liquid is identified above the echogenic line that represents the bone structure of the pelvis. 2: A second image of the uterine section is observed beyond the echogenic line of the pelvis. This "illegitimate" image results from the return of the reflected wave to the uterine horn at the very reflective surface of the pelvis. The returning echoes produced by the uterine horn are reflected again to the surface of the pelvis and then return to the probe. Due to the latency of the return of the echoes, the image of the uterine horn is reproduced beyond the pelvis.

Beam-width artifacts

The periphery of a large pocket of liquid or air, or even the entire volume of a small vesicle (follicle), has a grainy appearance due to filling of the nonechogenic area (liquid) by echogenic spot artifacts (Figure 1.22). This is due to a lateral resolution problem for the segment of the beam that simultaneously explores the fluid and the wall at a given depth. When two echoes

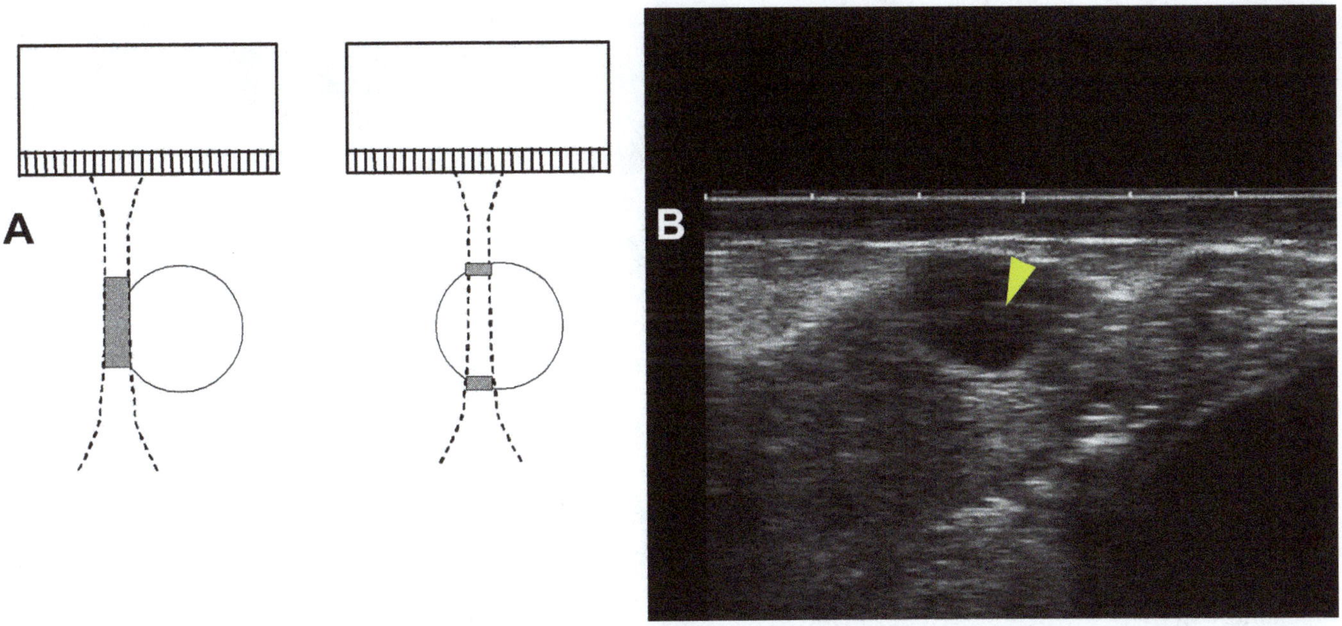

Figure 1.22. A beam-width artifact (adapted from Ginther 1995). A: When the beam hits a solid and a liquid area simultaneously, the two structures will be seen together. Part of the liquid area will therefore appear gray even though it is normally totally anechogenic. This gives the impression that the wall is not clear, and that it is somewhat fragmented by aggregates. This is due to the echoes coming from tissues adjacent to the liquid area. To the left, there are image artifacts on the lateral walls of the follicle. On the right, these image artifacts include the upper and lower areas of the follicle. B: On this ultrasound image, artifacts are observed in the follicular liquid (arrow), giving the impression that there is granular material inside (8.0 MHz probe; depth of 4 cm).

are captured by the probe at the same time they are treated as a single signal. These artifacts can suggest solid projections and wall disorganization, and may lead to an erroneous conclusion of atresia or death of the embryo.

References

1. Boyd JS (1995). Real-time diagnostic ultrasound in bovine reproduction. In: Goddard PJ (Ed.), Veterinary Ultrasonography. CAB International, Wallingford, pp. 1–19.
2. Carrière P, DesCôteaux L, Durocher J (2005). Ultrasonography of the reproductive system of the cow [CD-ROM]. Faculté de médecine vétérinaire, Université de Montréal, St-Hyacinthe, Québec.
3. Fishetti AJ, Scott RC (2007). Basic ultrasound beam formation and instrumentation. Clin Tech Small Anim Pract 22: 90–92.
4. Ginther OJ (1995). Ultrasonic Imaging and Animal Reproduction: Fundamentals. Equiservices Publishing, Wisconsin.
5. Goddard PJ (1995). General principles. In: Goddard PJ (Ed.), Veterinary Ultrasonography. CAB International, Wallingford, pp. 1–19.
6. Kossoff G (2000). Basic physics and imaging characteristics of ultrasound. World J Surg 24: 134–142.
7. Nyland TG, Mattoon JS, Wisner ER (1995). Physical principles, instrumentation, and safety of diagnostic ultrasound. In: Nyland TG, Mattoon JS (Eds.), Veterinary Diagnostic Ultrasound. WB Saunders Company, Philadelphia, pp. 3–18.
8. Penninck DG (1995). Imaging artifacts in ultrasound. In: Nyland TG, Mattoon JS (Eds.), Veterinary Diagnostic Ultrasound. WB Saunders Company, Philadelphia, pp. 19–29.
9. Pierson RA, Kastelic JP, Ginther OJ (1988). Basic principles and techniques for transrectal ultrasonography in cattle and horses. Theriogenology 29: 3–20.
10. Whittingham TA (2007). Medical diagnosis applications and sources. Prog Biophys Mol Biol 93: 84–110.

Points to Remember

- Probes are classified as either linear or sector.
- The frequencies used in medical imaging are between 2 and 10 megahertz (MHz).
- The speed of ultrasound wave propagation is independent of frequency and remains nearly constant in soft tissue (1540 m/s).

- The higher the frequency the shorter the wavelength, which results in better axial and lateral resolutions.
- The higher the frequency the smaller the penetrating distance of the ultrasound waves.
- The focal distances of the probes used in transrectal ultrasound are 7.0, 3.5, and 2.0 cm in depth with the respective frequencies of 3.5, 5.0, and 7.5 MHz.
- Good quality images can be obtained at up to twice the focal distance of the probe.
- The brightness of the different elements of the image varies according to the intensity of the echo: anechogenic liquid appears black, and highly echogenic structures appear white.
- Understanding the different types of artifacts is essential in improving the diagnostic value of echographic images.
- Specular reflections occur frequently in ultrasound examinations of the reproductive system.

Summary Questions

1. The penetration distance of ultrasound in tissues
   a. Increases with frequency
   b. Decreases with frequency
   c. Does not vary according to frequency
   d. Increases with focalization

2. Axial resolution increases when
   a. The wavelength decreases
   b. The wavelength increases
   c. The frequency decreases
   d. The amplitude decreases

3. The intensity of the reflected wave increases with
   a. Frequency
   b. Attenuation
   c. The incident angle
   d. The difference in acoustic impedance

4. At the soft tissue/bone interface, the ultrasound waves are
   a. Transmitted across the interface
   b. Strongly reflected
   c. Diffused
   d. Deviated

5. Compared to the ultrasound image on the left, the image on the right was obtained with
   a. Lower frequency
   b. Higher amplitude
   c. Higher frequency
   d. A longer wavelength

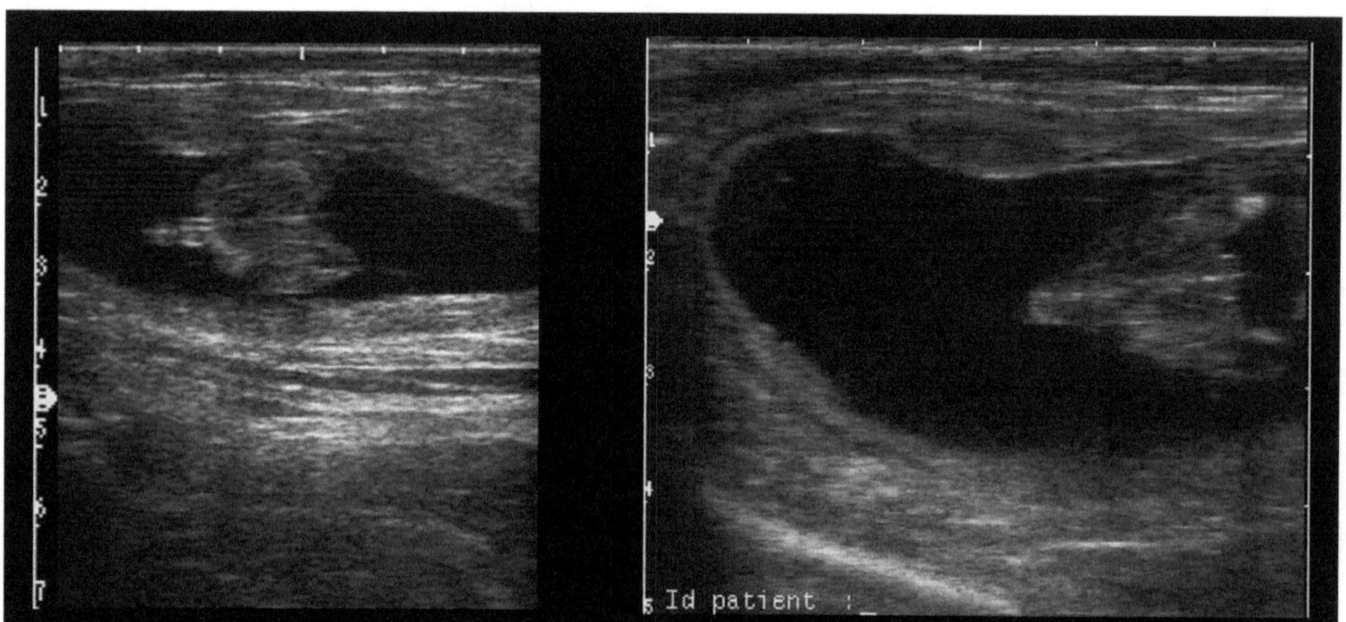

6. Ultrasound blocking by the ribs of the fetus can be explained by
   a. An increase in velocity and density
   b. A decrease in velocity combined with an increase in density
   c. An increase in velocity combined with a decrease in density
   d. A decrease in velocity and density

7. A nonspecular reflection is obtained when the ultrasound waves hit
   a. A large interface at a perpendicular angle
   b. A small interface
   c. A large interface at a nonperpendicular angle
   d. Gas

Answers

1. b
2. a
3. d
4. b
5. c
6. a
7. b

CHAPTER TWO

Scanning Techniques and Common Errors in Bovine Practice

Jill Colloton, Luc DesCôteaux, and Giovanni Gnemmi

Description of Scanning Technique

Equipment and methods to hold the linear probe

For reproductive examinations of cattle in the field, the 5MHz linear rectal probe is the most versatile and most commonly used[1-3]. Some researchers prefer 7.5MHz to 10MHz transducers, particularly when studying ovaries or very early pregnancies. Newer machines often come equipped with a "variable frequency" probe that adjusts from about 5–10MHz. Some ultrasonographers use a curvilinear[3] or sector probe, but these can be difficult to manipulate transrectally and have fallen out of favor in recent years so will not be discussed here.

All probe heads have a tactile way to determine whether the reading face is properly positioned. This indicator may be a groove, a raised dot, or a curved top. The probe may be held in the fingers (Figure 2.1A), or it may be rested in the palm with fingers free (Figure 2.1B).

One author prefers the palming method, finding it more relaxed. This method has the advantage of allowing the operator to retract the uterus while scanning if necessary. Experienced operators rarely need to manipulate the uterus while scanning. However, some operators feel more confident that they have thoroughly examined the entire reproductive tract if the uterus is retracted.

Position of the viewing device

The viewing device may be a monitor, a monocular eyepiece, or a binocular eyepiece. All must be positioned properly for the best image quality, particularly LCD devices. Cart-based monitors should be positioned on the opposite side of the palpating arm at an angle comfortable for the operator and safely out of the path of cow movement. Portable units worn on the person should be positioned to the side opposite the scanning arm. Positioning these units directly in front of the abdomen of the user obscures the view of the subject's hindlegs. In addition, special care must be taken when using binocular eyepieces because they limit the vision of the operator.

Manipulation of the Probe

Systematic method to scan the reproductive tract

Needless to say, the subject must be safely restrained to avoid injury to the operator or the equipment. Manure evacuation is necessary if the rectal wall is tight or when excellent image quality is required, such as for early pregnancy diagnosis and fetal sexing. It is most expedient to do this prior to introducing the probe.

The lubricated probe is then inserted into the rectum and a systematic examination of the entire

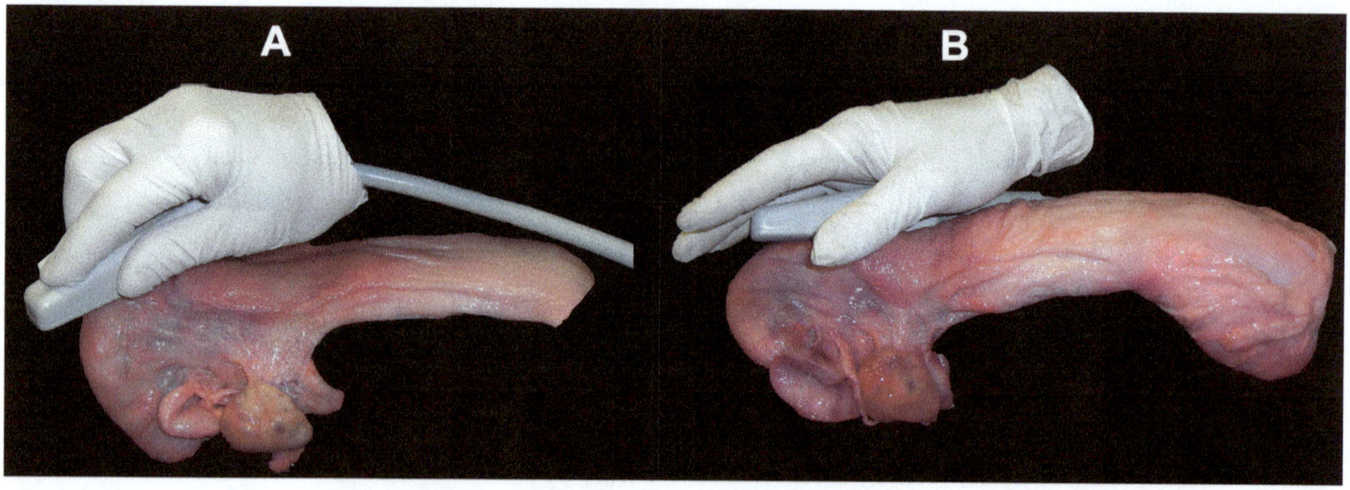

Figure 2.1. Controlled (on left) and palming (on right) methods of holding the ultrasound linear probe for transrectal examinations. A: Ultrasonographers who prefer not to manipulate the uterus often choose to hold the probe in a very controlled fashion; B: Note that the palming method frees the fingers for retraction of the uterus if necessary.

reproductive tract is performed. It is recommended that the same method is used with every examination[1]. The leading author prefers to examine the ovaries first, proceeding from the ovary to the tip of the uterine horn, continuing through the entire horn to the uterine body, and back up the contralateral horn to the other ovary. Great care must be taken to follow all the curves of the uterus, particularly at the tips of the horns. The angle of the probe on the tract is not important. Longitudinal, cross, or oblique sections are all acceptable as long as the entire tract is scanned. If the operator is unsure of the diagnosis after scanning the entire tract once, he or she must perform a second examination to verify the diagnosis. The cervix and vagina can be examined as the probe is withdrawn at the end of the examination.

Positioning for best image quality

Objects close to the face of the probe appear high on the monitor screen. This is desirable for the best image quality (Figure 2.2). Objects more than 8 cm away from the face of the probe will have poor detail. The probe can be manipulated into any position to visualize the desired object (see Chapter 7 on fetal sexing scanning technique).

Centering the object on the screen

An object under the tip (free end) of the probe may appear on either the right or the left side of the screen. This is a function of machine setting, not of position of the probe. Conventionally, most machines are set with the probe tip to the left. In this case, if the image is too

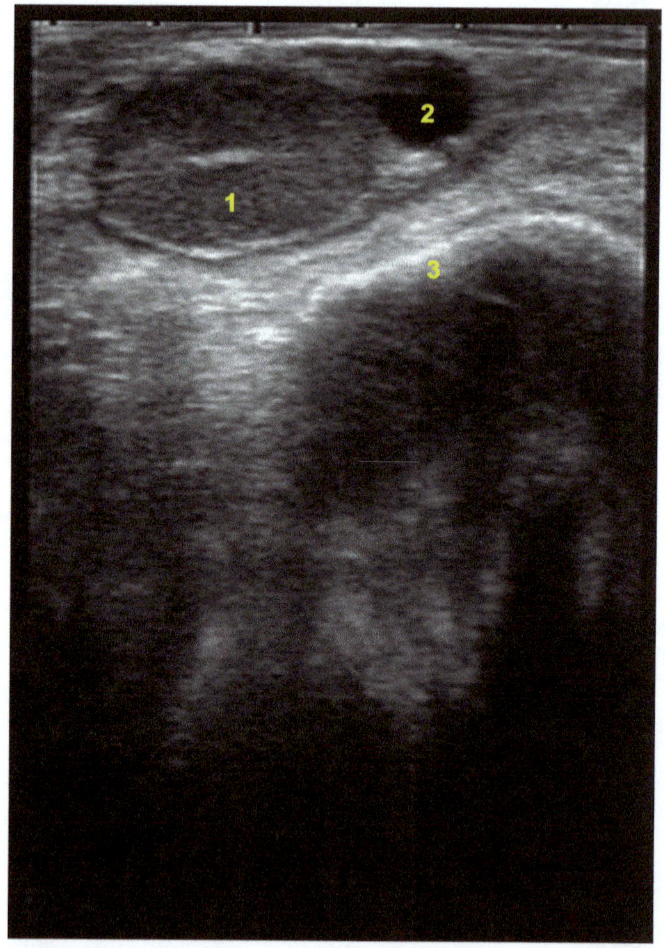

Figure 2.2. Good image quality produced by excellent scanning technique (5 MHz probe; depth of 7 cm). This sonogram of an ovary with a corpus luteum (1) and a follicle (2) demonstrates excellent image quality. The face of the probe is very close to the ovary so the image appears high on the screen; 3: pelvic bone.

far to the left of the screen the probe must be pushed forward to center it. Conversely, if the image is too far to the right the probe must be pulled back to center it. The opposite is true when the probe tip is set to the right of the screen.

Examining the object

Once the object is centered on the screen, the probe is moved side to side to fully examine it. These movements must be very small and slow. For small objects such as ovaries, some ultrasonographers prefer to slowly rock the probe in each direction rather than moving the entire probe. For larger objects, such as fetuses for sexing, the entire probe must be moved along the entire object. Because the image on the screen represents a very thin section of tissue (Figure 2.3), it is very important to scan in each direction until the object is no longer seen to avoid missing important structures. This is especially important when performing fetal sexing examinations because the male and female genital tubercles protrude away from the body and will be missed if the ultrasonographer stops short.

Figures 2.4 and 2.5 demonstrate probe position and the resultant image in a fetal sexing examination. Further discussion of fetal sexing methods is found in Chapter 7.

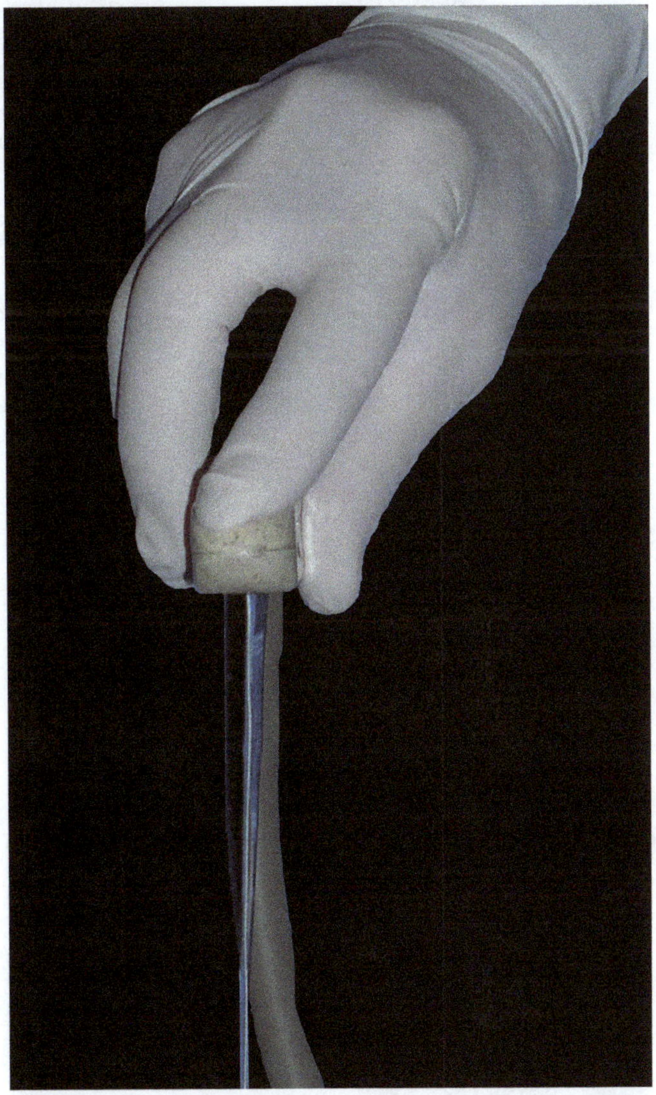

Figure 2.3. Demonstration of how the probe produces a thin section through tissue. Note that the image seen on the ultrasound monitor represents about a 2 mm section of tissue (see Figure 2.5).

Common Errors

Manure, gas, or finger interferences

The reading face of the probe must be firmly in contact with the rectal wall. Excessive manure (Figure 2.6), gas (Figure 2.7), or fingers will interfere with the scan. Gas (reverberation) artifacts are common when a plastic sleeve is used to protect the probe. This can be avoided by putting lubricant inside the sleeve as well as on the outside. See Chapter 1 for further information about artifacts.

Incomplete scan

Incomplete scans can occur when variations of the anatomy of the reproductive tract between animals are not considered. Depending on the age of the cow or the stage of pregnancy, the reproductive tract may be quite deep in the abdomen or completely in the pelvic cavity. Ovaries may be quite lateral to the uterine horns or nearly ventral to them. If the uterus is tightly curled the tips of the uterine horns may be lateral or even beneath the cervix, particularly in young animals. In older animals the uterine horns may extend cranially from the uterine body well into the abdomen.

Machine setting

Errors of improper machine settings include gain set too high or low, brightness set too high or low, focal points set at incorrect depths, or too many focal points. Chapter 1 discusses how to properly adjust the machine settings.

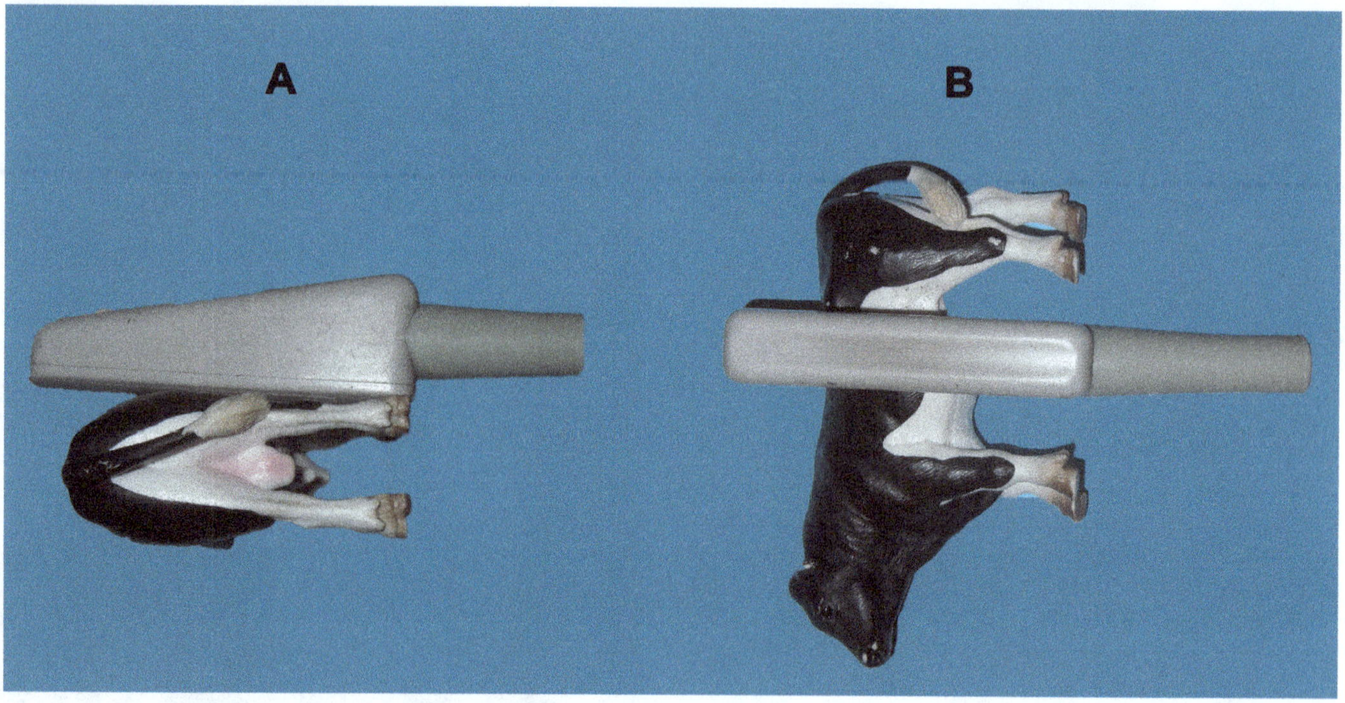

Figure 2.4. Position of the probe on a male fetus that produces the ultrasound image in Figure 2.5. Note that the structures seen on the ultrasound scan are exactly those one would expect to see in a thin section through this portion of a fetus.

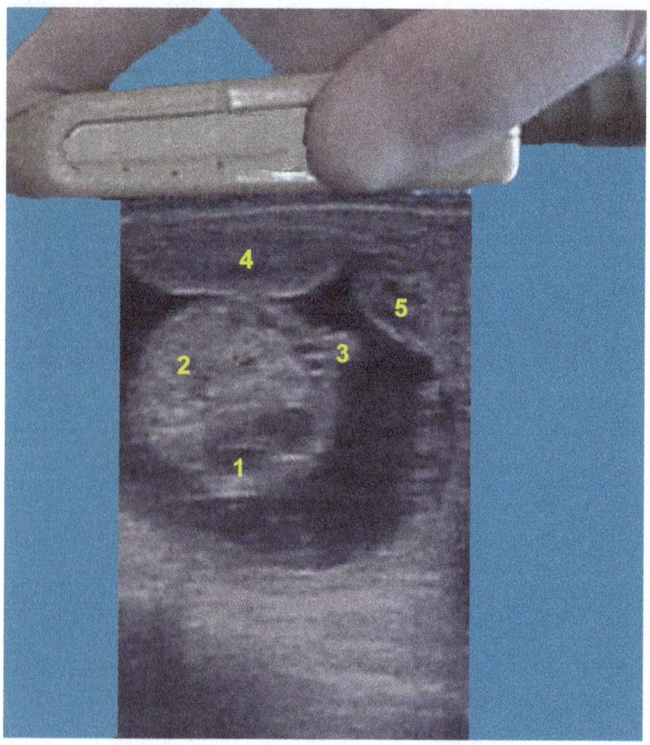

Figure 2.5. Fetal organs as seen in cross section through the abdomen when the probe is located just behind the umbilical cord of a 69-day-old male fetus (Figure 2.4). 1: Fetal stomach; 2: Liver; 3: Genital tubercle; 4: Placentome; 5: Umbilical cord in oblique section.

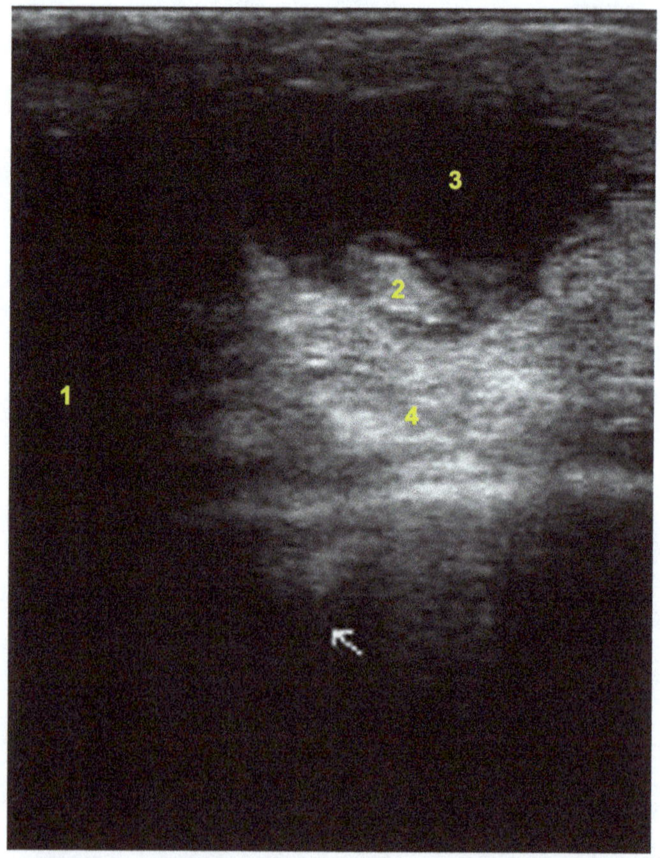

Figure 2.6. Manure interference with image quality (7.5 MHz probe; depth of 7 cm). 1: The dark area on the left side of this image results from poor contact on the probe on the rectal wall, most likely due to manure; 2: Embryo; 3: Allantoic fluid; 4: Enhancement artifact.

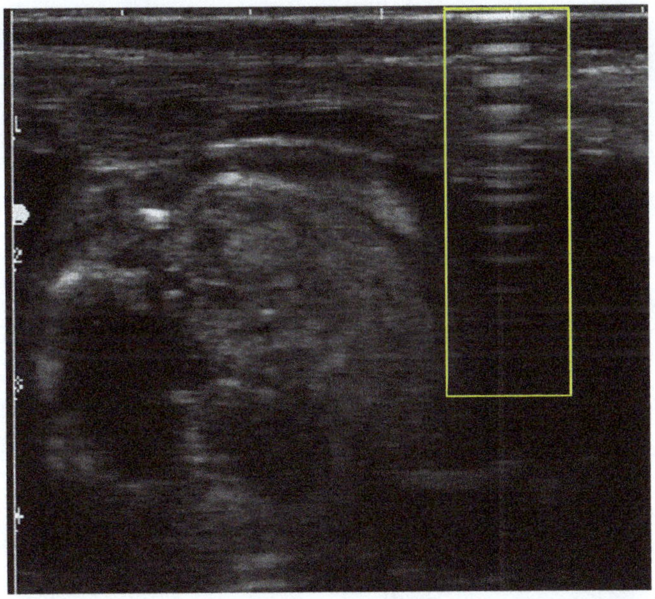

Figure 2.7. Gas interference with image quality produces reverberation artifacts (10 MHz probe; depth of 5 cm). The white half-moon shaped artifacts in the yellow square indicate gas between the face of the probe and underlying structures.

Bright environment

Inadequate shading of the monitor or eyepiece significantly reduces the ability of the operator to distinguish tissue densities. When working outdoors, the operator should shade the viewing device, even on cloudy days. This is also true if working indoors with bright lights.

References

1. Carrière P, DesCôteaux L, Durocher J (2005). Ultrasonography of the reproductive system of the cow. [CD-ROM]. Faculté de médecine vétérinaire, Université de Montréal, St-Hyacinthe, Québec.
2. Ginther OJ (1995). Ultrasonic Imaging and Animal Reproduction: fundamentals. Equiservices Publishing, Wisconsin.
3. Stroud B (1997). Bovine reproductive ultrasonogaphy [DVD]. Biotech Productions, Texas.

Points to Remember

- Various types of probes and viewing devices can be used for reproductive ultrasound examinations. Probes can be linear, curvilinear, or sector, with frequencies ranging from 5–10 MHz. Viewing devices include monitors, monocular eyepieces, or binocular eyepieces.
- Proper manipulation of the ultrasound probe across all portions of the reproductive tract is critical for complete examinations.
- It is recommended that the same method be used with every examination. The reproductive tract examination can start on one ovary, proceeding from the ovary to the tip of the uterine horn, continuing through the entire horn to the uterine body, and back up the contralateral horn to the other ovary.
- The most common errors in transrectal scanning are manure or gas interferences, incomplete scan of the reproductive tract, improper machine setting, and inadequate shading of the viewing device.

Summary Questions

1. Objects under the tip of the probe appear
   a. To the left of the screen
   b. To the right of the screen
   c. To either the left or right of the screen, depending on machine setting
   d. At the top of the screen

2. Retraction of the uterus is
   a. Necessary for all ultrasound examinations
   b. Necessary for fetal sexing examinations only
   c. Necessary for fetal sexing and early pregnancy exams only
   d. Usually not necessary for experienced operators

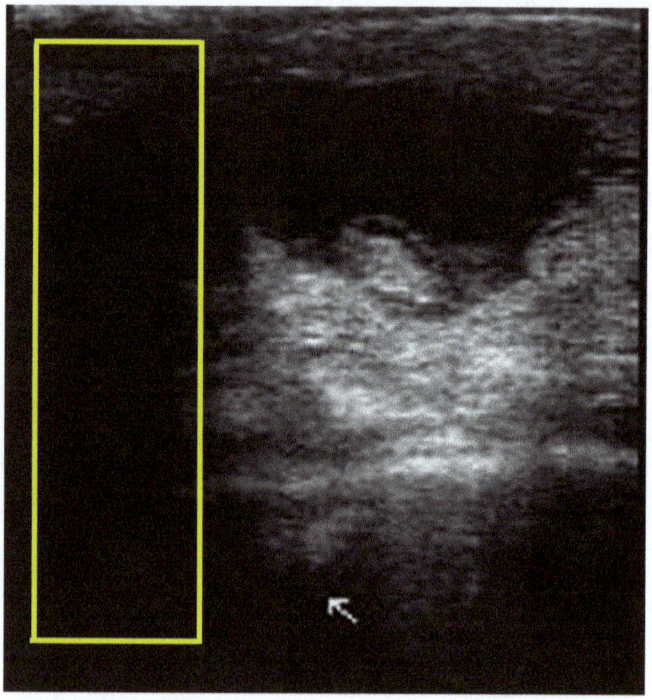

3. The dark area in the yellow rectangle on the following sonogram is most likely caused by
   a. Manure under the probe
   b. Air under the probe
   c. Incorrect machine settings
   d. Urine in the bladder

4. When examining a small object such as an ovary it is important to
   a. Position the ovary about 8 cm away from the probe
   b. Use the lowest frequency probe available
   c. Slowly rotate the probe across the entire ovary
   d. Hold the ovary with the fingers while examining it

Answers

1. c
2. d
3. a
4. c

CHAPTER THREE

Anatomy of the Reproductive Tract of the Cow

Réjean C. Lefebvre and Giovanni Gnemmi

Introduction

Real-time ultrasonography has become an essential diagnostic tool as well as a research tool in veterinary and animal sciences because it provides information beyond transrectal palpation of the reproductive organs. As a diagnostic aid ultrasonography is well suited for bovine practice, particularly for the examination of female and male reproductive tracts[1,3,6]. A 5.0 to 7.5 MHz transducer is preferable to obtain good quality and detailed images of the different tissues of the reproductive organs. This chapter reviews the anatomy of the female bovine reproductive tract essential for effective ultrasonography and clinical interpretation of the results.

Genital Tract

A thorough understanding of the structures of the reproductive tract, including the vagina, the cervix, the uterus, and the ovaries is essential for interpretation of the physiological changes occurring during the estrous cycle, and of pathological conditions (Figure 3.1). The dynamic changes observed with ultrasonographic technology mirror ovarian steroid changes and aid in the assessment of uterine function (see Chapters 4 and 5 for more details). Much attention is given to the ultrasonographic appearance and orientation of the tubal tract, requiring the sonographer to do a systematic and complete examination (Chapter 2).

Vagina

Anatomy

Except for obvious intravaginal or perivaginal anomalies (e.g., a mass), a vaginal examination by rectal palpation is difficult, not effective, and not routinely performed. In cases where a complete and detailed vaginal examination is indicated, an ultrasound examination, vaginoscopy, and/or digital evaluation should be performed.

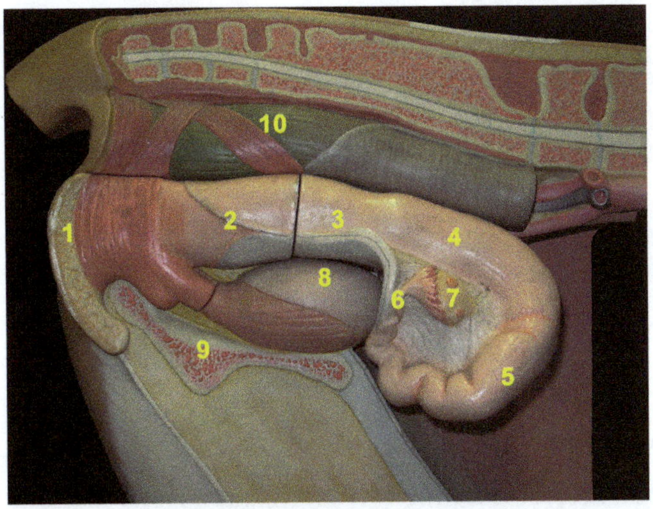

Figure 3.1. Anatomy of the reproductive tract of the cow. 1: Vulva; 2: Vagina; 3: Cervix; 4: Body of the uterus; 5: Right uterine horn; 6: Oviduct; 7: Ovary; 8: Urinary bladder; 9: Ischial bone (cut); 10: Rectum.

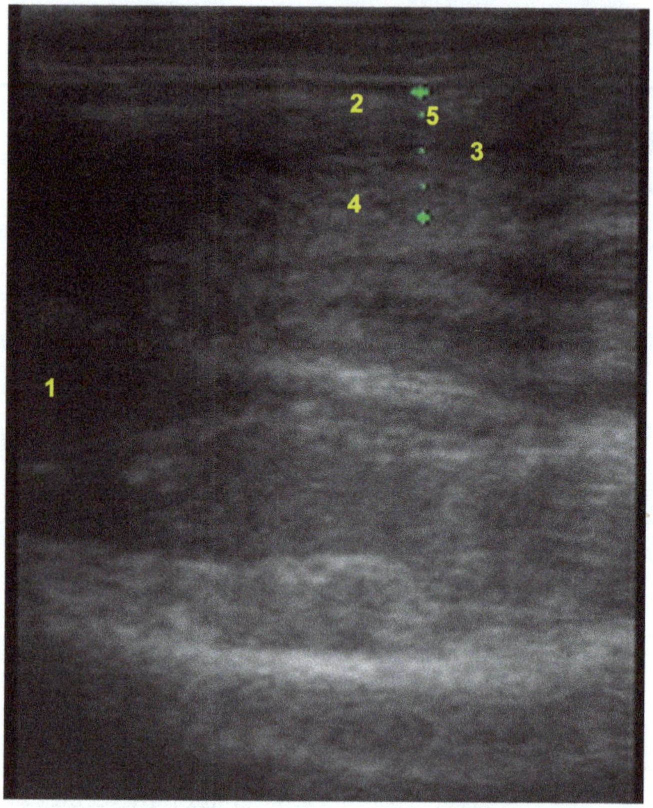

Figure 3.2. Ultrasonogram of a longitudinal view of the vagina of a cow (7.5 MHz probe; depth of 8 cm). The cranial portion of the vagina is observed as a longitudinal bright line when the transrectal transducer is applied to its dorsal surface. The bright line represents the apposition of both inner surfaces (dorsal and ventral) of the vaginal wall. When fluid is present in the cranial vagina an elliptical anechoic form, representing the lumen, appears. With the presence of fluid, the caudal portion of the cervix projecting in the cranial vaginal and the external urethra orifice can be identified. 1: Bladder; 2: Vaginal wall (dorsal aspect); 3: Apposition of the inner vaginal surfaces; 4: Vaginal wall (ventral aspect); 5: Thickness of the vagina between +–+.

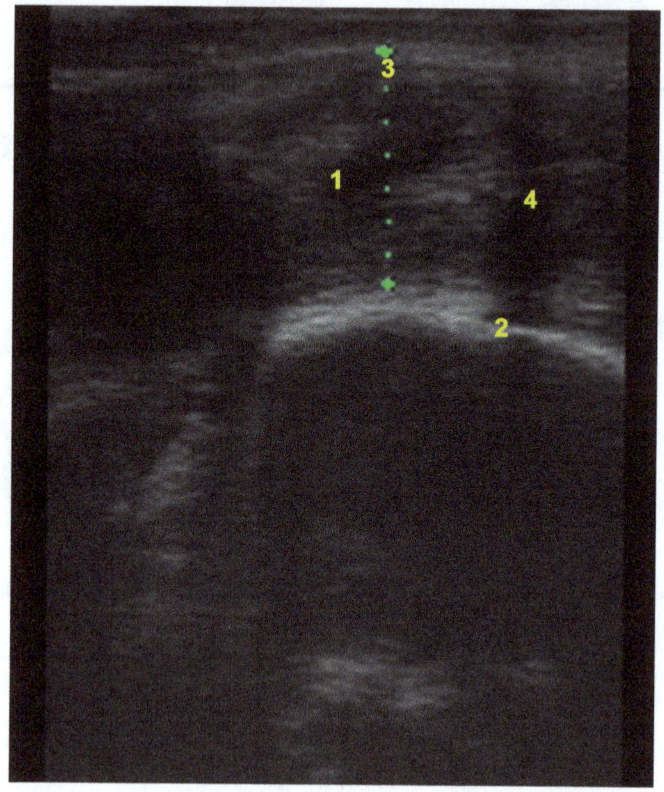

Figure 3.3. Ultrasonogram of the longitudinal view of the cervix (7.5 MHz probe; depth of 8 cm). A very distinctive heterogeneous cylindrical structure with various degrees of alternate acoustic shadows can be seen on the longitudinal image. The cervical rings appear more echoic than the intercervical spaces. It is difficult to recognize the internal os opening into the uterine body. The bones of the pelvic floor (hyperechoic) and the urinary bladder (anechoic) are frequently visible close to the cervix. The vaginal portion of the cervix projecting into the cranial vagina can be identified on the ultrasound image (4). 1: Cervical ring; 2: Ischial bone; 3: Cervix diameter (2.3 cm); 4: Vaginal portion of the cervix.

Ultrasound technique and imaging

Figure 3.2 presents the ultrasonographic appearance of the vagina in longitudinal view.

Cervix

Anatomy

The cervix is a firm, cylindrical, and mobile structure (7 to 10 cm long and 3 to 4 cm diameter) lying on the pelvic floor. Its size and location vary with age (parity) and reproductive status (postpartum or cycling). The lobulated appearance is explained by the presence of the three to four rings of the cervical mucosa. In a normal nonpregnant cow, the cervix is located in the pelvic cavity above the bladder.

Ultrasound technique and imaging

The veterinarian must advance the transducer or probe into the rectum and maintain it ventrally on the pelvic floor until the cervix is localized. Stabilizing the cervix with the other fingers may help visualize the structure (Figure 3.3).

Uterus

Anatomy

The bovine uterus has a short body (3.0 cm long) and two long uterine horns (30 to 40 cm) attached at the

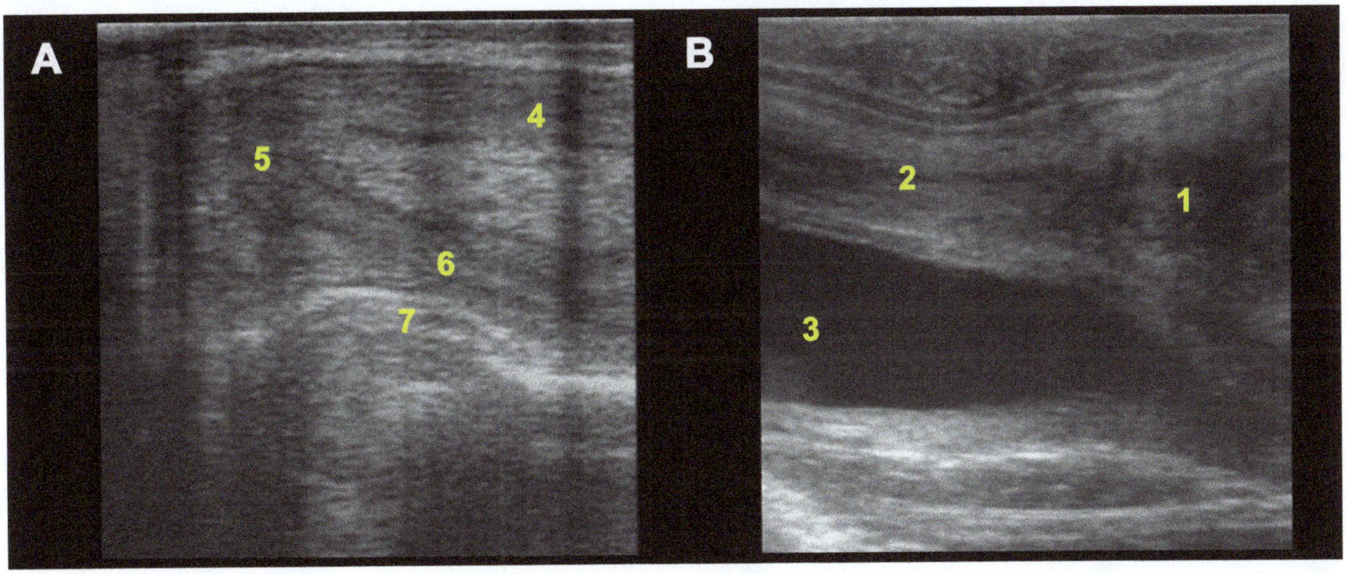

Figure 3.4. Ultrasonograms of a longitudinal view of the uterine horn (A) and of the uterine body and cervix (B) of a cow (7.5 MHz probe; depth of 6 cm). 1: Cervix; 2: Uterine body; 3: Bladder; 4: Uterine segment # 2; 5: Uterine segment # 3; 6: Uterine segment # 4; 7: Ischial bone.

bifurcation by the intercornual ligament. This ligament is divided into ventral and dorsal portions, forming a depression very useful for retraction of the uterus. The large and free convex curvature of the uterine horns faces dorsally and the small concave curvature, attached to the broad ligament, faces the abdominal cavity (Figure 3.1). The broad ligaments extend laterally and dorsally to join the dorsolateral abdominal wall. This anatomical arrangement gives a characteristic twisting and turning shape to the uterine horns. Landmarks for general orientation during transrectal palpation are the pelvic or pubic brim, the iliac shafts, and the obturator and sciatic foramens.

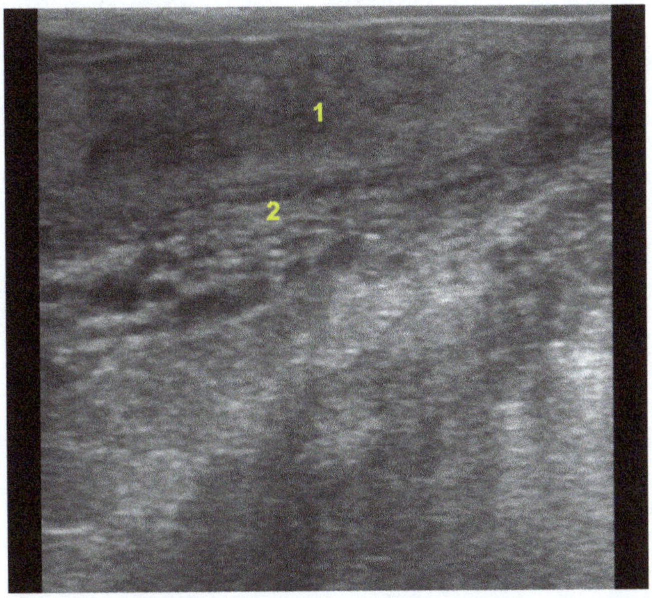

Figure 3.5. Ultrasonograms of the broad ligament (7.5 MHz probe; depth of 6 cm). 1: Uterine horn; 2: Broad ligament (multiple cross sections of vessels).

Ultrasound technique and imaging

From the cervix, the transducer is advanced into the rectum. The demarcation between the cervix and the uterine body is not as obvious as the one between the vagina and the cervix. Beyond the uterine body the characteristic echotexture of the uterus can be followed laterally to examine each horn. Dividing the uterine horn into arbitrary segments (1 to 5) as described by Ginther may help to designate the location of a structure during the examination of the uterine tract[2] (Figures 3.4, 3.5).

The ultrasonographic appearance of the uterine horns in the cow is characterized by different echotextures representing different layers. The peripheral part of the cross-sectional or longitudinal image of the uterine horn produces a hyperechoic signal. Under this hyperechoic surface a faint echoic line is observed representing vascular structures and the external and internal longitudinal circular muscular layers. Finally, the endometrium is characterized by an echoic appearance with nonspecular reflection so that dark and bright signals are seen within its thickness. In absence of fluid in the lumen, the dorsal and ventral endometrium join and appear as a bright line (see Chapter 5 for more details and images). The inner edge of the endometrium, or the bright line, is uneven and is thought to be due to the presence of uterine caruncles[1]. For the changes observed during the estrous cycle, readers are referred to Chapter 5.

Descriptive Terminology of the Ovary and Ovarian Structures

Reproductive ultrasonography is an indispensable tool for the evaluation of the reproductive tract of the cow. The ovary is readily examined and can be imaged in longitudinal and transverse sections[5]. Since the ovary is extremely mobile the sonographer may need to reposition the organ to obtain a clear image. When ultrasonography of the ovary is performed veterinarians must recognize the different structures and specify their locations. Follicles and corpora lutea may project from any part of the ovary surface. As with manual transrectal palpation, good terminology is important. Based on Zemjanis (1970), the ovary is ovoid and has one border attached ventrally to the mesovarium[7]. On the opposite side there is the free border. The posterior pole is in apposition to the tip of the uterine horns. The anterior pole is the portion closer to the abdominal wall. The medial face of the ovary is the surface facing the abdominal organs, and the lateral surface occupies the opposite position. The ovary is included in the broad ligament and is generally located against the ventral part of the iliac shaft at the level of the bifurcation of the uterine horns. The ovary is connected to the tip of the uterine horn by the oviduct, a narrow, hard, coiled tube of about 2 to 3 mm in diameter and 20 to 25 cm long. The diameter of the oviduct increases significantly at the anterior pole of the ovary forming the infundibulum, which is 4 to 6 cm deep and 8 to 12 cm wide. The mesosalpinx and the mesovarium ligaments join to form the ovarian bursa. The normal oviduct and infundibulum are not visible with field ultrasound units. Pathology, such as blockage of the oviduct or adhesions, can sometimes be identified, especially in cases of hydrosalpinx.

Ovary

Anatomy

The average size of an ovary without functional structures (corpus luteum or a dominant follicle) is about 4.0 cm long, 2.0 cm wide and 2.5 cm high. Cows have larger ovaries than heifers. The presence of a corpus luteum, ovarian cyst, or tumor increases the overall size of the ovary.

Ovaries must be routinely examined during all reproductive examinations. For pregnancy examinations ovarian evaluation enables the practitioner to determine the potential for pregnancy based on the presence or absence of a corpus luteum (CL), the probable location of the pregnancy, the presence of double ovulations (see twin section in Chapter 6), and the quality of the CL.

Ultrasound technique and imaging

The ovaries are found about 10 cm laterally from the midline and about 5 cm anterior and at the same level as the pelvic brim or external uterine bifurcation. If the ovaries are not located rapidly, the tips of the fingers can be used to locate the ovaries by grasping the anterior edge of the broad ligament (see Chapter 2 for more details on manipulations of the linear probe).

When the ovary is identified, the transducer can be slowly rotated to obtain different images (transverse or longitudinal). The sonographer must identify all sections of the ovary. Overlying intestinal gas, feces, and other organs can interfere with the visualization of the ovaries, but an adequate window can usually be found by repositioning the transducer or by evacuating fecal material. The transducer is positioned as closely as possible over the ovary and pointed toward the anterior pole of the ovary. By moving laterally or medially the ultrasonographer directs the transducer toward the anterior or posterior pole of the ovary, respectively.

Inactive ovaries are oval and have a fairly uniform echogenicity that is equal to or slightly greater than the cervix (see Chapter 4 for more details). Structures of the ovary that are easily observed on ultrasonography are the ovarian stroma, follicles (small: <4 mm; medium: 4–7 mm; large: ≥8 mm; and cystic), corpora hemorrhagica and diestrous corpora lutea (with or without a cavity), and ovarian vessels peripheral to the ovary (Figures 3.6–3.8). The structures present on the ovary make it easier to find. Without large active structures such as corpora lutea and large follicles, small and medium follicles are present within the outer portion of the ovarian stroma called the *cortex*. The stroma occupies the central portion (medulla) of inactive ovaries (in anestrus) and surrounds significant structures such as corpora hemorrhagica, corpora lutea, or

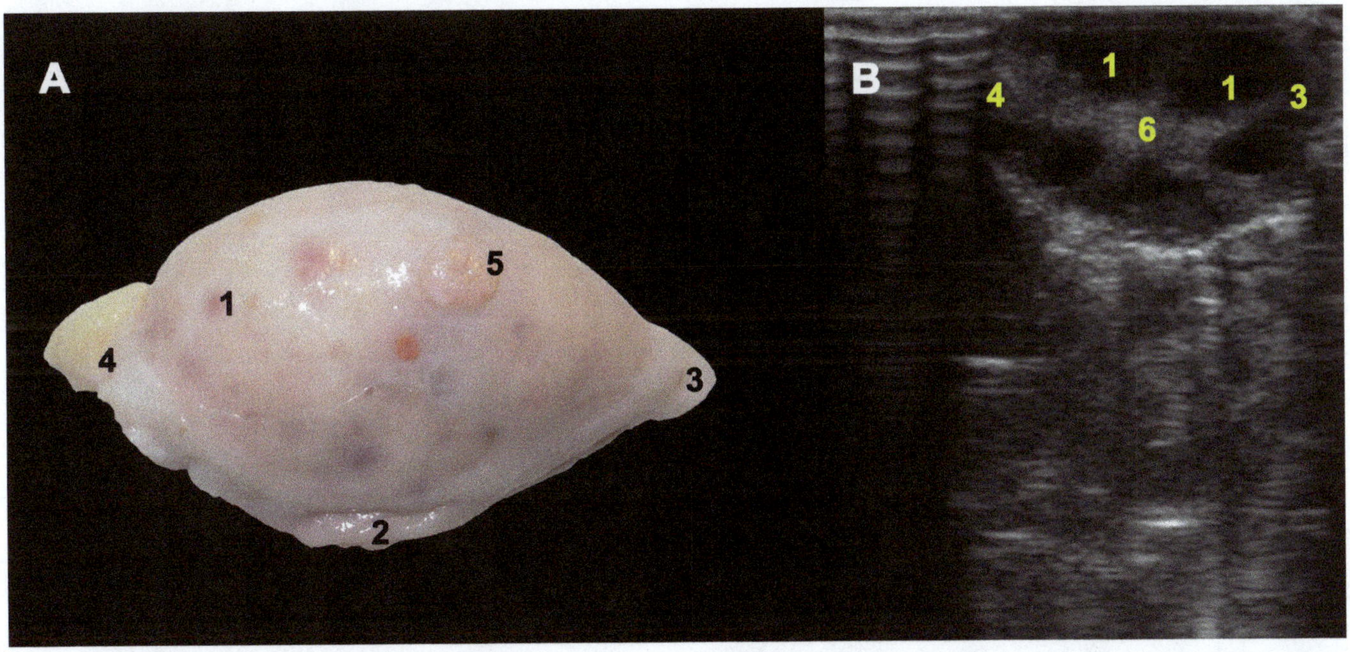

Figure 3.6. Anatomy (A) and ultrasonographic image (B) of an inactive ovary in anestrous cow (7.5 MHz probe; depth of 6 cm). 1: Small follicle; 2: Attached border of the ovary; 3: Posterior pole; 4: Anterior pole; 5: Corpus albican; 6: Ovarian stroma.

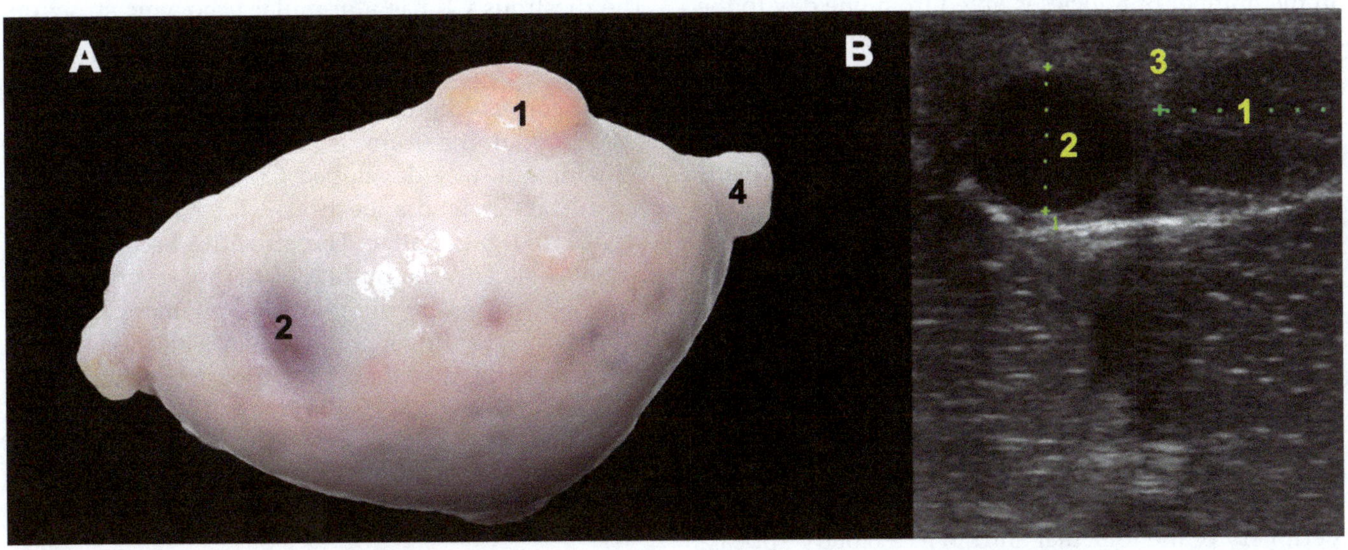

Figure 3.7. Anatomy (A) and ultrasonographic image (B) of an active ovary with a corpus luteum and a large dominant follicle (7.5 MHz probe; depth of 6 cm). The follicle is recognized by its smooth, round raised surface on the ovary. 1: Corpus luteum (1.8 cm); 2: Dominant follicle (1.4 cm); 3: Ovarian stroma; 4: Posterior pole of the ovary.

large follicles of active ovaries. The stroma is echoic and easily recognized with a good quality ultrasound unit.

Follicle

Figure 3.7 shows the anatomy (A) and ultrasonographic image (B) of an active ovary with a corpus luteum and a large dominant follicle.

Ultrasound appearance

Follicles appear as anechoic structures of various sizes. The line between the follicular wall and the follicular antrum is always smooth and well defined. The dominant follicle increases in size until the end of a follicular wave or the day before the ovulation (see Chapter 4 for more details). Ovulation may be detected by the disappearance of the preovulatory follicle, by the much

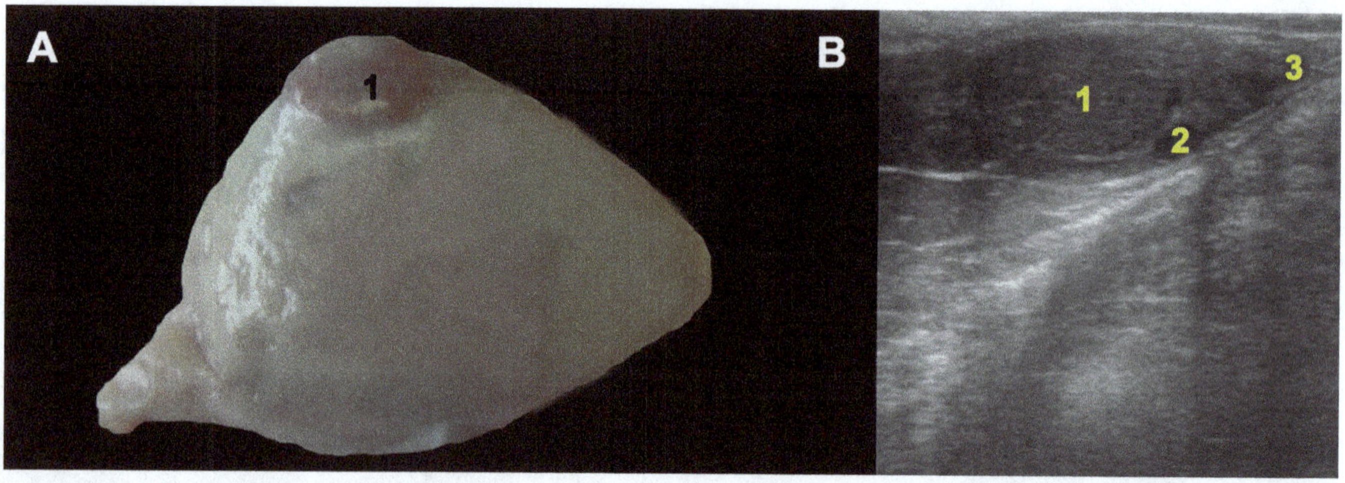

Figure 3.8. Anatomy (A) and ultrasonographic appearance (B) of the ovary with the presence of a mature corpus luteum (7.5 MHz probe; depth of 6 cm). 1: Corpus luteum (2.5 cm); 2: Follicle (4 mm); 3: Posterior pole of the ovary.

diminished size of a specific follicle, or when a decrease in the number of follicles is noted from one day to the next in superovulated cows (see Chapter 8 for examples). The borderline between the follicular wall and the surrounding stroma is not identifiable, except in images of large preovulatory follicles, just before ovulation. All follicles are not uniformly spherical. This is possibly a result of transducer pressure on large follicles or of pressure created by neighboring follicles. A small follicle adjacent to a larger follicle frequently appears as a convex impingement on the surface of the larger follicle. A bright straight line may appear between adjacent follicles, resulting from opposed walls when its thickness is within the range of the resolution of the transducer. However, opposing walls of several follicles are too thin to be detected, causing only irregular forms. Other artifacts appear in the periphery of the follicular antrum as a cloudy appearance and are caused by the width of the ultrasonographic beam. Echoing of the sound waves from the side of a curved surface may obscure the follicular outline parallel to the direction of beams[4]. See Chapter 1 for more information on artifacts.

Corpus luteum

Ultrasound appearance

On the ultrasonographic image, the diestrous corpus luteum (CL) may appear to be imbedded in the ovary or may appear to protrude from the ovary (Figure 3.8). The diestrous CL has a granular echogenic structure, which intensifies during the luteal phase (see Chapter 4 for more details on ultrasonographic particularities of the corpus luteum during the estrous cycle). The distortion of the form is more marked in ovaries containing a fully developed CL. At about day 17 of the estrous cycle, the diestrous CL begins to decrease in size and gets flatter. The structure becomes more hyperechoic and the outline of the regressing corpus luteum is not easily differentiated anymore from the ovarian stroma. In general, corpora albicantia are not discernible, because they have the same echogenicity as the stroma and are small (Figure 3.6).

Blood vessels

When viewed in cross section, blood vessels may be confused with small follicles. Extended blood vessels are seen during the luteal phase as a result of an increased blood flow to the corpus luteum (see the color Doppler section in Chapter 4). Large vessels enter the posterior pole of the ovary where they are imaged as two or three anechoic structures of 2 to 5 mm in diameter[1]. They can be identified by moving the transducer (Figure 3.9). Blood vessels, unlike follicles, can be traced over a longer distance and are generally seen on the border of the ovary, in the ovarian hilus, and around the CL.

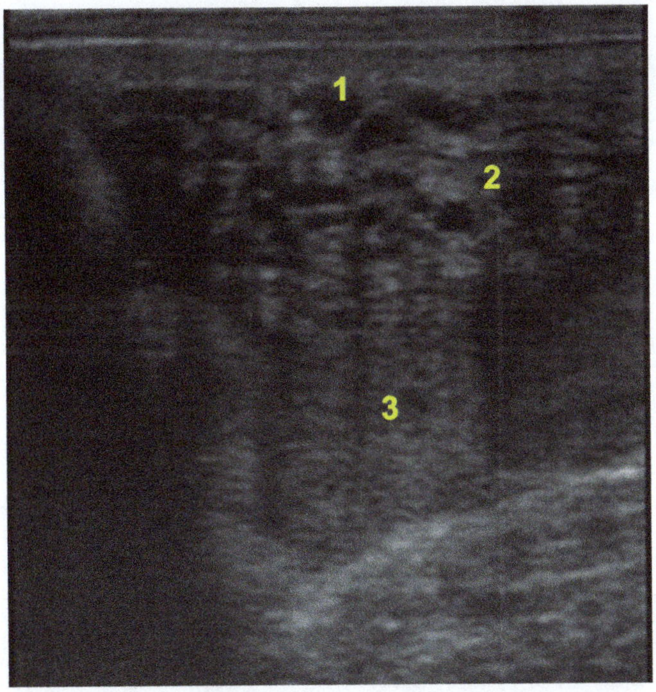

Figure 3.9. Ultrasound image of the broad ligament near the attached border of the ovary (7.5 MHz probe; depth of 6 cm). 1: Blood vessels near the broad ligament; 2: Fibrous tissues of the ligament; 3: Small intestine.

References

1. Boyd JS, Omran SN (1991). Diagnostic ultrasonography of the bovine female reproductive tract, Practice 13: 109–118.
2. Ginther OJ (1998). Ultrasonic Imaging and Animal Reproduction: Cattle. Equiservices Publishing, Wisconsin, pp. 232–246.
3. Kh Abdel-Razed A, Ali A (2005). Development changes of bull (*Bos taurus*) genitalia as evaluated by calliper and ultrasonography, Reprod Dom Anim 40: 23–27.
4. Pierson RA, Ginther OJ (1988). Ultrasonic imaging of the ovaries and uterus in cattle, Theriogenology 29: 21–37.
5. Pieterse MC (1989). Ultrasonic characteristic of physiological structures on bovine ovaries. In: Taverne MAM, Willemse AH (Eds.). Diagnostic Ultrasound and Animal Reproduction. Kluwer Academic Publisher, London, pp. 37–52.
6. Weber JA, Hilt CJ, Woods GL (1988). Ultrasonographic appearance of bull accessory sex glands, Theriogenology 29: 1347–1355.
7. Zemjanis R (1970). Diagnostic and Therapeutic Techniques in Animal Reproduction, 2nd ed. William and Wilkins Company, Baltimore, pp. 55–77.

Points to Remember

- The veterinarian must advance the transducer or probe into the rectum and maintain it ventrally on the pelvic floor until the cervix is localized. Stabilizing the cervix with the other fingers may help the visualization of the structure.
- Dividing the uterine horn into arbitrary segments may help to designate the location of a structure during the examination of the uterine tract.
- Follicles appear as anechoic structures of various sizes, and the line between the follicular wall and the follicular antrum is always smooth and well defined.
- The corpus luteum has a granular echogenic structure, which intensifies during the luteal phase.
- The regressing corpus luteum is not easily differentiated from the ovarian stroma.

Summary Questions

1. What is the ultrasonographic distinction between the appearance of the vascular layer and the endometrium of the uterus?
   a. The vascular bed of the uterine wall appears as a faint echoic line compared to the endometrium and is characterized by an echoic appearance with nonspecular reflection so that dark and bright signals are seen within the thickness.
   b. There is no distinction between the appearance of the vascular layer and the endometrium of the uterus.
   c. The vascular bed of the uterine wall between the serosa and the muscle tissues appears as a hyperechoic line compared to the endometrium.
   d. The ultrasonographic distinction between the vascular layer and the endometrium of the uterus is visible only in uterine infection (endometritis) and appears as a hyperechoic line compared to the endometrium.

2. What are the anatomic features and ultrasonographic characteristics of an inactive ovary?
   a. Without functional structures such as large follicles, the ovarian stroma is enhanced and the ovary has a heterogenic echogenicity.
   b. An inactive ovary has an echogenic appearance similar to that of a functional ovary.
   c. Without functional structures, the inactive ovary is almond-shaped and firm and has a uniform echogenicity that equals to or is slightly greater than the cervix.
   d. An inactive ovary is firm on transrectal palpation and has a heterogenic appearance with different anechoic structures (follicles) and hyperechoic areas (ovarian stroma).

Answers

1. a
2. c

CHAPTER FOUR

Bovine Ovary

Paul D. Carrière, Giovanni Gnemmi, Luc DesCôteaux, Motozumi Matsui, Akio Miyamoto, and Jill Colloton

Introduction

The bovine ovary is a fascinating structure that produces a single ovulatory follicle and corpus luteum (CL) at regular intervals. Correct interpretation of the nature of ovarian structures observed by ultrasonography is a complex issue because follicles and CLs are continuously growing or regressing. The challenge for the practitioner is to determine in a limited number of observations whether the developmental process leading to ovulation and production of a CL is proceeding normally to ensure fertilization and pregnancy. The first section of this chapter reviews the endocrinology and normal ovarian structures observed in the bovine ovary with emphasis on the identification of the CL at different stages of development. The second section reviews the principal ovarian anomalies and differential diagnosis. The third section introduces a new frontier in the understanding of ovarian physiology using color Doppler. This technique will allow the practitioner to characterize the hemodynamic changes that occur during the cyclical remodeling of the ovary. The last section discusses the use of ovarian ultrasound in reproduction synchronization protocols for dairy cattle.

Endocrinology and Ovarian Structures in Pubertal Cows

Endocrinology

In the pubertal heifer and adult cow, growth of antral follicles occurs continuously throughout the estrous cycle. The speed of follicular growth increases exponentially as follicles increase in size. It has been estimated that small antral follicles grow from 1.5 mm to 3.8 mm in 30 days and larger follicles grow from 4 to 8 mm in less than 1 week[33]. In the absence of gonadotropin stimulation, follicles grow up to 4 mm but fail to grow beyond this size and will regress and disappear by the process of atresia[13]. Growth of ovarian follicles beyond 4 mm requires FSH and LH stimulation. Throughout the estrous cycle a transient increase in plasma FSH occurs periodically every 7–10 days, and is responsible for the recruitment of a cohort of follicles known as the follicular wave[4,48] (Figure 4.1). Among the recruited follicles of a follicular wave, a single dominant follicle (exceptionally two) will be selected over the next few days[18]. Selection is a term used to describe the point of divergence in growth between the largest and second largest follicle. In Holstein heifers, when the largest follicle grows from 8.5 to 9.5 mm a slower rate of growth of the second largest follicle can be measured by ultrasound. This difference in growth rate results in a significant difference in size between the largest and the second largest follicle and is referred to as deviation[23]. Selection of the dominant follicle corresponds to the time of deviation, and the terms *selection* and *deviation* are used synonymously. The largest follicle is called *dominant* because for a certain period of time no other follicle >4 mm can be observed in its presence. Plasma FSH values reach maximum when the future dominant follicle is about 5 mm and reach low levels by the time of deviation[30]. Exogenous FSH delays or overrides deviation.

Although FSH, LH, estradiol, and progesterone are key players in follicular development (Figure 4.2), many other factors are involved, including insulin, IGF, and locally produced growth factors of the TGF-beta superfamily, and other endocrine, paracrine, and autocrine factors. It is important to realize that follicular waves are produced continuously during the

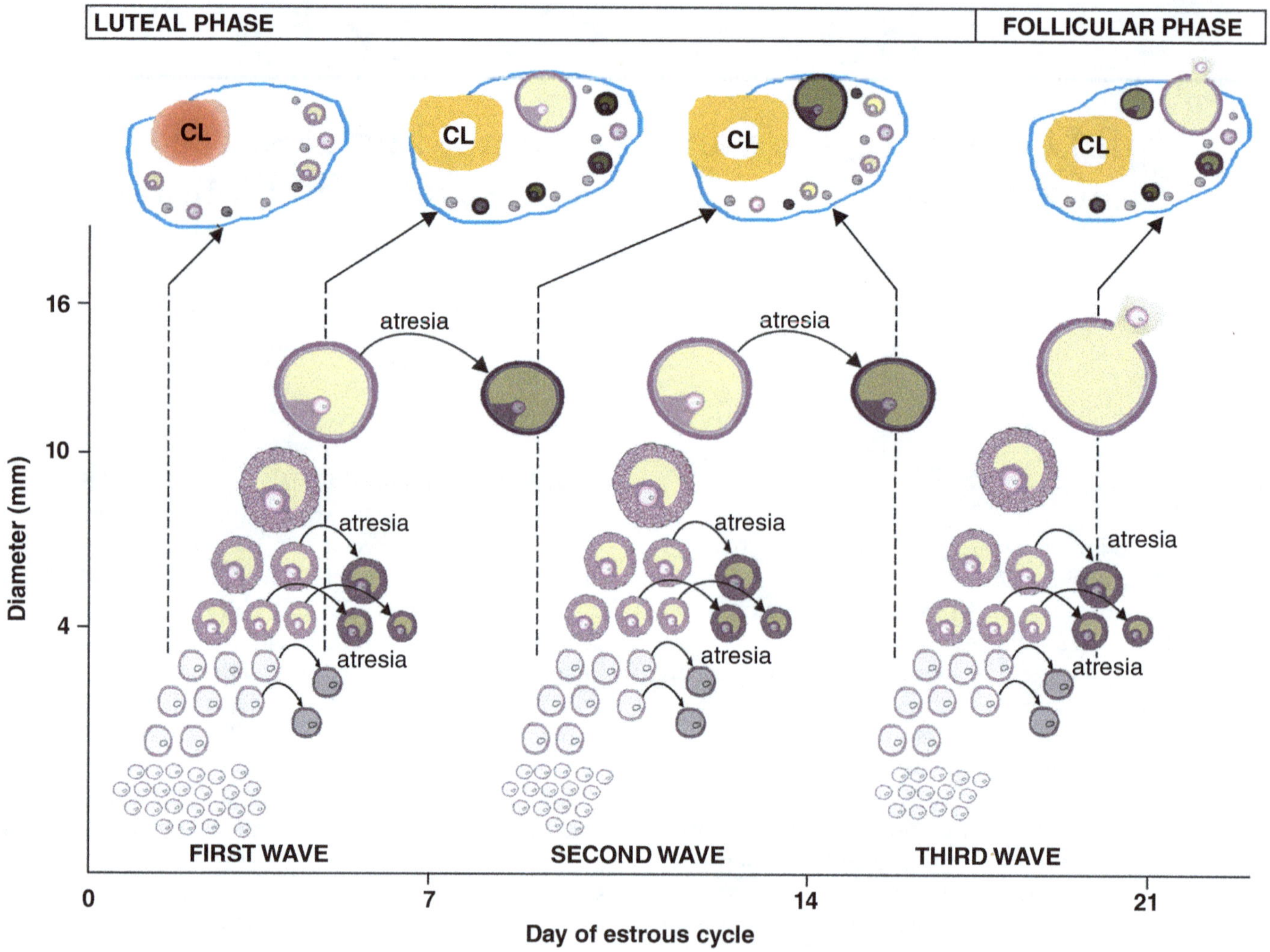

Figure 4.1. Follicular waves and corpus luteum development during the bovine estrous cycle with three follicular waves (illustration by Dr. Xiaofeng Zheng). During the estrous cycle of 18 to 24 days, usually two or three (and occasionally four) follicular waves will develop and from each wave will emerge a single large dominant follicle of 12–15 mm. During the luteal phase, the dominant follicle of the first wave will regress slowly by atresia and only the dominant follicle emerging from the last wave of the cycle will become the ovulatory follicle. The dominant follicle of the last wave grows in the presence of declining progesterone concentration (due to luteolysis), which stimulates an increase in LH pulse secretion and induces a rapid rise in estradiol. The combination of low progesterone with high estradiol will stimulate the hypothalamus and pituitary for generation of the LH surge (Figure 4.2). The LH surge causes a decrease in estradiol secretion and a sudden rise in progesterone secretion from the granulosa cells of the preovulatory follicle. The rise in follicular progesterone will initiate the activation of the enzymes responsible for the degradation of the follicular wall and will favor ovulation[16]. In this figure atretic follicles are darker compared to healthy follicles.

follicular and luteal phases and also during pregnancy in the cow.

During antral follicular growth, the proportion of follicles undergoing atresia increases dramatically and the rate of atresia doubles between 2 and 8 mm[33]. Atresia of subordinate follicles in favor of the dominant follicle is a physiological process that is necessary for selection of the dominant follicle and is associated with a decrease in circulating concentrations of FSH. Administration of exogenous FSH to induce superovulation can overcome the natural process of selection and induce multiple ovulations (see Chapter 8).

Ovarian structures

Ultrasound imaging is considered the most accurate diagnostic method to identify ovarian and uterine structures. Transrectal palpation is a complement to

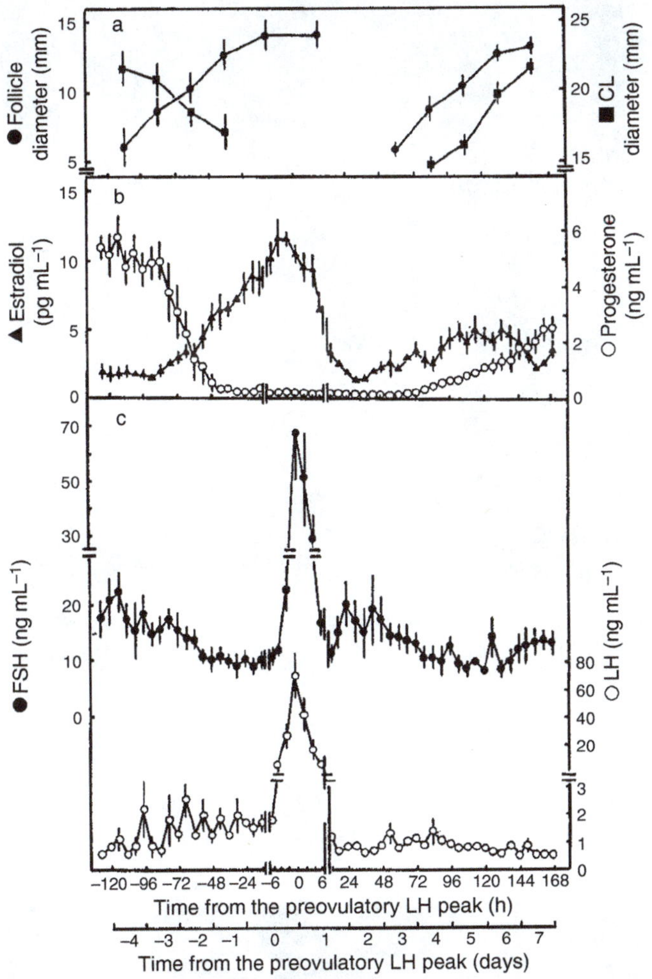

Figure 4.2. Mean diameters of dominant follicles and corpora lutea (CL), plasma concentrations of estradiol and progesterone, and plasma concentrations of FSH and LH during the spontaneous luteal-follicular transition, ovulation, and early luteal phase in five cows (mean ± SEM). From Kaneko et al. (1991)[27], with permission of CSIRO PUBLISHING accessible at http://www.publish.csiro.au/nid/45/issue/2331.htm.

the ultrasound examination and remains a practical means of evaluating the contours and texture of these organs.

Follicles

The follicle can be easily identified on the screen and appears black due to hypoechogenic follicular fluid. The ultrasound appearance of ovarian follicles is shown in Figure 4.3. During the ultrasonographic evaluation of the ovaries, it is important to be able to distinguish a follicle from a blood vessel. A cross-sectional view of an ovarian blood vessel resembles the image of a spherical segment of a follicle. However, when moving the probe in the direction that will allow a longitudinal section rather than a cross section of the blood vessel, the initial spherical image will become elongated, contrary to the follicle, which becomes a smaller sphere and simply disappears from view when the probe is moved away. Due to the continuous production of follicular waves throughout the estrous cycle, large follicles >8 mm are always present in bovine ovaries (except for the first few days of the cycle), and thus it can be misleading to attempt to predict the time of ovulation based solely on the size of the largest follicle. We therefore need to rely on other signs, such as changes in ultrasound echogenicity of the uterine wall (see Chapter 5) and CL, increased uterine tone, the presence of endometrial secretion within the uterus, the presence of cervical mucus, and the cow's behavioral changes.

Corpus luteum

In bovine reproduction, it is very important to be able to recognize the presence of the corpus luteum (CL). The presence of a CL confirms that a heifer has attained puberty. Localization of the CL on the left or right ovary can indicate to the practitioner in which uterine horn the presence of an embryo or fetus needs to be confirmed for pregnancy diagnosis. Defining the age of the CL could be helpful in deciding when to start a synchronized ovulation protocol (OvSynch) or to propose treatment with prostaglandin. It is also possible in these cases to verify the presence of a large follicle (≥8 mm) in order to better predict the response and success of the proposed synchronization reproduction protocol (see the last section of this chapter for more details). Correct identification of the bovine CL is a real challenge to the practitioner because, depending on the stage of development, this structure can present many different morphological appearances.

The mature CL is hypoechogenic (darker) compared to the ovarian stroma due to extensive vascularization. Echographically we can distinguish differences between a mature compact corpus luteum and a mature cavitary corpus luteum (CCL). The ovaries can contain more than one CL and these can be compact and/or with a cavity (Figure 4.4). The size of the cavity can vary considerably and echogenic fibrin strands are occasionally observed within the fluid-filled cavity (Figure 4.4).

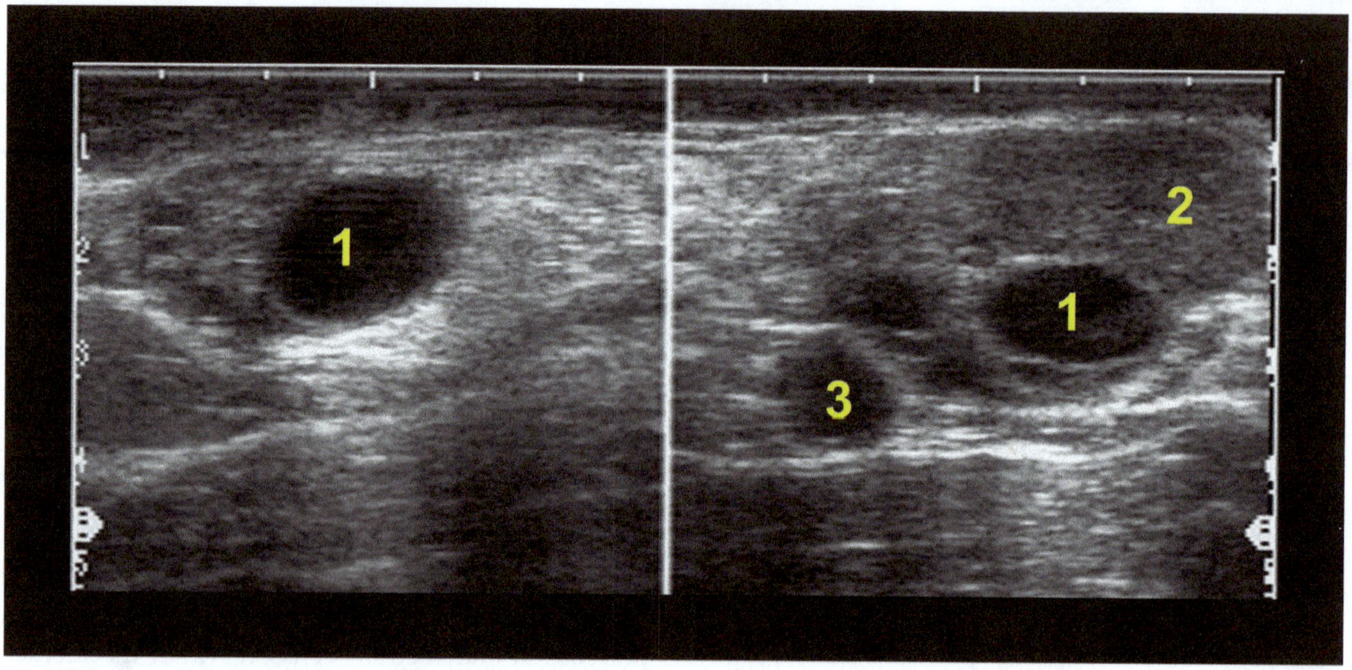

Figure 4.3. Ultrasound images in BB-mode of both ovaries in a cow in diestrus (probe 8 MHz; depth 5 cm). Notice the presence of a single 16 mm follicle on the left ovary. A 2.5 cm CL and an 11 mm follicle are present on the right ovary. 1: Follicle; 2: Corpus luteum (CL); 3: Blood vessel.

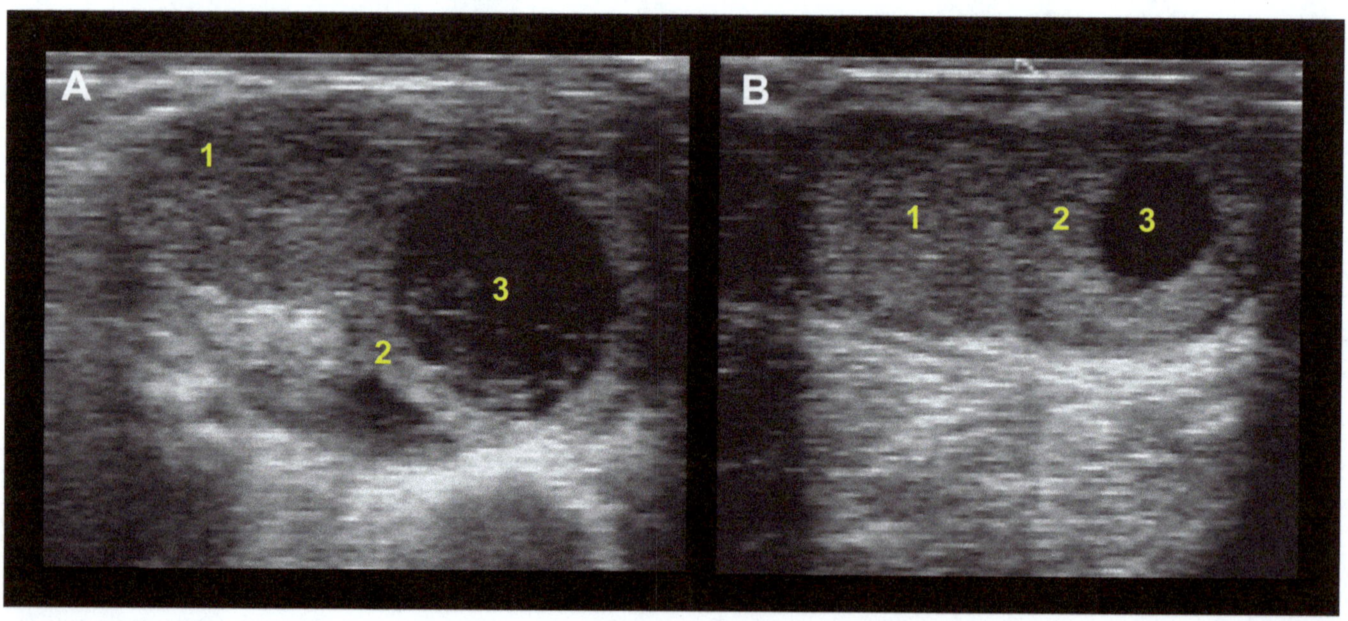

Figure 4.4. Ultrasonograms of two ovaries that present cavitary and compact corpora lutea (CL) in the same ovary (7.5 MHz probe; depth of 5 cm). 1: Compact CL; 2: Luteal tissue of a cavitary CL (CCL); 3: Cavity of a CCL. Echogenic fibrin strands are also observed in the cavity of the CCL (A).

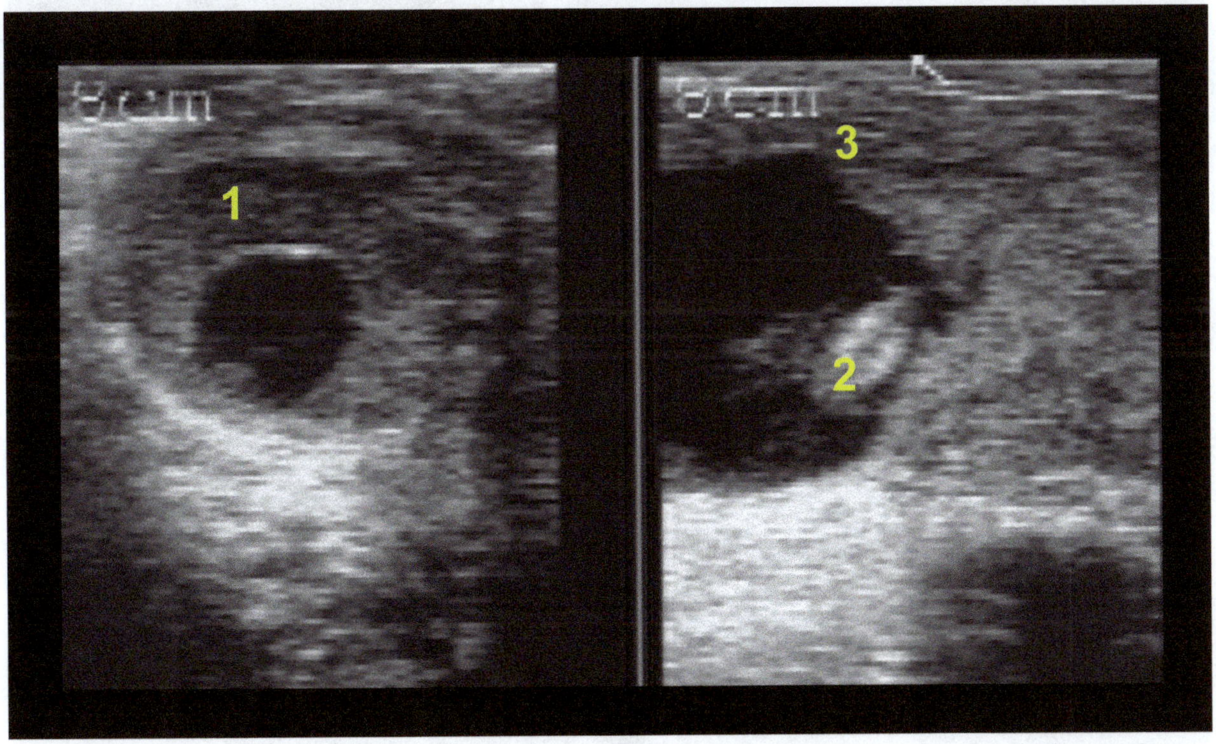

Figure 4.5. Presence of a cavitary corpus luteum (CCL) in a 32-day pregnant dairy cow (7.5 MHz probe; depth of 5 cm). 1: CCL; 2: Embryo proper; 3: Endometrium.

Under field conditions with a portable unit (5 to 7.5 MHz) a well-defined border of the CL is visible after 3–4 days. During the first 10 days of the ovarian cycle, 30–50% of all corpora lutea will develop a cavity[25,29,41]. A CCL is considered a normal structure producing normal progesterone levels[25]. It does not alter the length of the ovarian cycle, or reduce the likelihood of pregnancy[25,28,41]. Occasionally a CCL will be seen in a pregnant cow[25,26,29]. In pregnant cows, it is rare (but not impossible) to find a CCL beyond day 30 of gestation[28] (Figure 4.5). It is likely that the volume of luteal tissue is more important than the presence or absence of a cavity.

The cavity in the CL can be central or eccentric and we can find more than one cavity in the same CL and in some cases only partial incomplete luteinization of the follicular wall[25] (Figure 4.6). Between the 10th and 15th day of the cycle, most CCLs lose their cavity[25,41]. The cavity can be substituted by new echogenic tissue. Filling of the cavity can take many different forms:

1. In some cases, uniform hyperechogenic tissue completely fills the cavity[22,25,26,42] (Figure 4.7). The exact nature of this tissue is unknown but might be due to specular reflexions of new lutal tissue intermixed with fibrin strands, which are known to be very echogenic.
2. In some cases, the filling of the cavity occurs gradually and can be partial or complete[42] (Figure 4.8).
3. The cavity can be completely substituted by luteal tissue leaving only a hyperechogenic line or scar[22,25] (Figure 4.9).
4. The cavity stays but an evident hyperechogenic ring appears surrounding the same cavity (Figure 4.10).

Follicles and CL at proestrus, estrus, and metestrus

The resolution of the corpus luteum changes according to the phase of the estrous cycle. The luteal tissue is more difficult to recognize during proestrus, estrus,

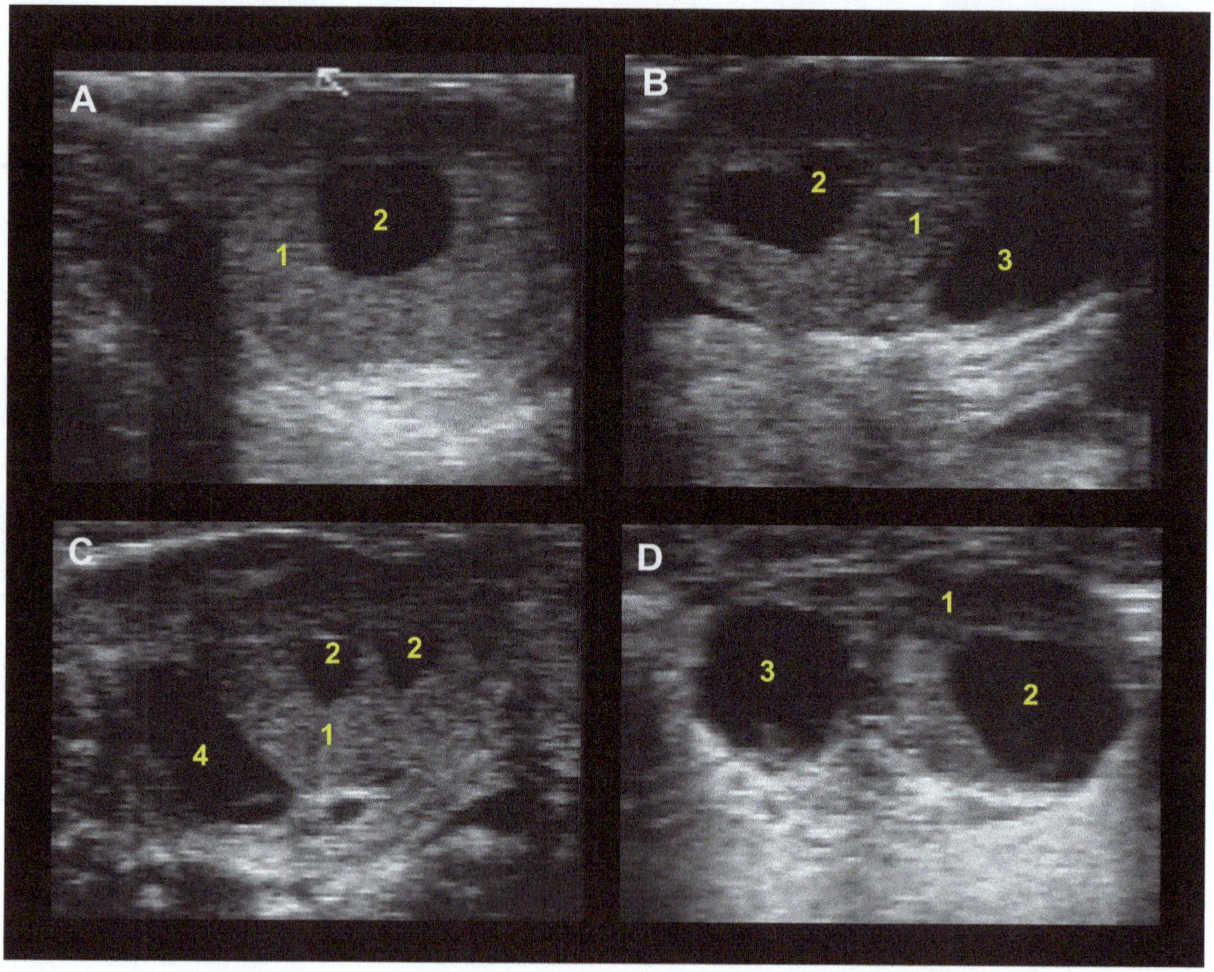

Figure 4.6. Cavitary corpus luteum (CCL) with central, eccentric, and double cavities and CCL with incomplete luteinization (7.5 MHz probe; depth of 5 cm). A: CCL with a central cavity; B: CCL with an eccentric cavity; C: CCL with two cavities; D: CCL with incomplete luteinization. 1: Luteal tissue; 2: Cavity; 3: Follicle; 4: Blood vessel.

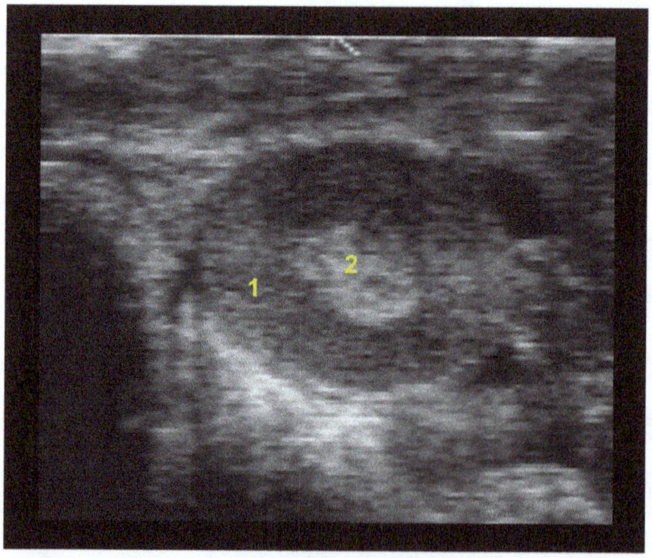

Figure 4.7. Cavitary corpus luteum (CCL) in which the cavity disappeared and is replaced by hyperechogenic tissue after 10 days of the estrous cycle (7.5 MHz probe; depth of 5 cm). 1: Luteal tissue; 2: Hyperechogenic zone.

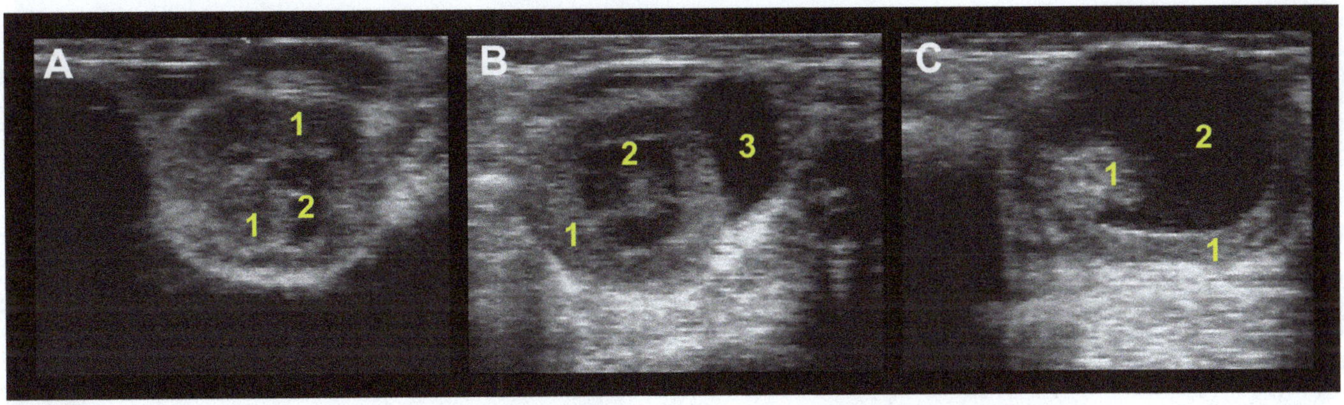

Figure 4.8. Cavitary corpus luteum (CCL) with different filling patterns of the cavity (7.5 MHz probe; depth of 4.5 cm). A: CCL with central filling; B: CCL with eccentric filling; C: CCL with eccentric incomplete filling. 1: Luteal tissue; 2: Cavity; 3: Follicle.

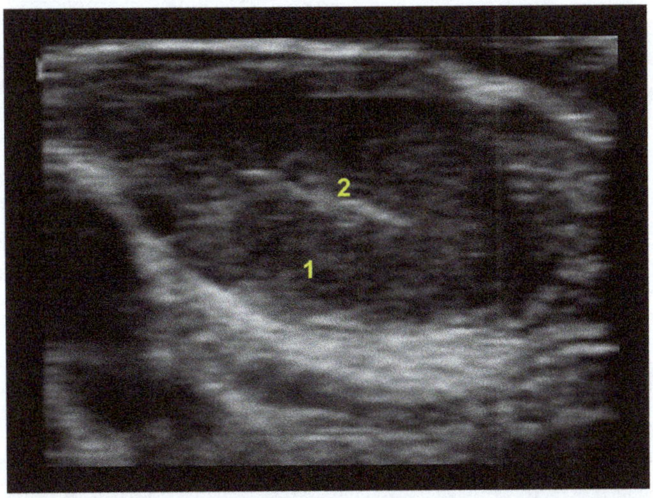

Figure 4.9. Cavitary corpus luteum in which the cavity was replaced by white hyperechogenic line or scar at approximately 10 days of the estrous cycle (7.5 MHz probe; depth of 4.5 cm). 1: Luteal tissue; 2: Central scar.

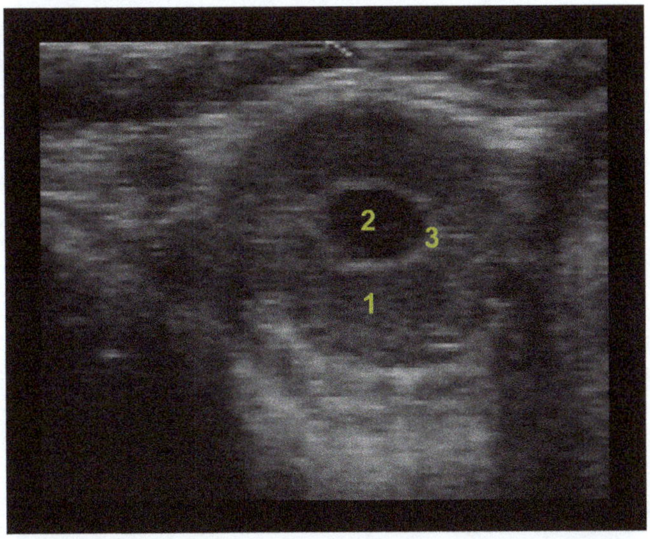

Figure 4.10. Cavitary corpus luteum in which the cavity is surrounded by a hyperechogenic ring (7.5 MHz probe; depth of 4.5 cm). 1: Luteal tissue; 2: Cavity; 3: Hyperechogenic ring.

and metestrus than it is during diestrus because the CL is isoechogenic compared to the surrounding stroma. During metestrus, the echogenicity of the CL depends on newly formed angiotrophic tissue of the corpus hemorrhagicum, and during proestrus it depends on the abundance of connective tissue[22]. This distinction is very difficult to obtain under field conditions with current commercially available units. For this reason the age determination of a CL must be assisted by considering the differences in follicular structures that occur during the follicular waves in addition to the ultrasonographic appearance of the uterus during the cycle (see Chapter 5).

At estrus (day 0), the most obvious structure is the dominant ovulatory follicle, which has an average internal diameter of 13 mm, with a range between 11 and 16 mm[10]. The regressing CL is sometimes difficult to observe during the follicular phase (Figure 4.11). During transition from proestrus to estrus, other signs such as changes in echogenicity of the uterine wall (see Chapter 5), increased uterine tone at palpation, the presence of endometrial

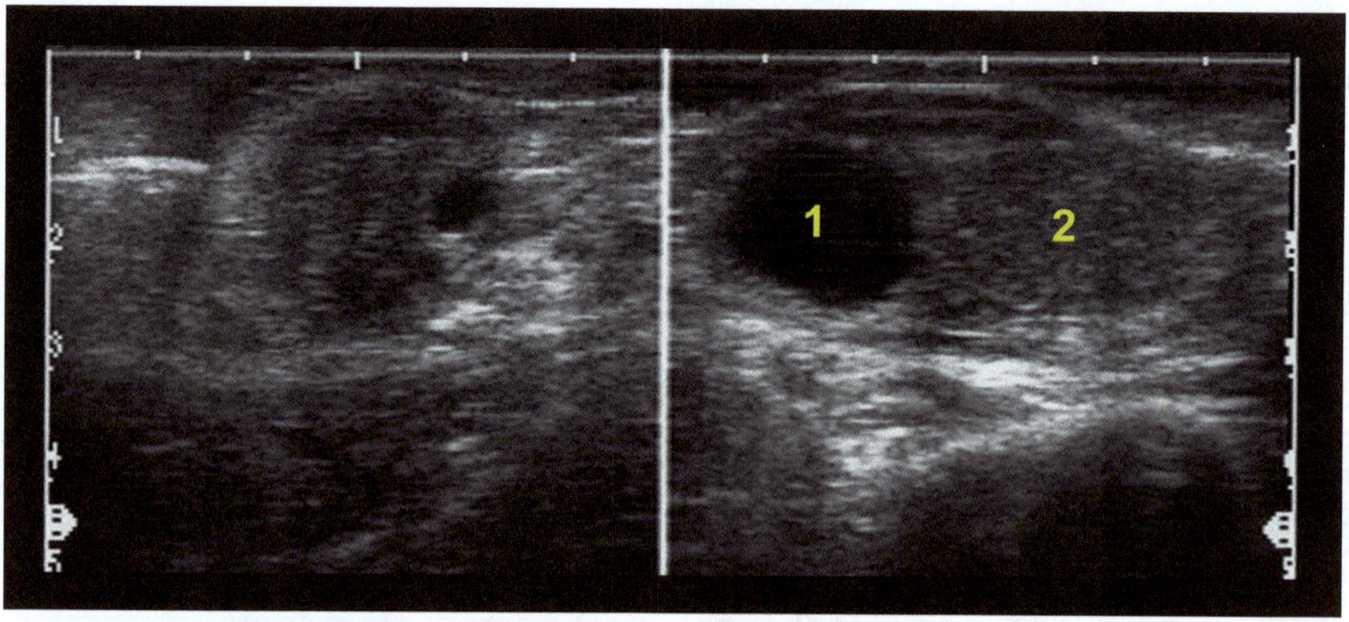

Figure 4.11. Ultrasonogram of both ovaries in BB-mode during estrus with the presence of a regressing corpus luteum (CL) and a dominant preovulatory follicle on the right ovary and of an inactive left ovary which shows a small follicle. 1: Dominant preovulatory follicle (14 mm); 2: Regressing CL. Note the scale on this image is 1 cm per line.

secretion within the uterus, the presence of cervical mucus, and estrus behavior of the cow are needed to confirm that the animal is truly approaching estrus.

Ovarian Anomalies and Differential Diagnosis

Inactive ovaries

Inactive ovaries are associated with anestrus and are characterized by the absence of large follicles, no CL, and the presence of small follicles less than 4 mm in diameter (Figure 4.12).

Ovarian cysts

Ovarian follicular cysts in cattle are characterized by the persistence of large anovulatory structures for various periods of time in the absence of corpora lutea, with interruption of normal estrous cycles. Although traditionally cysts have been defined as follicular structures of 25 mm or greater, more recently a

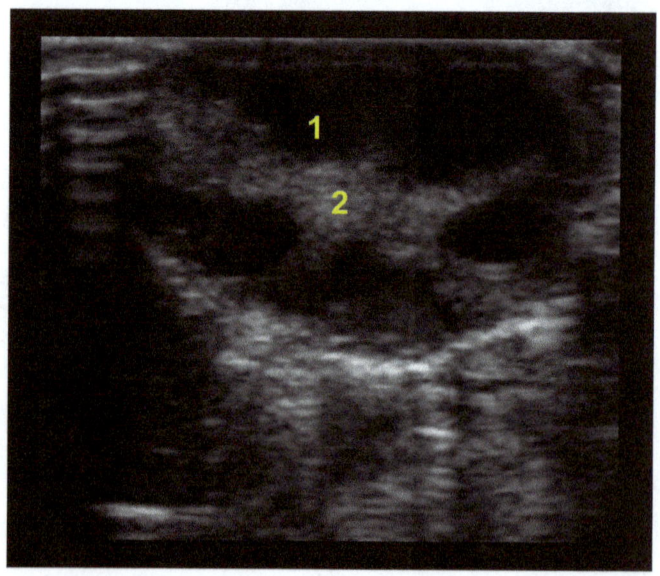

Figure 4.12. Ultrasound image of an inactive ovary (probe 7.5 MHz; depth 2.5 cm). Notice the presence of many small follicles (less than 4 mm) around the ovarian stroma. 1: Follicle; 2: Ovarian stroma.

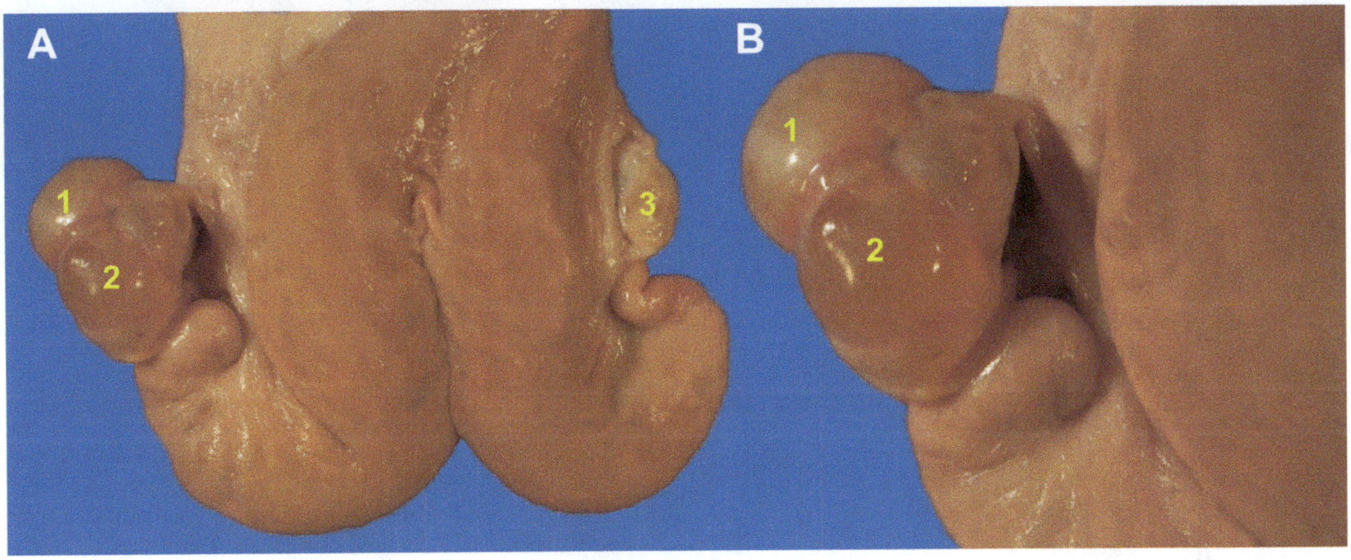

Figure 4.13. Reproductive tract of a cow in anestrus showing a polycystic right ovary and a left inactive ovary. 1: Follicular cyst #1 (3.7 cm); 2: Follicular cyst #2 (3.0 cm); 3: Inactive ovary. (Photo, Dr. Luc DesCôteaux.)

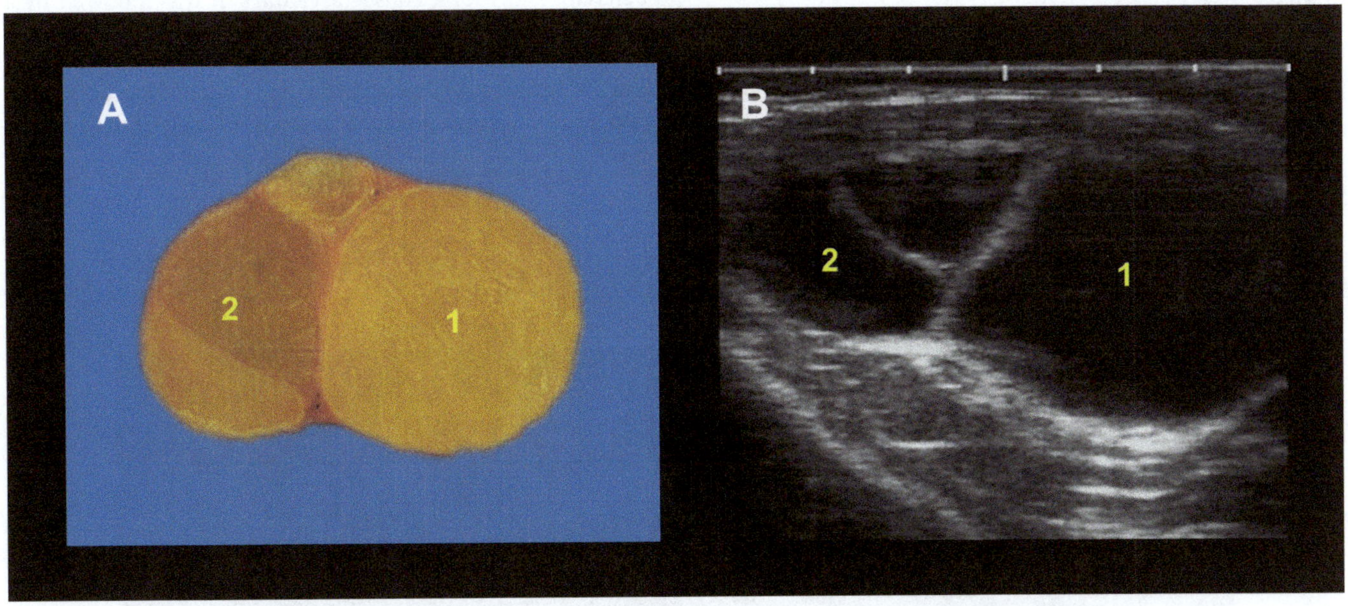

Figure 4.14. Multiple follicular cysts: (A) cut section of the frozen ovary from Figure 4.13 and its ultrasonographic appearance (B) (probe 8 MHz; depth 5 cm). (Photo, Dr. Luc DesCôteaux.) 1: Follicular cyst #1 (3.7 cm); 2: Follicular cyst #2 (3.0 cm).

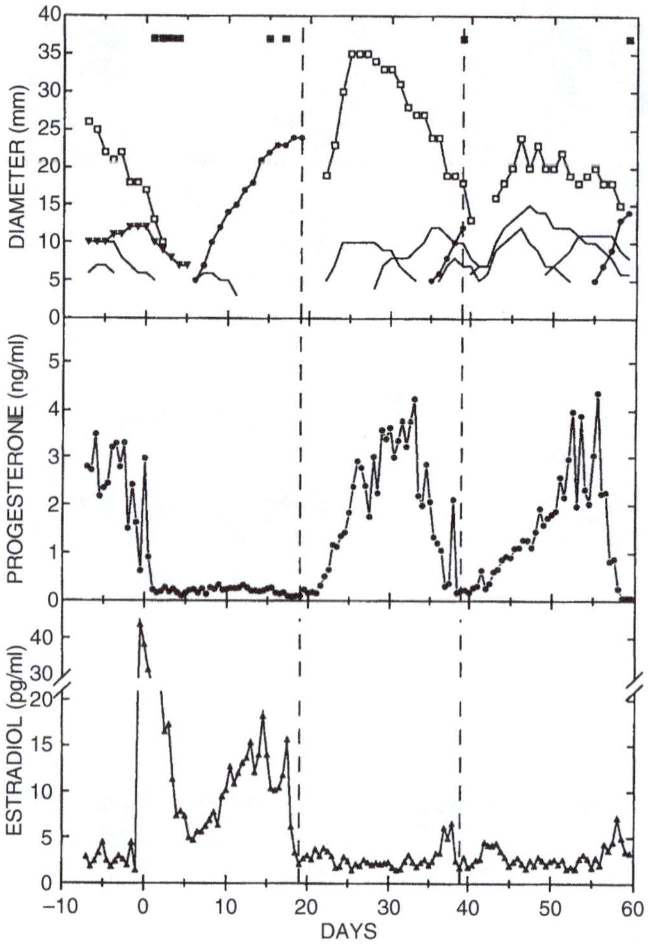

Figure 4.15. Estrous behavior, follicular growth pattern, plasma estradiol, and progesterone profile in a heifer (#79) injected with estradiol valerate and PG (day 0) during the follicular phase, which produced a follicular cyst that ovulated and developed into a large cavitary CL. From Carrière et al. (1995)[10]. Top panel shows diameter of the CLs (open squares), recruited anovulatory follicles (simple lines), ovulatory follicle (black circles), and broken vertical line representing day of ovulation. Black squares at top indicate estrous behavior signs. Middle and bottom panels show plasma progesterone and estradiol profiles. Note the increase in estradiol production due to the injection of estradiol valerate at day 0, which inhibited growth of the dominant follicle (inverted black triangles of top panel) and stimulated estrous behavior signs for 4 consecutive days. It was followed by a second increase in estradiol secretion produced by the growing follicular cyst. This heifer presented interrupted estrous behavior signs, and then the follicular cyst ovulated spontaneously and produced a large cavitary CL (see Figure 4.16).

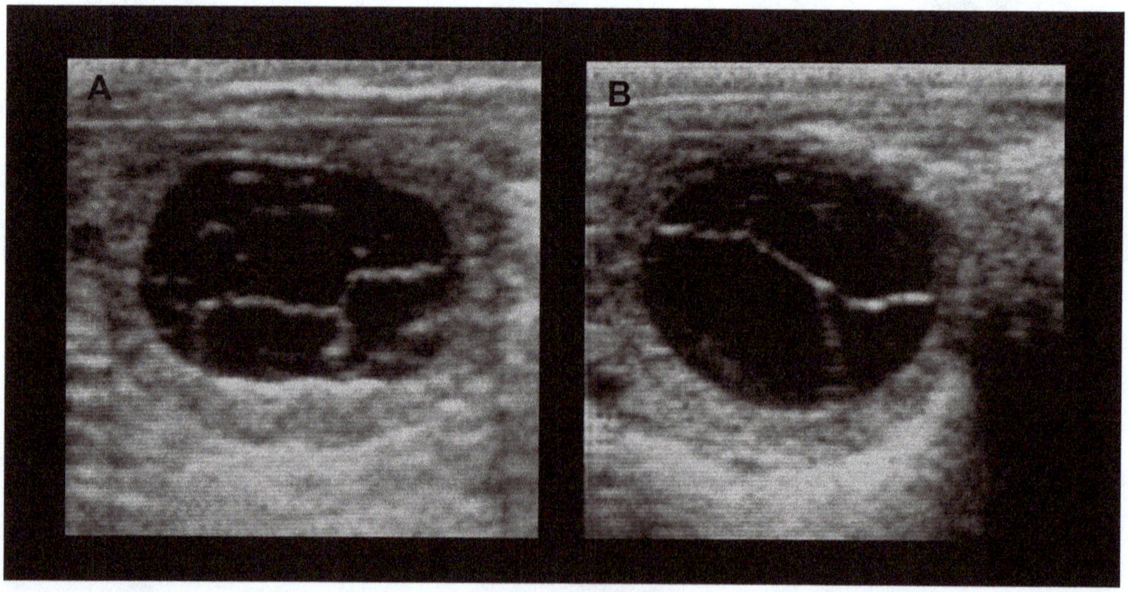

Figure 4.16. Ultrasonogram of a large cavitary CL with a 30 mm cavity that developed following spontaneous ovulation of an experimentally induced follicular cyst in two heifers. A: Cavitary CL with fibrin trabecula of heifer #79; B: Cavitary CL with fibrin trabecula of heifer #89. From Carrière et al. (1995)[10]; Amaya D (1994)[5]. Master's thesis. Université de Montréal.

diagnosis of ovarian follicular cyst was based on a diameter greater than 16 or 17 mm[10,21,47]. Cystic ovaries, ovarian cysts, and cystic ovarian degeneration are terms used synonymously with ovarian follicular cysts. The condition causes economic losses to the dairy industry by extending the interval from calving to conception. The macroscopic and ultrasonographic appearances of multiple follicular cysts on the same ovary are shown in Figures 4.13 and 4.14.

It is important to recognize that ovarian cysts are dynamic structures. During an experimental study, heifers received an injection of estradiol and prostaglandin during the follicular phase and subsequently developed a single large follicular cyst in the absence of a corpus luteum[10]. There were several different outcomes in response to treatment. In the first scenario, in two heifers, a dominant follicle emerged 5 days after treatment and continued to grow until it ovulated 10 to 14 days later at a diameter of 19 and 24 mm, respectively, (mean diameter in control heifers: 13.4 ± 2 mm). Preceding ovulation, both animals exhibited prolonged or split estrus lasting several days. The estrous behavior, plasma concentrations of progesterone and estradiol, and diameter of the CL and follicles during and after spontaneous recovery of one of these heifers are shown in Figure 4.15. The ovulation of the follicular cyst subsequently developed into a cavitary CL, with a very large 30 mm cavity that was traversed by echogenic fibrin trabecula (Figure 4.16). This large cavitary CL regressed spontaneously during a normal interval, and this was followed by a regular estrous cycle with normal ovarian structures (Figure 4.15).

In the second scenario, the follicular cyst failed to ovulate, partially luteinized, and regressed. In the third scenario, several successive waves producing a follicular cyst developed and the heifer failed to ovulate for 52 days. Each wave produced an active estradiol-secreting follicular cyst that reached maximum size in 5–10 days and then regressed slowly over 30 days[10]. The estrous behavior, plasma concentrations of progesterone and estradiol, and follicle dynamics of this heifer are shown in Figure 4.17.

Based on this experimental study[10] and others[50], active follicular cysts secreting estradiol may retain the capacity to ovulate. Ovulation of a follicular cyst in the estradiol-treated model was shown to result in the formation of a large cavitary CL with traversing fibrin strands visible after 2–4 days[5,10] (Figure 4.16). The morphological appearance of these large cavitary CLs was indistinguishable from the morphological appearance of so-called luteal cysts, which are believed to

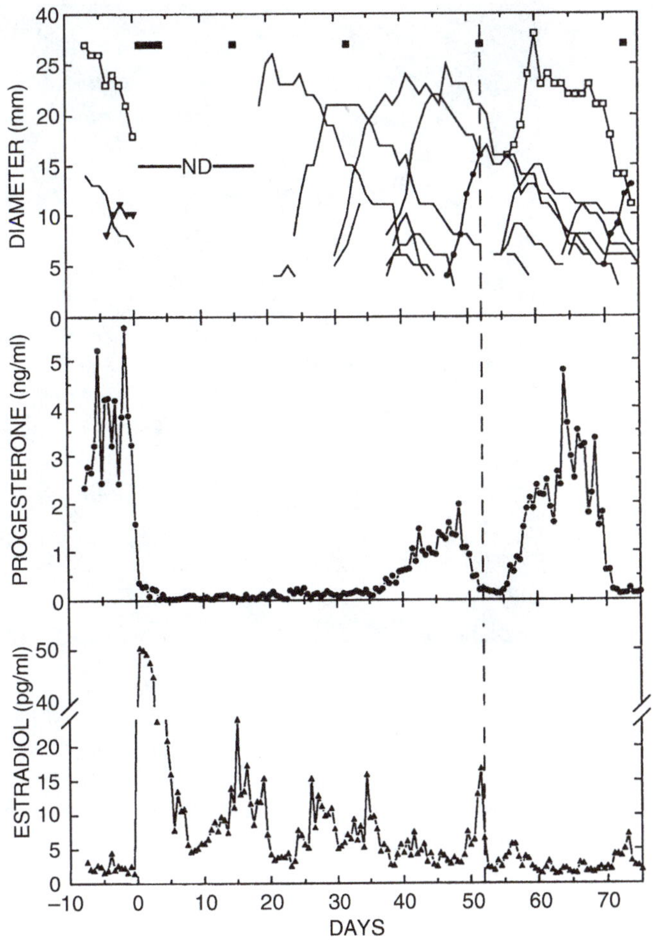

Figure 4.17. Estrous behavior, follicular growth pattern, plasma estradiol, and progesterone profile in a heifer injected with estradiol valerate and PG (day 0). This heifer developed several successive follicular cysts and failed to ovulate for 52 days. From Carrière et al. (1995)[10]. Top panel shows diameter of the CLs (open squares), recruited anovulatory follicles (simple lines), ovulatory follicles (black circles), and the broken vertical line representing day of ovulation. Black squares at top indicate estrous behavior signs. ND indicates that ultrasonography was not performed for the first 20 days to allow this heifer to recover from rectal fissures. Middle and bottom panels show plasma progesterone and estradiol profiles. Note the increase in estradiol production due to the injection of estradiol valerate at day 0 followed by subsequent increases in estradiol secretion produced by the growing follicular cysts. The four successive follicular cysts that were observed did not ovulate and regressed slowly. From day 35 of treatment, one of the follicles luteinized spontaneously and the first ovulation occurred 52 days after treatment.

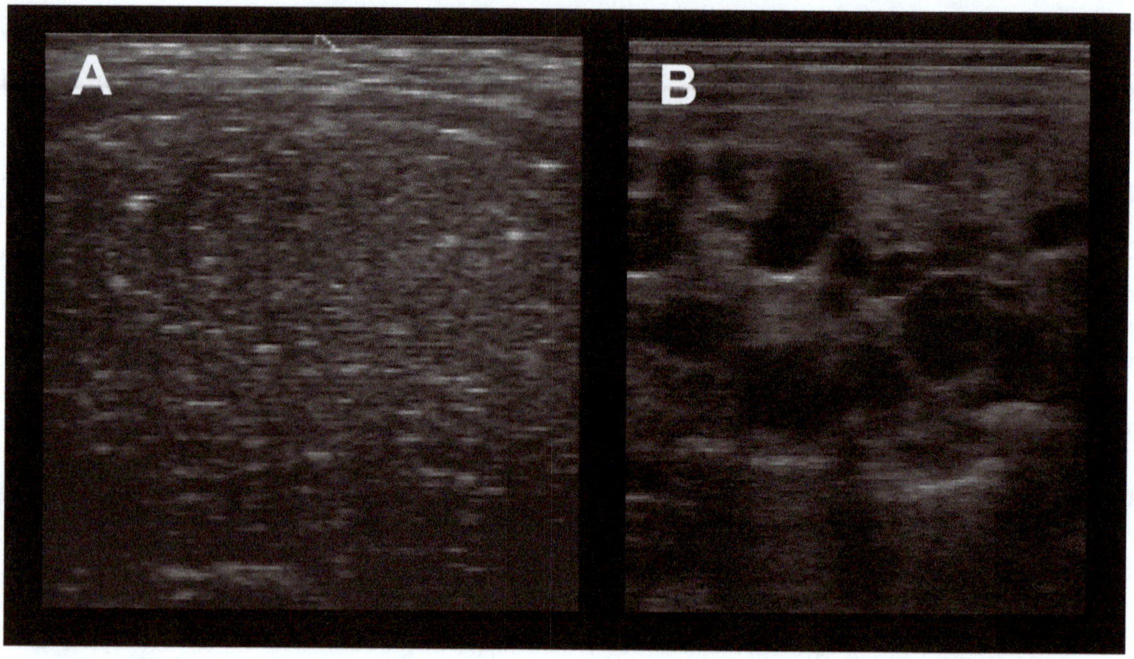

Figure 4.18. Ultrasonographic appearances of granulosa cell tumors in cows. Granulosa cell tumors (GCT) in the cow are usually unilateral and the gross appearance varies considerably. The surface may be smooth or coarsely lobulated. The cut surface may be solid, consist predominantly of cysts of varied size, consist of a mixture of solid and cystic tissue, or consist of a single large cyst. Structurally, a GCT is generally heterogeneous, some parts may be echogenic, others anechogenic. In some cases areas of calcification or necrosis may be found (A), as well as fluid-filled spaces (or cavities) (B), in the stroma of the tumor. Ultrasound images are courtesy of Dr. Giovanni Gnemmi (A) and Dr. T.A.E. Stout of Utrecht University, The Netherlands (B).

result from lutenization of follicular cysts that have failed to ovulate. Morphologically, it may not be possible to differentiate with certainty between a large cavitary CL and a luteal cyst unless daily ultrasound sessions have proved that the expulsion of follicular fluid at ovulation had actually taken place. Nevertheless, these academic distinctions do not in any way modify the course of action to follow when the structures are identified. Prostaglandins can be used to lyse the structure and induce a new estrus within the same time frame of 2–7 days after injection, just as with a normal or cavitary CL. Also, synchronization protocols of the ovulation such as OvSynch can be used effectively in the presence of luteal tissue originating from either a cavitary CL or a luteal cyst. Follicular cysts are treated with GnRH. However, based on the above, the practitioner should be aware that follicular cysts are often benign; they may have become inactive and are slowly regressing during a normal cycle and can be seen in pregnant cows.

Granulosa cell tumor

Although ovarian tumors are rare in the cow, granulosa cell tumors are the most common. Granulosa cell tumors are characterized by unilateral ovarian enlargement greater than 10 cm in diameter. The surface of the ovary may be smooth or coarsely lobulated. The behavior of the cow can range from anestrus to nymphomania. In some cases udder development and lactation occur in heifers. The ultrasound appearance of a granulosa cell tumor is shown in Figure 4.18.

Differential diagnosis of corpus luteum

It is very important to correctly distinguish ultrasound images that resemble a CL. In the following figures, various images are presented in order to avoid misdiagnosis of CL structures with placentomes, ovarian abscesses or transverse uterine horn sections (Figures 4.19–4.21).

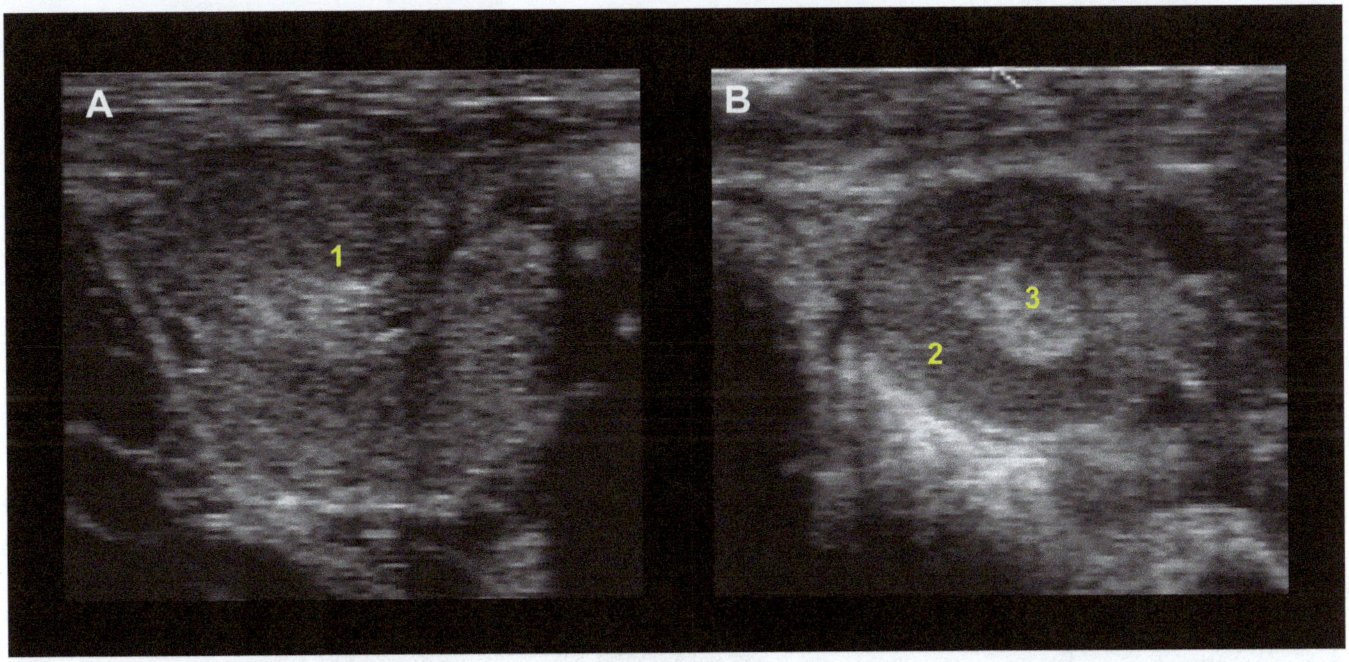

Figure 4.19. Differential diagnosis of corpus luteum with a placentome (7.5 MHz probe; depth of 5 cm). A: Placentome; B: CL; 1: Placentome; 2: Luteal tissue; 3: Echogenic central zone.

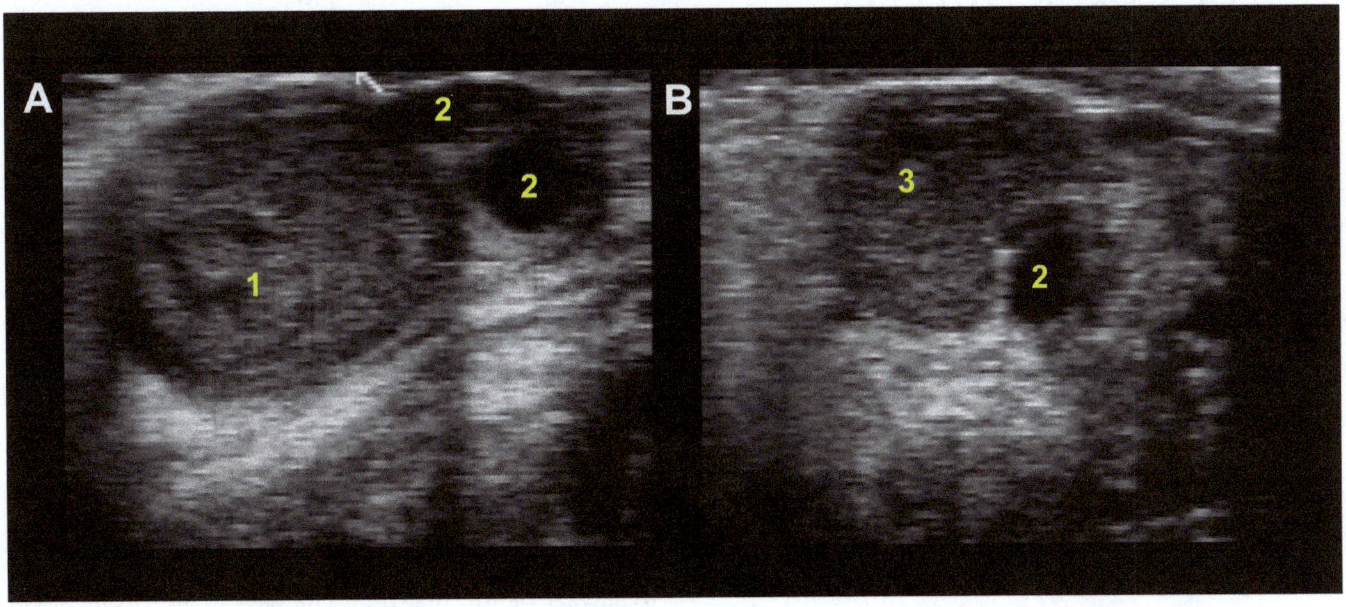

Figure 4.20. Differential diagnosis of corpus luteum with an ovarian abscess (7.5 MHz probe; depth of 5 cm). A: Ovarian abscess; B: CL; 1: Abscess; 2: Follicle; 3: Corpus luteum.

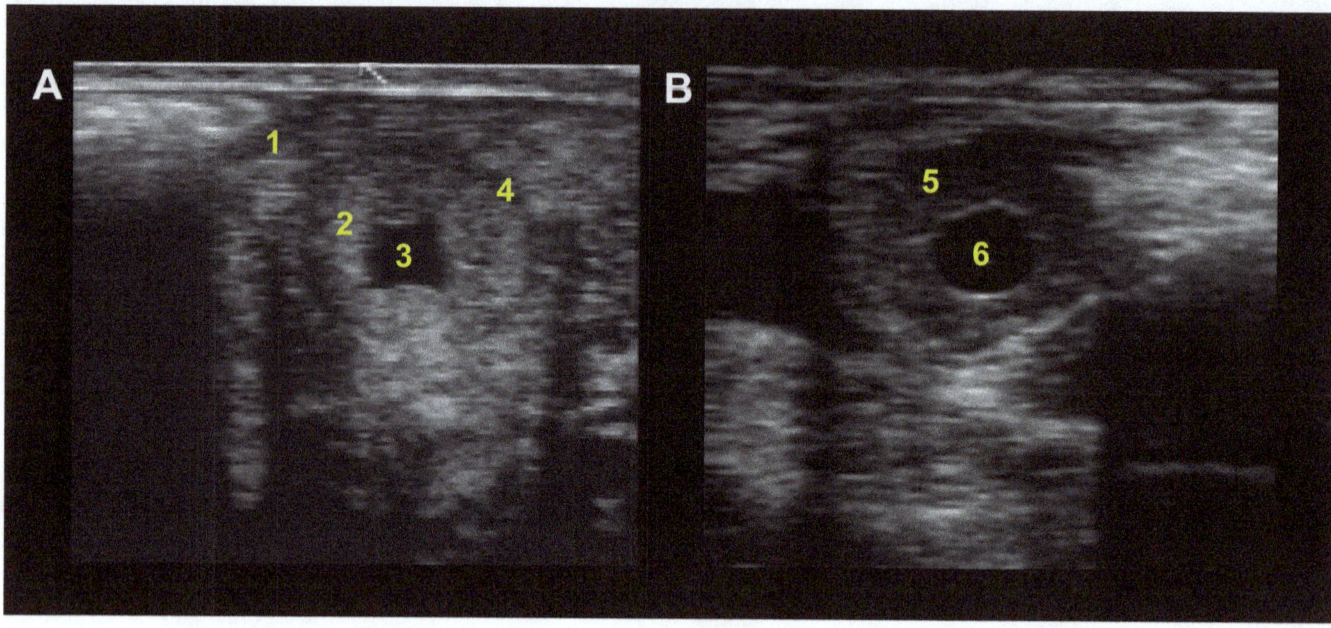

Figure 4.21. Differential diagnosis of cavitary corpus luteum (CCL) with the uterine horn in transverse section (7.5 MHz probe; depth of 5 cm). A: Transverse section of the uterus in the estrous phase; B: CCL; 1: Myometrium; 2: Endometrium; 3: Uterine lumen with anechoic liquid; 4: Vascular layer of the myometrium; 5: Luteal tissue; 6: Cavity of the CL.

Use of Color Doppler to Monitor Ovarian Blood Flow

Physiological angiogenesis plays an essential role in the female reproductive system. Hemodynamic changes are involved in the cyclical remodeling of ovarian tissue that occurs during final follicular growth, ovulation, and development of a new corpus luteum (CL)[3,9,12].

Color Doppler ultrasonography is a useful, noninvasive technique for evaluating ovarian vascular function, allowing a visual observation of the blood flow in a delimited area in the wall of the preovulatory follicle[9,36] or within the corpus luteum[3,36,38].

In this section, recent observations of real-time changes in the ovarian blood flow during the estrous cycle will be described using data that investigated hemodynamic changes in the local blood flow in individual follicles and CL of the cow using color Doppler ultrasonography.

Changes in the ovarian blood flow

Follicular growth

A recent study, which examined the presence of blood flow for each follicle >2.5 mm in diameter during the first follicular wave in cycling cows, demonstrated that the percentage of follicles with detectable blood flow in the subsequently determined largest follicle was not different from that in the second largest follicle before follicular deviation[1] (Figure 4.22). In the second largest follicles, the percentage of follicles with detectable blood flow significantly decreased after follicular deviation. From 1 day before the occurrence of follicular deviation, the diameter of small follicles with detectable blood flow was larger than those without detectable blood flow[1] (Figure 4.23). The data suggest that the change of blood supply to an individual follicle closely relates to follicular growth, selection, and atresia.

Ovulation

Ovulation or rupture of the follicular wall is one of the most dramatic morphological changes in the ovary. Analysis of the real-time changes in the local blood flow detected in the theca externa of preovulatory follicles showed that blood flow rapidly increased around the initiation of the LH surge and reached its maximum before ovulation[2] (Figure 4.24). The data suggest that a synchronous increase in local blood flow within the follicular wall concomitant with the initiation of the LH surge may be closely associated with the structural and functional changes of the follicular wall during the process of ovulation.

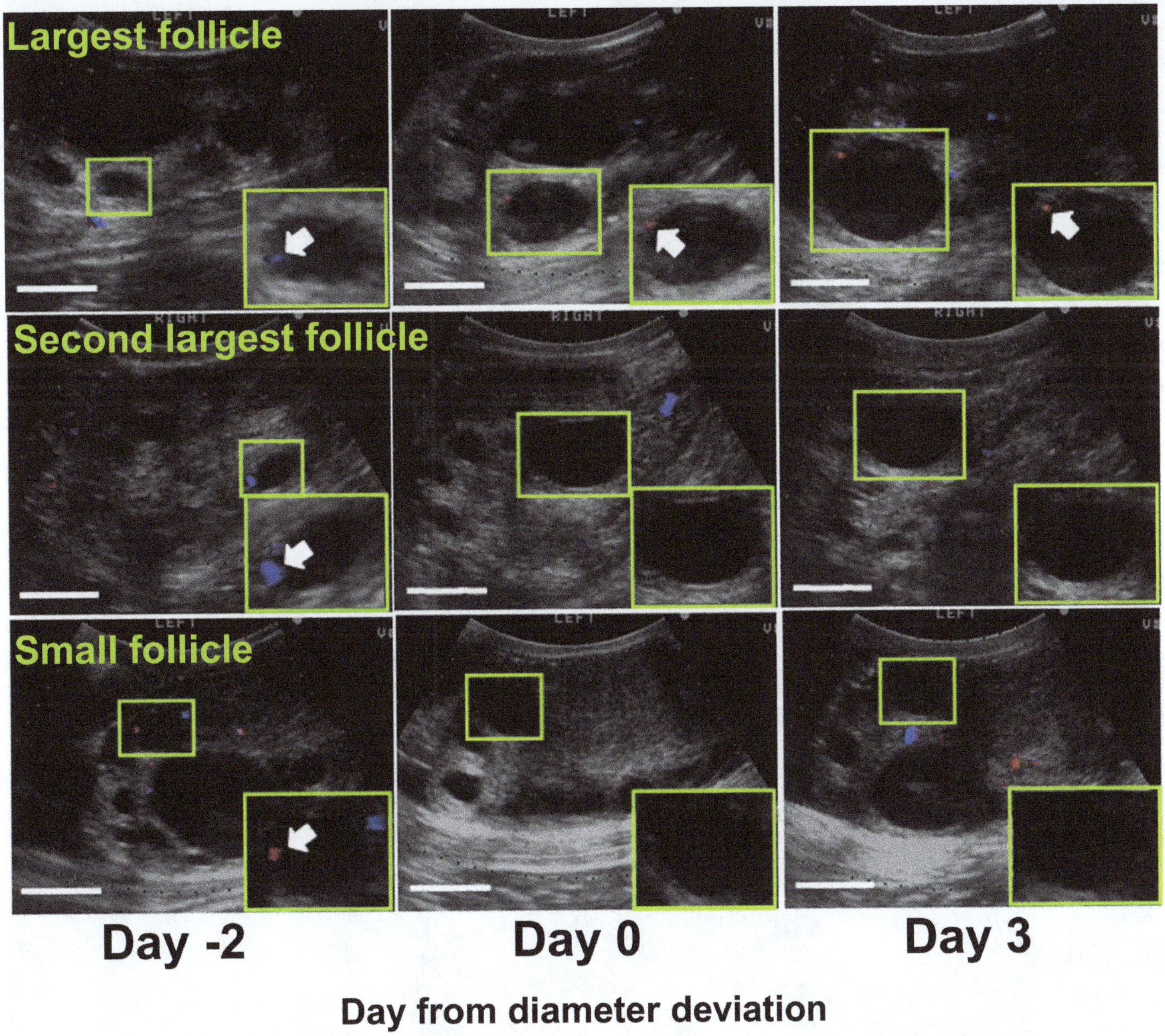

Figure 4.22. Color Doppler images of the ovary around the days of follicular deviation. Boxed areas show the largest (upper panel), second largest (middle panel) and small follicles (lower panel) at days −2, 0, and 3 from follicular deviation. Note that the very large follicle shown in days −2 and 0 of upper left panel was a regressing dominant follicle of a previous wave. Enlarged boxed images in the lower right show typical changes in detectable blood flow. Arrow indicates areas with detectable blood flow within the follicle wall. Before follicular deviation (day −2), blood flow was detected in the largest, second largest, and small follicles. After follicular deviation (days 0 and 3), blood flow disappeared in the second largest follicle and small follicle. Scale bar represents 1 cm. Reproduced with permission of the Society of Reproduction and Development from Acosta et al. (2005)[1].

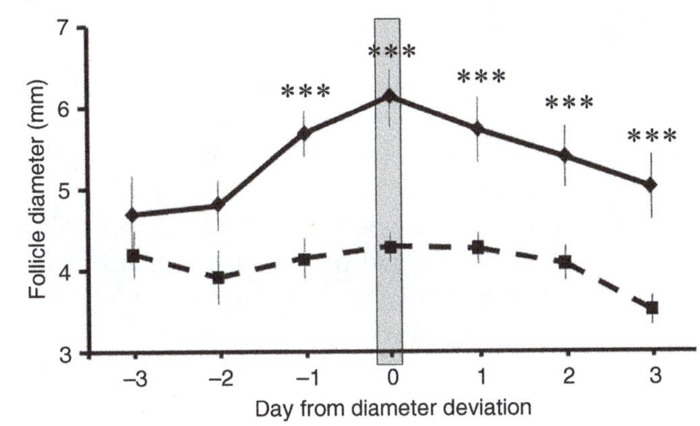

Figure 4.23. Changes in the follicular diameter and blood flow of small follicles around the day of follicular deviation. Diameter of the follicle with detectable blood flow (diamonds) and with undetectable blood flow (squares). Data are means ± SEM for each time period. Asterisks ***: $p < 0.001$ versus values of small follicles with detectable blood flow. Reproduced with permission of the Society of Reproduction and Development from Acosta et al. (2005)[1].

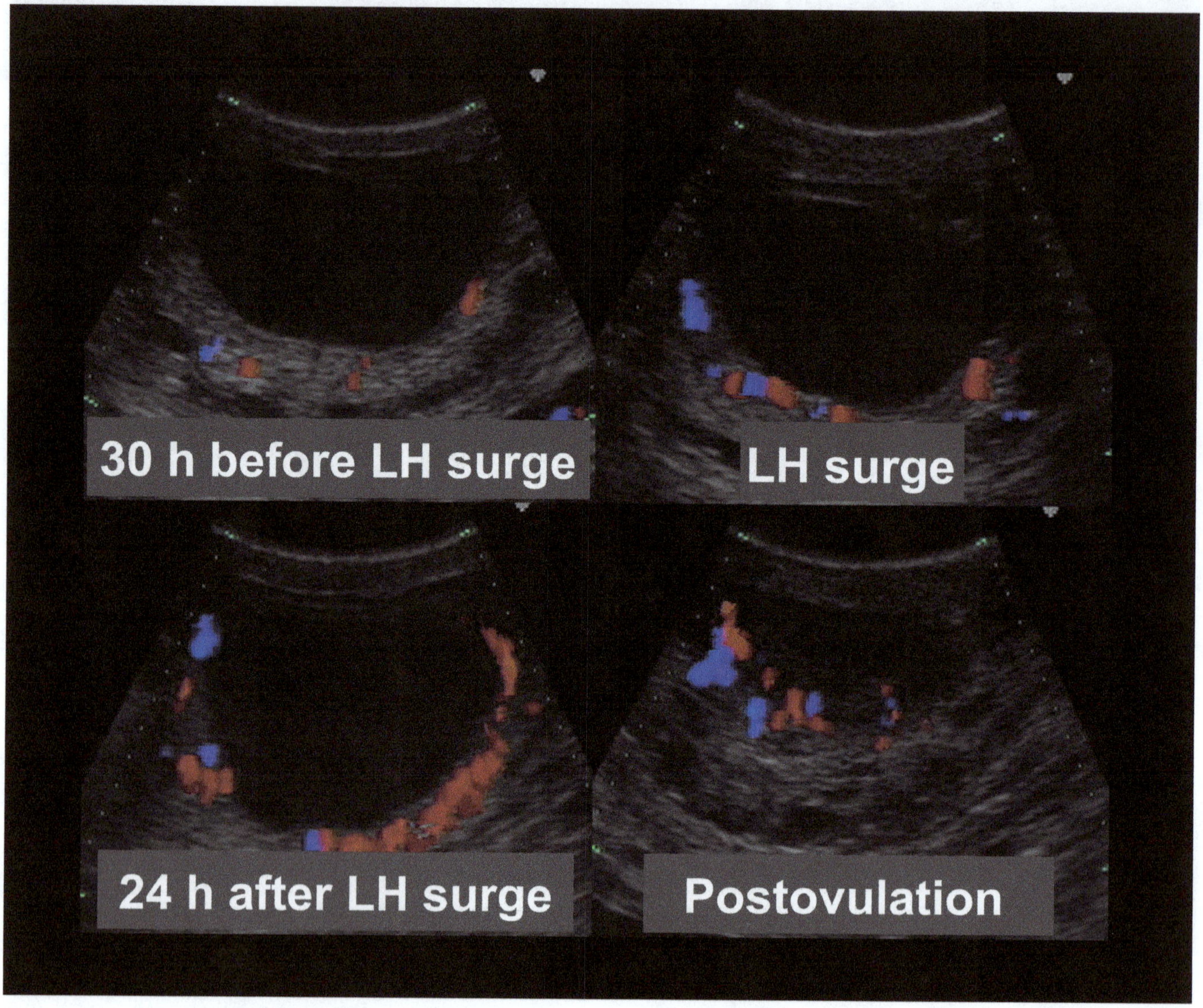

Figure 4.24. Images of the time-related changes in blood flow in the preovulatory follicle with spontaneous ovulation. Images were obtained at 30 h before LH surge, LH surge, 24 h after LH surge, and postovulation. At 24 h after LH surge, highly active blood flow surrounding the preovulatory follicle was observed. Reproduced with permission of BioScientifica from Acosta et al. (2003)[2].

CL development

The CL is one of the most highly vascularized organs and receives the greatest rate of blood flow per gram of tissue of any organ in the body[54]. During CL development, the blood flow surrounding an early corpus luteum gradually increases in parallel with the increase in CL volume and plasma progesterone concentration[2]. The data suggest that blood flow is closely associated with the potential to produce and release progesterone.

CL regression

Studies, which evaluated the ratio of the colored area in a sectional image of the CL as a quantitative index of the changes in blood flow, demonstrated that a clear increase in blood flow surrounding the CL was observed on days 17–18 after estrus, followed by a decrease in plasma progesterone level 1 day later[37,45] (Figure 4.25). This increase in luteal blood flow coincided with an acute increase in plasma levels of PGFM, a metabolite of prostaglandin $F_{2\alpha}$ ($PGF_{2\alpha}$)[24,45] (Figure

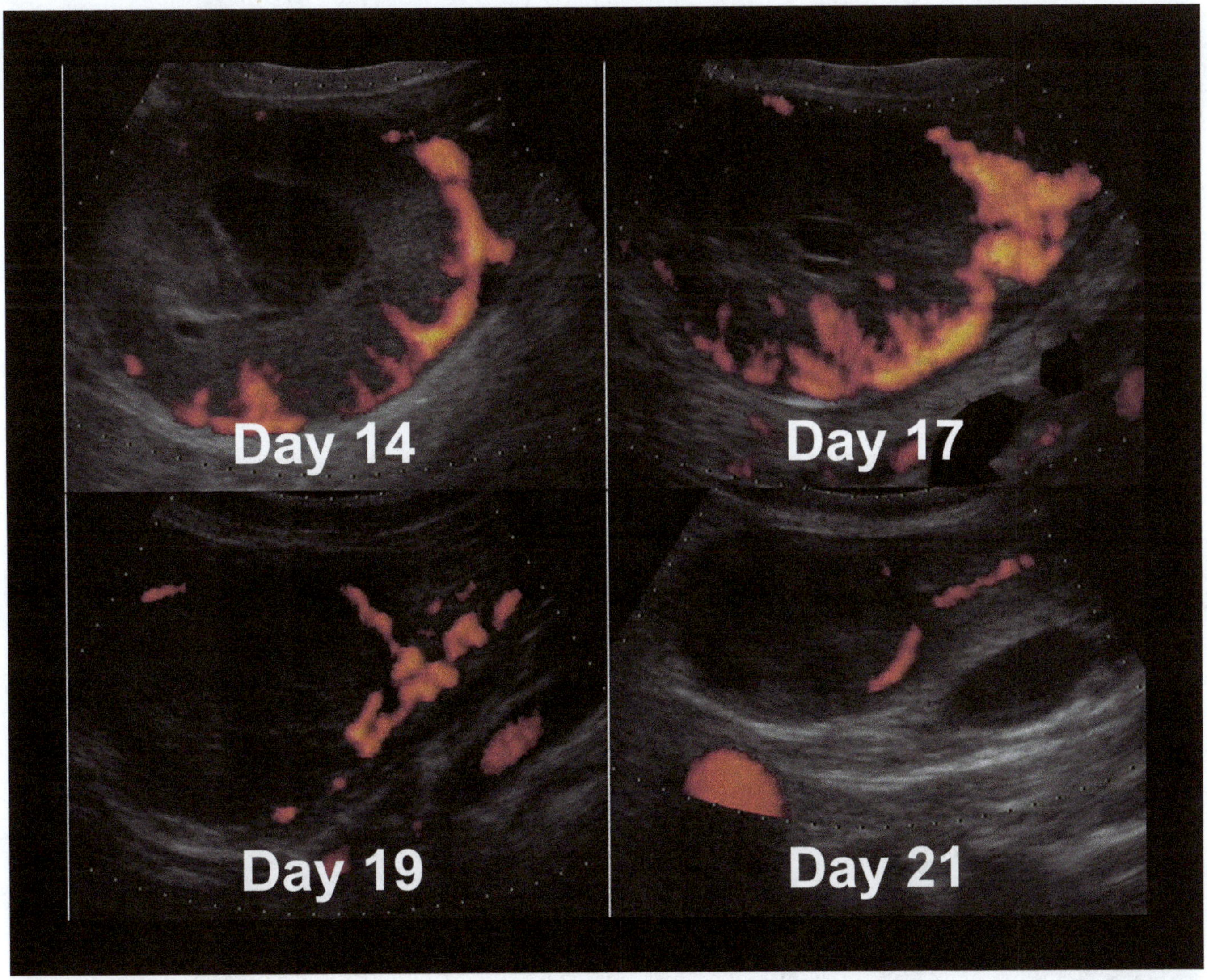

Figure 4.25. Images of the luteal blood flow during spontaneous luteolysis. Images were obtained at day 14, 17, 19, and 21 of the estrous cycle. Clear increase in blood flow surrounding the corpus luteum was observed at day 17. Reproduced with permission of the Society of Reproduction and Development from Miyamoto et al. (2006)[36].

4.26). Furthermore, blood flow within the midcycle CL acutely increased within 30 min after injection of a luteolytic dose of $PGF_{2\alpha}$, and remained high up to 2 h after $PGF_{2\alpha}$ injection[3] (Figure 4.27). These results clearly suggest that the drastic increase in luteal blood flow, which was induced by $PGF_{2\alpha}$ released from the uterus, is a key phenomenon of the onset of luteal regression. Changes in ovarian blood flow (BF) during the estrous cycle of cows are summarized in Figure 4.28.

Cystic ovarian degeneration

A mature follicle may fail to ovulate but continue to grow and persist for 10 days or more, at which point it is considered a cyst. These may be follicular cysts with a thin follicular wall, or luteinized cysts with thicker luteal walls[15]. Generally, gonadotropin releasing hormone (GnRH) analog or human chorionic gonadotrophin (hCG) is used to treat follicular cysts

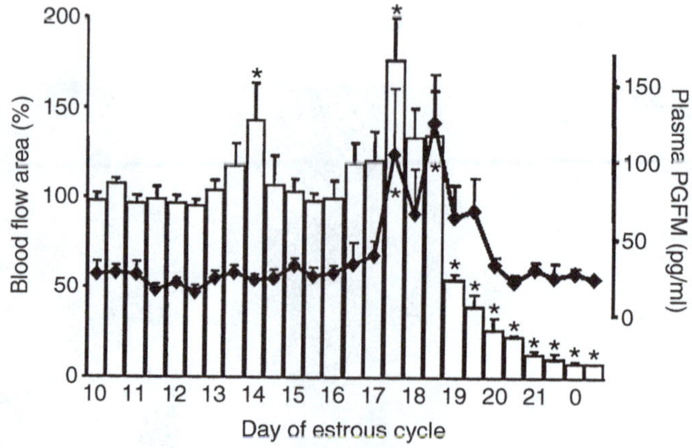

Figure 4.26. Changes in luteal blood flow area and plasma PGFM during spontaneous luteolysis. Luteal blood flow area is denoted with bars, and PGFM concentrations are marked with a solid line. Means ± SEM are presented. Asterisks indicate values statistically different compared with baseline ($p < 0.05$). Reproduced with permission of BioScientifica from Shirasuna et al. (2008)[45].

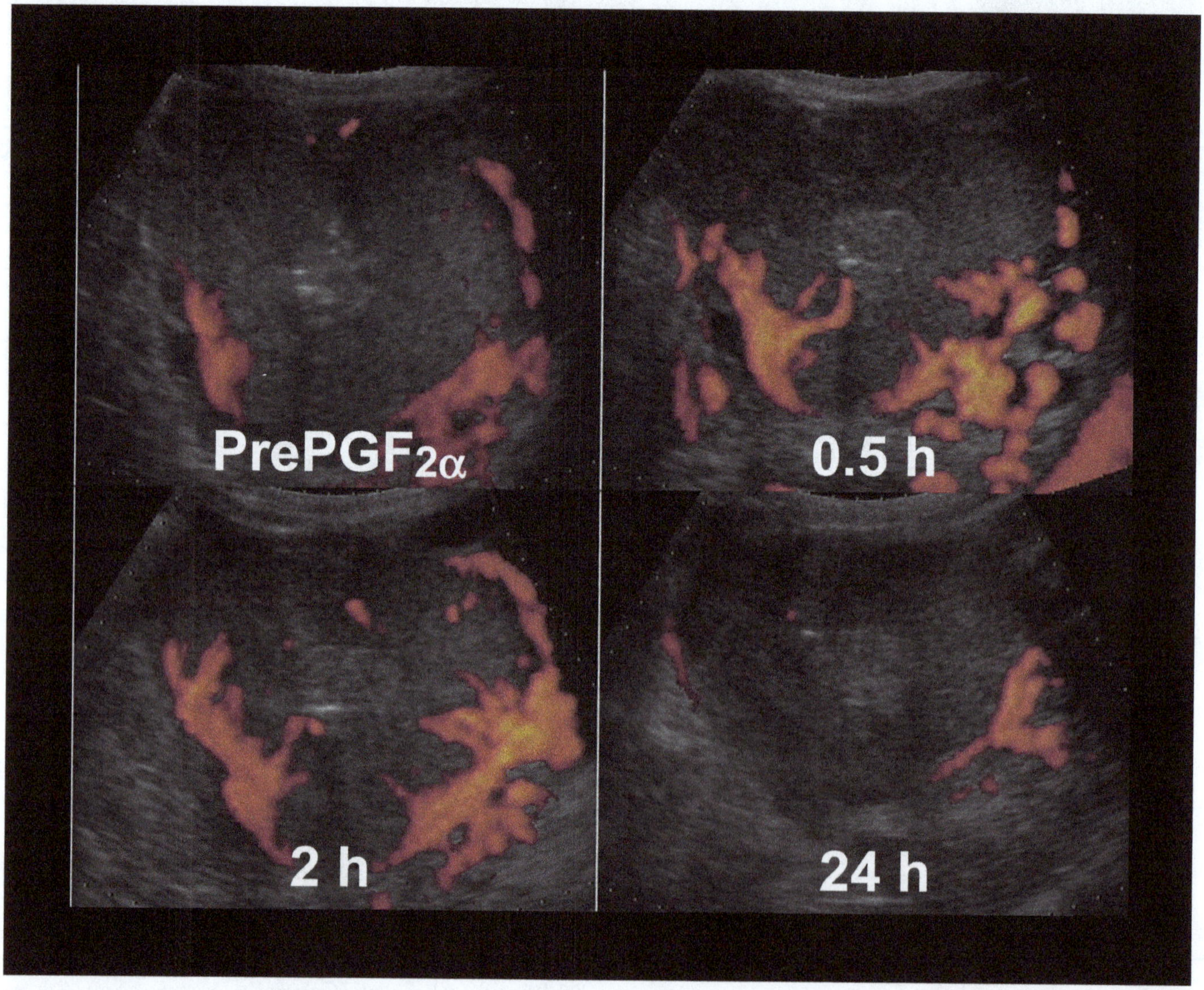

Figure 4.27. Images of the luteal blood flow during $PGF_{2\alpha}$-induced luteolysis. Images were obtained at pre-$PGF_{2\alpha}$, 0.5, 2, and 24h after $PGF_{2\alpha}$ administration on day 10 of the estrous cycle. Increase in blood flow surrounding the corpus luteum was observed at 0.5 and 2h after $PGF_{2\alpha}$. Reproduced with permission of the Society of Reproduction and Development from Miyamoto et al. (2006)[36].

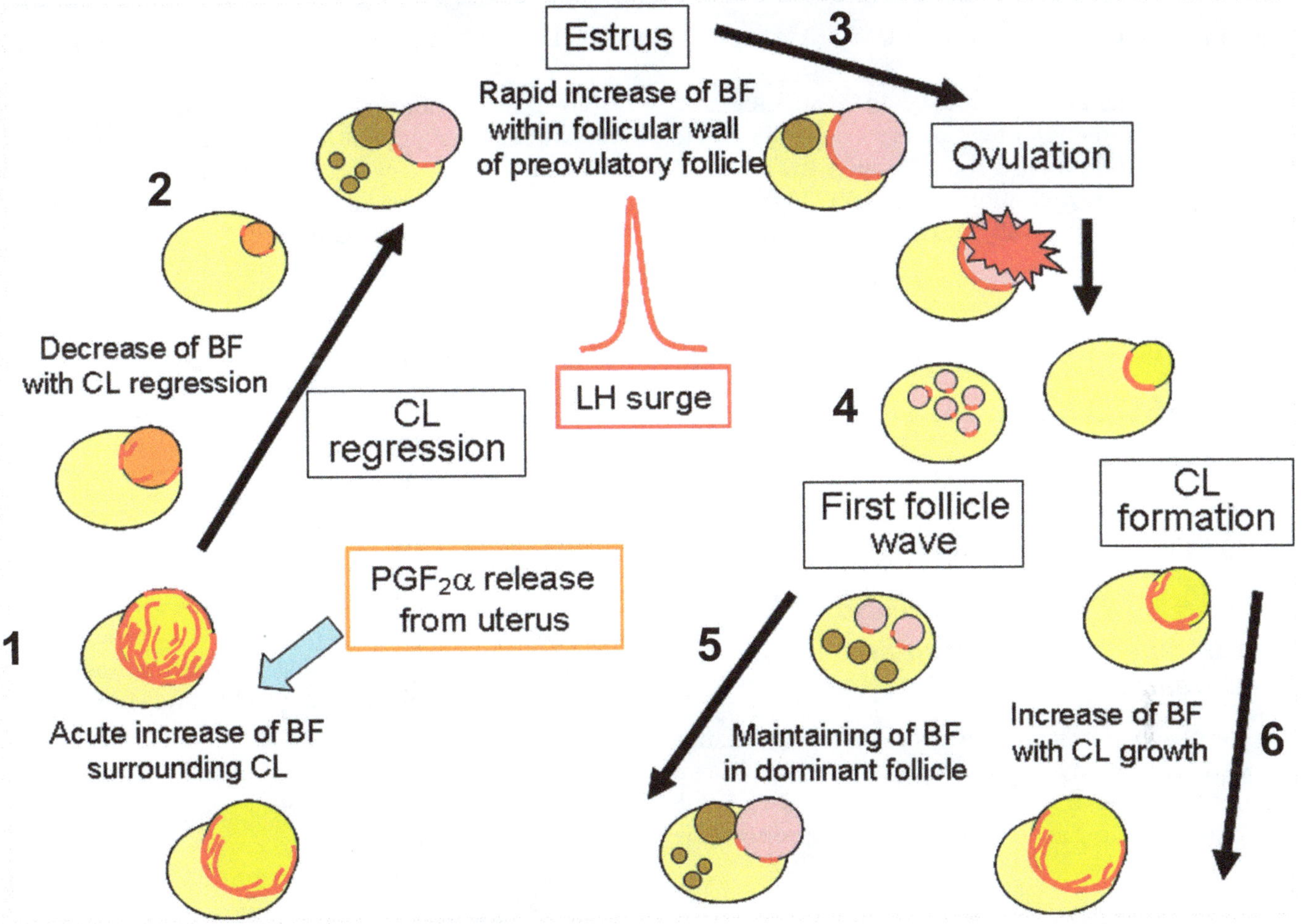

Figure 4.28. Changes in ovarian blood flow (BF) during the estrous cycle. 1) BF surrounding the CL increases acutely in response to $PGF_{2\alpha}$ released from the uterus at 17–18 days after estrus. This acute increase in BF is a sign of initiation of luteal regression. 2) Decrease in BF surrounding the CL is observed during luteal regression. 3) After the LH surge, BF rapidly increases within the follicular wall of the preovulatory follicle. 4) Detectable BF surrounding the follicle is also observed in the developing follicles of the first follicular wave. 5) However, unselected follicles lose BF and become atretic. 6) During CL formation, a gradual increase in BF surrounding the early CL is concomitant with an increase in plasma progesterone level.

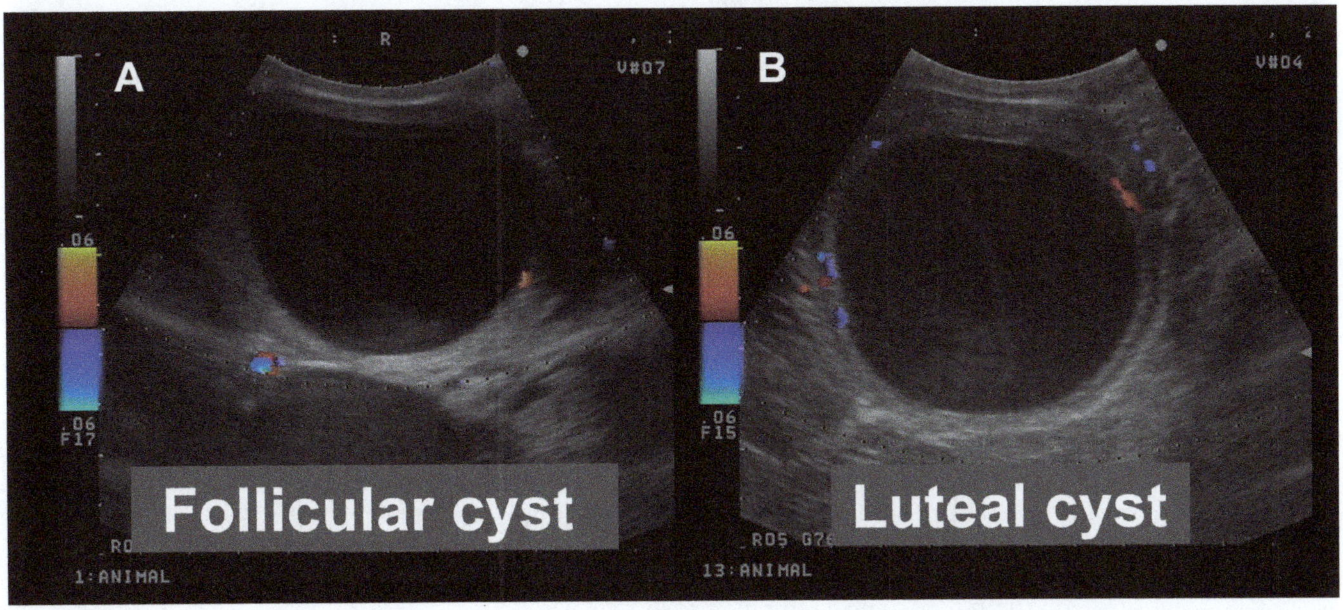

Figure 4.29. Color Doppler images of a follicular cyst (A) and a luteal cyst (B). Note the clear luteinized wall of the luteal cyst between the cavity and the detectable blood flow. In follicular cysts, blood flow appears very close to the cystic cavity. Reprinted with permission from Elsevier, from Matsui and Miyamoto, Evaluation of ovarian blood flow by color Doppler ultrasound: Practical use for reproductive management in the cow. Vet Journal (2008).

and $PGF_{2\alpha}$ or its analog are used to treat luteinized cysts. Since treatment for ovarian cysts depends on the classification of the cyst, a color Doppler US is one of the most effective applications to confirm the thickness and blood flow of the wall of ovarian cystic structures (Figure 4.29).

Ultrasound Use in Reproduction Synchronization Protocols for Dairy Cattle: Two Perspectives

First perspective (Colloton and DesCôteaux)

The use of synchronization protocols has dramatically changed breeding management for dairy cattle. These authors believe that ultrasound can be used to great advantage to improve results in synchronization programs.

Reproductive tract health

Ultrasound is a more accurate assessor of uterine and ovarian health than palpation[17,34,46,53]. Naturally, animals with reproductive tract pathology will have poor conception regardless of the synchronization method used. An ultrasound examination prior to beginning a synchronization protocol will identify these animals before time and money is spent on drugs and insemination. These authors believe that on farms with excellent cow health, good management, and good records, postpartum examinations can be reserved only for cows with a history of dystocia, retained placenta, metritis, or metabolic disease.

Anovular cows

Ultrasound can help estimate the proportion of anovular cows at breeding time, particularly when a presynchronization protocol (PreSynch) is used[7,46]. A typical PreSynch protocol is to give cows two prostaglandin (PG) injections at 2-week intervals prior to beginning the OvSynch program (GnRH-PG-GnRH) 12 to 14 days after the second prostaglandin injection. Under this protocol almost all cycling cows should have a CL on the day the OvSynch portion of the protocol is started. Ultrasound is a very accurate method to detect the presence or absence of a CL[34,46]. High rates of anovular cows indicate herd management problems that must be addressed to improve fertility.

Protocol selection

Ultrasound can help choose which synchronization protocol is most appropriate[6–8]. There is considerable evidence that the presence of progesterone improves response to ovulation synchronization protocols[7,11,35,49,52]. Healthy cows in good condition, but with no CL, benefit from the inclusion of an intravaginal progesterone releasing device in the protocol[52]. Cows with a CL likely will not benefit from adding the expense and inconvenience of such a device. This was demonstrated in a study from Galvao et al. (2007)[20] and summarized in the following:

- For cows with CL and ovulation at the first injection of GnRH (G1), the 38-day pregnancy rate was 42.2%.
- When the CL was present but no ovulation was recorded at G1, pregnancy rate was 37.7%.
- For cows that had no CL at G1 but had ovulated after G1, pregnancy rate was 27.6%.
- When no CL and no ovulation were recorded at G1, the pregnancy rate was only at 15.4%[20].

Pregnancy diagnosis

Early pregnancy examinations with ultrasound can return open cows to the breeding pool as quickly as possible. Data from the University of Wisconsin[19] indicates that approximately 32 days postbreeding is an optimal time to resynchronize open cows.

Limitations

There is evidence indicating improved conception rates if the first GnRH injection (G1) of the OvSynch protocol produces an ovulation[20]. Ultrasound can be used to determine whether there is a potentially ovular follicle (greater than 8 mm) on the day of G1. However, these authors do not feel that this is an accurate predictor of whether an ovulation will indeed occur. Because of this, and since the presence or absence of a CL appears to be more significant than whether an ovulation occurs after G1, these authors feel it is simpler and saves time to base protocol selection only on the presence or absence of a CL.

As ultrasound units improve, particularly with the addition of a color Doppler component, it may be possible in the future to more accurately assess ovulation potential of follicles. Also, as more synchronization of ovulation research is done new ways may be found to utilize ultrasound to improve results.

Second perspective (Gnemmi)

Many scientists and practitioners consider routine postpartum examinations useless. This author, however, considers ultrasonographic evaluation of the reproductive tract before implementing any synchronization program essential to improve the pregnancy rate of dairy herds.

Reproductive tract health in the postpartum period

The first ultrasonographic evaluation must be done after 10 days postpartum in order to assess the uterine condition (presence/absence of metritis/endometritis) and, most importantly, to determine whether ovarian activity has resumed. The higher precision of the ultrasound exam compared to manual palpation for identification of a CL after 25 days of the postpartum period enables a higher success rate of the PreSynch protocol. Moreover, identifying the presence of dominant follicles is not possible without ultrasound.

European Union restrictions regarding hormone use impose serious questions

Without precise ovarian evaluations too many progesterone devices are used in cycling cows with already high progesterone levels. This empiric method causes animal welfare problems and public health concerns. Beginning in October 2006, European Union restrictions regarding hormone use stimulated serious challenges. Can the use of hormones be optimized? Is it possible to establish when prostaglandin, GnRH, or slow progesterone release devices are really necessary in cows?

Protection of the health of consumers and respect of the animal welfare guidelines must push researchers and practitioners to look for new strategies. Using ultrasonography in synchronization programs is definitely a great approach to reconcile ethical, medical, and economic concerns and guarantee the production of good quality products through carefully limited use of hormone treatments.

Protocol selection with the use of ultrasonographic examinations

There are two basic types of synchronization programs:

1. Synchronization of estrus
2. Synchronization of ovulation

Synchronization of estrus is generally obtained with the use of prostaglandins followed by timed insemination. The time elapsing between the administration of prostaglandin and estrus depends on the diameter of the dominant follicle at the time of administration. In animals with two or three follicular wave cycles, the deviation of the first dominant follicle generally occurs 4 or more days after ovulation, when the follicle has a diameter of 8 mm. This is considered the minimum size for the follicle to ovulate since the quantities of LH receptors are sufficient to respond to LH. Manual identification of an 8 mm follicle is difficult, which justifies the use of ultrasonography.

Synchronization of ovulation can be induced using programs that combine the use of GnRH, prostaglandin, and sometimes a progesterone releasing device (OvSynch, PreSynch, CIDRsynch and similar protocols). Cows treated with OvSynch have similar conception rates to those obtained by insemination after natural heat recognition[40,43]. To use this system of synchronization it is best to have a cycling cow with an active CL that remains functional for at least 7 days between the administration of the first GnRH (G1) and the prostaglandin. Moreover, the cow needs the presence of a functional dominant follicle to ovulate after the first GnRH administration. About 30% of all cows treated with OvSynch do not synchronize and therefore will not get pregnant[14,40,52]. Such a synchronization protocol works best in cows with two follicular wave cycles. Thus OvSynch is more appropriate in dairy cows and water buffalo but it is not as suitable for beef cows and zebu with three follicular waves per cycle.

If it is true that the presence of a CL is crucial, it is also true that the conception rate with OvSynch varies notably according to the age of the CL[43] (Table 4.1). Therefore, it is important to combine ultrasonographic examinations with the use of the OvSynch protocol.

From this table we note that the ovulatory response after the first GnRH injection changes according to the age of the CL and dimensions/age of the dominant follicle. During the first 4 days of the ovarian cycle,

Table 4.1.
Ovulatory response after the first GnRH injection at the start of an OvSynch protocol according to days after ovulation (adapted from Pursley, Michigan State University)

Age of the Corpus Luteum	Ovulatory Response at First Injection of GnRH
1–4 days	23%
5–10 days	96%
11–16 days	54%
17–21 days	77%

recruitment of follicles takes place in the absence of a dominant follicle. The presence of only small follicles (<8 mm) is responsible for the low ovulation response typical of this period[39,44,52]. After day 4, follicular deviation takes place by which one dominant (two in the case of codominance) follicle grows more than the other follicles. Between day 5 and day 10 of the cycle there is usually a dominant follicle larger than 10 mm and, of course, a CL, which explains the high ovulation rate to GnRH given at this time. This is the best moment to start a synchronized ovulation program like OvSynch. The synchronization response is optimal when all prerequisite conditions for successful fertilization have been met[39,44,52].

Between day 11 and day 16 of the estrous cycle the ovulation response to GnRH is variable because the dominant follicle of the first or second follicular wave may or may not ovulate if atresia has begun. During this period, it is very easy to detect the mature CL by transrectal palpation only, since it has reached its maximum diameter. However, the presence of a large CL can make transrectal identification of relatively smaller follicles (even 8–13 mm) more difficult. The presence of follicles ≥8 mm and precise assessment of their size by ultrasound examination can be used to estimate their ovulation potential. This window of time is the period where the OvSynch protocol gives minimal results because most dominant follicles have become atretic. It also explains why cows do not come into heat rapidly after a single injection of prostaglandin at this time.

After day 16 of the cycle, there will again be a dominant follicle that responds to GnRH, but the ovulatory response is inferior to the one detected between day 5 and day 10 of the cycle, probably due to the drop in the progesterone level.

The PreSynch program can be used provided that the cow is cycling, particularly when begun in the presence of a CL. Normally the PreSynch protocol is started after day 25–28 after calving. The fact that we obtain three heats in a 35–38-day period makes this synchronization method suitable for therapeutic use in cows with endometritis[32,51,55]. When using the PreSynch protocol the overall pregnancy rate rises. The reason for this improvement is that the double prostaglandin injections lead to starting the OvSynch program with a CL of 5–10 days, which is the optimal period to start a synchronized ovulation protocol with GnRH. Note that only one single administration of prostaglandin 10 days before the start of OvSynch does not improve reproductive performance[31].

On the international market, slow-release progesterone devices are sold in different varieties and with different recommendations for their use. They are one of the best systems to guarantee high conception rates in animals in real anestrus or with cystic ovarian degeneration. These devices can be inserted intravaginally or under the skin of the ear. There are some objective limits to their use, including the expense; the anatomical conditions of the site of insertion, which may lead to irritations and infections; and other restrictions on their use by the European legislation.

For all these reasons, this author favors the use of ultrasonographic examinations as early as 10 days after parturition of all cows in order to make specific recommendations on the use of rational therapeutic or synchronization protocols.

References

1. Acosta TJ, Hayashi KG, Matsui M, Miyamoto A (2005). Changes in follicular vascularity during the first follicular wave in lactating cows. J Reprod Dev 51: 273–280.
2. Acosta TJ, Hayashi KG, Ohtani M, Miyamoto A (2003). Local changes in blood flow within the preovulatory follicle wall and early corpus luteum in cows. Reproduction 125: 759–767.
3. Acosta TJ, Yoshizawa N, Ohtani M, Miyamoto A (2002). Local changes in blood flow within the early and mid-cycle corpus luteum after prostaglandin F(2 alpha) injection in the cow. Biol Reprod 66: 651–658.
4. Adams GP, Matteri RL, Kastelic JP, Ko JC, Ginther OJ (1992). Association between surges of follicle-stimulating hormone and the emergence of follicular waves in heifers. J Reprod Fertil 94: 177–188.
5. Amaya D (1994). Étude échographique et endocrinologique d'un modèle expérimental de dégénérescence ovarienn kystique chez la vache. MSc Université de Montréal, St-Hyacinthe, Québec, Canada, p. 94.

6. Bartolome JA, Silvestre FT, Kamimura S, Arteche AC, Melendez P, Kelbert D, McHale J, Swift K, Archbald LF, Thatcher WW (2005). Resynchronization of ovulation and timed insemination in lactating dairy cows I: use of the Ovsynch and Heatsynch protocols after non-pregnancy diagnosis by ultrasonography. Theriogenology 63: 1617–1627.
7. Bartolome JA, Sozzi A, McHale J, Melendez P, Arteche AC, Silvestre FT, Kelbert D, Swift K, Archibald LF, Thatcher WW (2005). Resynchronization of ovulation and timed insemination in lactating dairy cows, II: assigning protocols according to stages of the estrous cycle, or presence of ovarian cysts or anestrus. Theriogenology 63: 1628–1642.
8. Bartolome JA, Sozzi A, McHale J, Swift K, Kelbert D, Archbald LF, Thatcher WW (2005). Resynchronization of ovulation and timed insemination in lactating dairy cows III. Administration of GnRH 23 days post AI and ultrasonography for nonpregnancy diagnosis on day 30. Theriogenology 63: 1643–1658.
9. Brannstrom M, Zackrisson U, Hagstrom HG, Josefsson B, Hellberg P, Granberg S, Collins WP, Bourne T (1998). Preovulatory changes of blood flow in different regions of the human follicle. Fertil Steril 69: 435–442.
10. Carrière PD, Amaya D, Lee B (1995). Ultrasonography and endocrinology of ovarian dysfunctions induced in heifers with estradiol valerate. Theriogenology 43: 1061–1076.
11. Chebel RC, Santos JE, Cerri RL, Rutigliano HM, Bruno RG (2006). Reproduction in dairy cows following progesterone insert presynchronization and resynchronization protocols. J Dairy Sci 89: 4205–4219.
12. Collins W, Jurkovic D, Bourne T, Kurjak A, Campbell S (1991). Ovarian morphology, endocrine function and intra-follicular blood flow during the peri-ovulatory period. Hum Reprod 6: 319–324.
13. Crowe MA, Kelly P, Driancourt MA, Boland MP, Roche JF (2001). Effects of follicle-stimulating hormone with and without luteinizing hormone on serum hormone concentrations, follicle growth, and intrafollicular estradiol and aromatase activity in gonadotropin-releasing hormone-immunized heifers. Biol Reprod 64: 368–374.
14. DeJarnette JM, Salverson RR, Marshall CE (2001). Incidence of premature estrus in lactating dairy cows and conception rates to standing estrus or fixed-time inseminations after synchronization using GnRH and PGF(2alpha). Anim Reprod Sci 67: 27–35.
15. Douthwaite R, Dobson H (2000). Comparison of different methods of diagnosis of cystic ovarian disease in cattle and an assessment of its treatment with a progesterone-releasing intravaginal device. Vet Rec 147: 355–359.
16. Drummond AE (2006). The role of steroids in follicular growth. Reprod Biol Endocrinol 4: 16.
17. Farin PW, Youngquist RS, Parfet JR, Garverick HA (1992). Diagnosis of luteal and follicular ovarian cysts by palpation per rectum and linear-array ultrasonography in dairy cows. J Am Vet Med Assoc 200: 1085–1089.
18. Fortune JE, Rivera GM, Evans AC, Turzillo AM (2001). Differentiation of dominant versus subordinate follicles in cattle. Biol Reprod 65: 648–654.
19. Fricke PM, Caraviello DZ, Weigel KA, Welle ML (2003). Fertility of dairy cows after resynchronization of ovulation at three intervals following first timed insemination. J Dairy Sci 86: 3941–3950.
20. Galvao KN, Sa Filho MF, Santos JE (2007). Reducing the interval from presynchronization to initiation of timed artificial insemination improves fertility in dairy cows. J Dairy Sci 90: 4212–4218.
21. Garverick HA (2007). Ovarian follicular cysts. In: Rudolph P (Ed.), Current Therapy in Large Animal Theriogenology. Saunders Elsevier, St. Louis, MO, pp. 379–383.
22. Ginther OJ (1998). Ultrasonic imaging and animal reproduction. Equiservices Publishing, Cross Plains, Wisconsin.
23. Ginther OJ, Beg MA, Bergfelt DR, Donadeu FX, Kot K (2001). Follicle selection in monovular species. Biol Reprod 65: 638–647.
24. Ginther OJ, Silva LA, Araujo RR, Beg MA (2007). Temporal associations among pulses of 13,14-dihydro-15-keto-PGF2alpha, luteal blood flow, and luteolysis in cattle. Biol Reprod 76: 506–513.
25. Kahn W, Volkmann D (1994). Veterinary Reproductive Ultrasonography. Mosby Wolfe, London, Toronto.
26. Kahn WL (1989). Ultrasonic characteristics of pathological conditions of the bovine uterus and ovaries. In: Taverne MAM, Willemse AH (Eds.), Diagnostic Ultrasound and Animal Reproduction. Dordrecht, Kluwer Academic, Boston, pp. 53–65.
27. Kaneko H, Terada T, Taya K, Watanabe G, Sasamoto S, Hasegawa Y, Igarashi M (1991). Ovarian follicular dynamics and concentrations of oestradiol-17 beta, progesterone, luteinizing hormone and follicle stimulating hormone during the periovulatory phase of the oestrous cycle in the cow. Reprod Fertil Dev 3: 529–535.
28. Kastelic JP, Pierson RA, Ginther OJ (1990). Ultrasonic morphology of corpora lutea and central luteal cavities during the estrous cycle and early pregnancy in heifers. Theriogenology 34: 487–498.
29. Kito S, Okuda K, Miyazawa K, Sato K (1986). Study on the appearance of the cavity in the corpus luteum of cows by using ultrasonic scanning. Theriogenology 25: 325–333.
30. Kulick LJ, Kot K, Wiltbank MC, Ginther OJ (1999). Follicular and hormonal dynamics during the first follicular wave in heifers. Theriogenology 52: 913–921.
31. LeBlanc SJ, Leslie KE (2003). Short communication: presynchronization using a single injection of PGF2alpha before synchronized ovulation and first

timed artificial insemination in dairy cows. J Dairy Sci 86: 3215–3217.
32. Lewis GS, Wulster-Radcliffe MC (2001). Lutalyse can up-regulate the uterine immune system in the presence of progesterone. J Anim Sci 79: 116.
33. Lussier JG, Matton P, Dufour JJ (1987). Growth rates of follicles in the ovary of the cow. J Reprod Fertil 81: 301–307.
34. McDougall S, Rhodes FM (1999). Detection of a corpus luteum in apparently anoestrous cows by manual palpation, transrectal ultrasonography and plasma progesterone concentration. NZ Vet J 47: 47–52.
35. Melendez P, Gonzalez G, Aguilar E, Loera O, Risco C, Archbald LF (2006). Comparison of two estrus-synchronization protocols and timed artificial insemination in dairy cattle. J Dairy Sci 89: 4567–4572.
36. Miyamoto A, Shirasuna K, Hayashi KG, Kamada D, Awashima C, Kaneko E, Acosta TJ, Matsui M (2006). A potential use of color ultrasound as a tool for reproductive management: New observations using color ultrasound scanning that were not possible with imaging only in black and white. J Reprod Dev 52: 153–160.
37. Miyamoto A, Shirasuna K, Wijayagunawardane MP, Watanabe S, Hayashi M, Yamamoto D, Matsui M, Acosta TJ (2005). Blood flow: a key regulatory component of corpus luteum function in the cow. Domest Anim Endocrinol 29: 329–339.
38. Miyazaki T, Tanaka M, Miyakoshi K, Minegishi K, Kasai K, Yoshimura Y (1998). Power and colour Doppler ultrasonography for the evaluation of the vasculature of the human corpus luteum. Hum Reprod 13: 2836–2841.
39. Moreira F, de la Sota RL, Diaz T, Thatcher WW (2000). Effect of day of the estrous cycle at the initiation of a timed artificial insemination protocol on reproductive responses in dairy heifers. J Anim Sci 78: 1568–1576.
40. Peters MW, Pursley JR (2003). Timing of final GnRH of the Ovsynch protocol affects ovulatory follicle size, subsequent luteal function, and fertility in dairy cows. Theriogenology 60: 1197–1204.
41. Pierson RA, Ginther OJ (1988). Ultrasonic imaging of the ovaries and uterus in cattle. Theriogenology 29: 21–37.
42. Pieterse MC (1994). Clinical use of ultrasound in bovine reproduction. Embryo Transfer Society Annual Meeting, Oct. 29–30. Verona: Italy.
43. Pursley JR, Wiltbank MC, Stevenson JS, Ottobre JS, Garverick HA, Anderson LL (1997). Pregnancy rates per artificial insemination for cows and heifers inseminated at a synchronized ovulation or synchronized estrus. J Dairy Sci 80: 295–300.
44. Sartori R, Fricke PM, Ferreira JC, Ginther OJ, Wiltbank MC (2001). Follicular deviation and acquisition of ovulatory capacity in bovine follicles. Biol Reprod 65: 1403–1409.
45. Shirasuna K, Watanabe S, Asahi T, Wijayagunawardane MP, Sasahara K, Jiang C, Matsui M, Sasaki M, Shimizu T, Davis JS, Miyamoto A (2008). Prostaglandin F2alpha increases endothelial nitric oxide synthase in the periphery of the bovine corpus luteum: the possible regulation of blood flow at an early stage of luteolysis. Reproduction 135: 527–539.
46. Silva E, Sterry RA, Fricke PM (2007). Assessment of a practical method for identifying anovular dairy cows synchronized for first postpartum timed artificial insemination. J Dairy Sci 90: 3255–3262.
47. Silvia WJ, Hatler TB, Nugent AM, Laranja da Fonseca LF (2002). Ovarian follicular cysts in dairy cows: an abnormality in folliculogenesis. Domest Anim Endocrinol 23: 167–177.
48. Sirois J, Fortune JE (1988). Ovarian follicular dynamics during the estrous cycle in heifers monitored by real-time ultrasonography. Biol Reprod 39: 308–317.
49. Stevenson JS, Pursley JR, Garverick HA, Fricke PM, Kesler DJ, Ottobre JS, Wiltbank MC (2006). Treatment of cycling and noncycling lactating dairy cows with progesterone during Ovsynch. J Dairy Sci 89: 2567–2578.
50. Stock AE, Fortune JE (1993). Ovarian follicular dominance in cattle: relationship between prolonged growth of the ovulatory follicle and endocrine parameters. Endocrinology 132: 1108–1114.
51. Thatcher WW, Wilcox CJ (1972). Postpartum estrus as an indicator of reproductive status in the dairy cow. J Dairy Sci 56: 608–610.
52. Vasconcelos JL, Silcox RW, Rosa GJ, Pursley JR, Wiltbank MC (1999). Synchronization rate, size of the ovulatory follicle, and pregnancy rate after synchronization of ovulation beginning on different days of the estrous cycle in lactating dairy cows. Theriogenology 52: 1067–1078.
53. Walsh RB, Leblanc SJ, Duffield TF, Kelton DF, Walton JS, Leslie KE (2007). The effect of a progesterone releasing intravaginal device (PRID) on pregnancy risk to fixed-time insemination following diagnosis of non-pregnancy in dairy cows. Theriogenology 67: 948–956.
54. Wiltbank MC, Dysko RC, Gallagher KP, Keyes PL (1988). Relationship between blood flow and steroidogenesis in the rabbit corpus luteum. J Reprod Fertil 84: 513–520.
55. Wulster-Radcliffe MC, Seals RC, Lewis GS (2001). Lutalyse alters the immune response in sows after intrauterine inoculation with bacteria. J Anim Sci 79: 115.

Points to Remember

- Throughout the estrous cycle a transient increase in plasma FSH occurs periodically every 7–10 days and is responsible for the recruitment of a cohort of follicles known as the *follicular wave*.
- Growth of ovarian follicles beyond 4 mm requires FSH and LH stimulation.
- During the estrous cycle of 18 to 24 days, two or three follicular waves will develop, and from each wave will emerge a single dominant follicle (exceptionally two) of 11–16 mm.
- Follicular waves are produced continuously during the follicular phase and luteal phase and also during pregnancy in the cow.
- If the dominant follicle of the last wave grows in the presence of declining progesterone concentration due to luteolysis, it will become the ovulatory follicle.
- Follicles over 8 mm generally have sufficient quantities of LH receptors to ovulate after GnRH/LH treatment. Manual determination of an 8 mm follicle is difficult, thus justifying the use of ultrasonography.
- Detectable blood flow surrounding a dominant follicle is maintained throughout follicular deviation. However, unselected follicles lose blood flow and become atretic follicles.
- After an LH surge, blood flow within the follicular wall of a preovulatory follicle rapidly increases.
- During CL development, a gradual increase in blood flow surrounding the early CL is concomitant with an increase in plasma progesterone level.
- Blood flow surrounding a CL acutely increases in response to $PGF_{2\alpha}$ released from the uterus at 17–18 days after estrus. This acute increase in blood flow is a sign of initiation of luteal regression.
- Decrease in blood flow surrounding a CL is observed during luteal regression.
- During the first 10 days of the ovarian cycle, 30–50% of all corpora lutea will develop a cavity.
- A cavitary corpus luteum (CCL) is considered a normal structure producing normal progesterone levels. It does not alter the length of the ovarian cycle, or reduce the likelihood of pregnancy.
- Using ultrasonography in synchronization programs is a great approach to reconcile ethical, medical, and economic concerns and guarantee the production of good quality products through carefully limited use of hormone treatments.

Summary Questions

1. Which statement is false?
   a. Large follicles >8 mm are always present in active bovine ovaries except for the first few days of the cycle.
   b. FSH is responsible for recruitment of a cohort of follicles known as the *follicular wave*.
   c. Selection of a single dominant follicle is associated with a rise in circulating FSH.

2. Which statement is true? The corpus luteum of the bovine ovary
   a. Is visible by ultrasound at days 3–4 of the estrous cycle
   b. Is rarely seen with a cavity (10–20%)
   c. Produces less progesterone when a cavity is present

3. Which of the following structures can be misdiagnosed as a corpus luteum?
   a. Follicle
   b. Blood vessel
   c. Transverse section of a uterine horn

4. When does the second largest follicle during the first follicular wave lose detectable blood flow?
   a. Beginning of follicular emergence
   b. After follicular deviation
   c. When the dominant follicle reaches maximum size

5. When is the drastic increase in blood flow surrounding a corpus luteum observed?
   a. During luteal formation (3–4 days after estrus)
   b. Mid-luteal phase (11–14 days after estrus)
   c. Onset of luteal regression (17–18 days after estrus)

Answers

1. c
2. a
3. c
4. b
5. c

CHAPTER FIVE

Bovine Uterus

Luc DesCôteaux, Sylvie Chastant-Maillard, Giovanni Gnemmi, Jill Colloton, and Heinrich Bollwein

Introduction

Ultrasound examination provides veterinarians with the most rapid, thorough, and least invasive method of evaluating the health of the uterus[4,28]. Ultrasound is more accurate and objective than transrectal palpation alone[4].

Before carrying out ultrasound evaluations of the uterus it is vital to have adequate knowledge and understanding of the anatomical location and structures of the uterus (see Chapter 3). One must also remember the normal physiological changes that the uterus undergoes during the estrous cycle (tone, vascular changes, edema, endometrial folds, etc.),[12,24] and in the postpartum period[14,18,22]. One of the most important uses of this examination is to be able to diagnose uterine abnormalities and provide follow-up assessment after treatment to ensure that the uterus returns to a normal state.

In this chapter the most important ultrasound images of the uterus in both longitudinal and transverse sections during the estrous cycle and the postpartum period are presented, and the major diseases of the bovine uterus are also presented. The advantages of color Doppler ultrasound are discussed to provide a comparison between this increasingly available technology and traditional ultrasound of the bovine uterus. Finally, the advantages of incorporating a routine uterine and ovarian ultrasound evaluation in the postpartum period are discussed because this method provides a much more accurate and objective evaluation of the postpartum reproductive tract than palpation.

Ultrasound of the Uterus During the Estrous Cycle and Normal Postpartum Period

Main section views of the uterus

Transverse section (Figure 5.1)

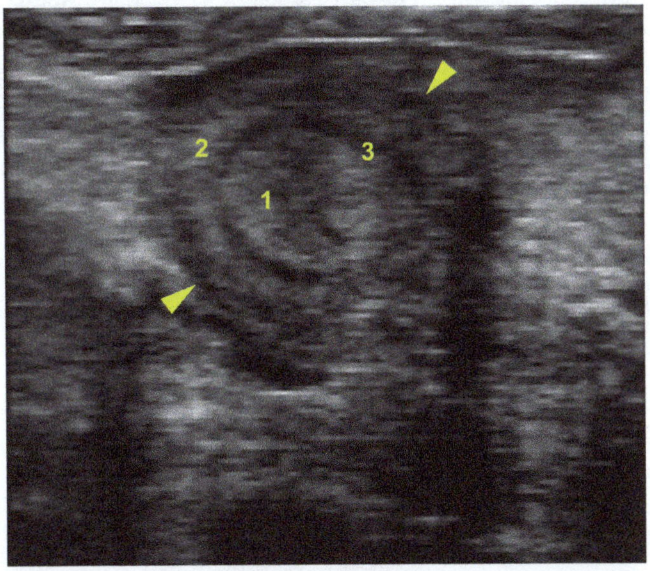

Figure 5.1. Ultrasonographic image of a transverse section of the uterine horn (probe 7.5 MHz; depth 5 cm). 1: Endometrium; 2: Myometrium; 3: Vascular portion of the uterus; Arrowheads: Edge of the uterus.

Longitudinal section (Figure 5.2)

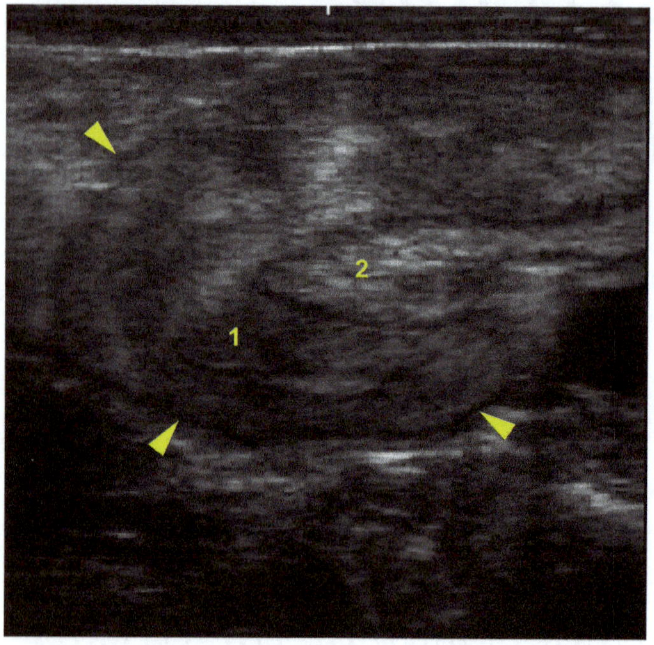

Figure 5.2. Ultrasonographic image of a longitudinal section of the uterine horn (probe 8 MHz; depth 6 cm). 1: Endometrium; 2: Myometrium; Arrowheads: Edge of the uterus.

Ultrasound appearance of the bovine uterus during the estrous cycle

The cyclical variations in circulating levels of progesterone and estrogen (Chapters 3 and 4) are responsible for the changes in the ultrasound appearance of the uterus during the estrous cycle.

Periestrus (proestrus, estrus, and beginning of metestrus)

During this period (–3 days to +4 days from estrus), which is characterized by a high level of circulating estrogen, the cervix partially opens, the uterus has increased tone, its walls are thicker, and the apex of the uterine horns unfold or are longer than during diestrus[3,8,12,23]. These modifications of the uterus are even more noticeable in camelids (Chapter 12).

These changes are caused by the following:

1. Increased blood circulation in the uterus (see section on color Doppler ultrasound later in this chapter)
2. Secretion of mucus by cells of the endometrial glands during proestrus and estrus[4,8]; this mucus facilitates the transfer of sperm to the oviducts[4]
3. Edema of the uterus that normally decreases between 4 and 5 days after estrus[3,23]

On the ultrasound monitor these physiological phenomena translate into less uniform gray tones or more heterogenicity as well as a swollen or swirled appearance of the uterine wall. There are also more areas of the uterus showing dark, anechogenic zones that denote areas of edema and increased vascularity under the endometrium (Figures 5.3–5.5) as compared to the uterus in diestrus (Figures 5.6, 5.7). During periestrus it is also possible to view a small to moderate quantity of mucus in the uterine lumen that appears as a rosette due to the presence of transverse sections of endometrial folds. At the center of the rosette is a thin, star-shaped anechogenic zone, approximately 1–2 mm, that denotes the presence of liquid in the uterus. Then the endometrium itself appears as an approximately 1 cm thick gray circle. Finally, an anechogenic area is seen under the mucosa. Thus, the entire rosette is seen on the screen as three concentric layers of black-gray-black (Figure 5.10). In some places the lumen may appear linear in the shape of a fine, wavy thread (Figures 5.5, 5.23).

During estrus the endometrial mucosa becomes especially echogenic[3] (Figures 5.3–5.5). Also, the limit between the endometrium and the myometrium is more obvious because the vascular portion increases in size,[8] and the uterine lumen may show a greater accumulation of mucus over a longer segment of the uterine horns[3,8,23] (Figure 5.5). This accumulation of liquid may be located in one of the uterine horns for up to 48 hours after estrus and give a false impression of early gestation (Figure 5.3). To avoid a false positive diagnosis of pregnancy the ovaries should be examined for the presence of a corpus luteum, the breeding history should be consulted, and the typical ultrasound evidence of gestation must be validated (see Chapter 6) before making a final diagnosis[4].

Some of these typical images of the uterus in periestrus may also be encountered with a follicular cyst. This will have to be confirmed by an ultrasound examination of both ovaries (Chapter 4).

Diestrus

During diestrus the circulating progesterone levels bring the uterus back to a state of calm, preparing it for the implantation of an embryo if fertilization occurred during estrus (see Chapter 6). The uterus loses its tone, becomes thinner and normally loses the endometrial liquid. Figures 5.6 and 5.7 show the normal

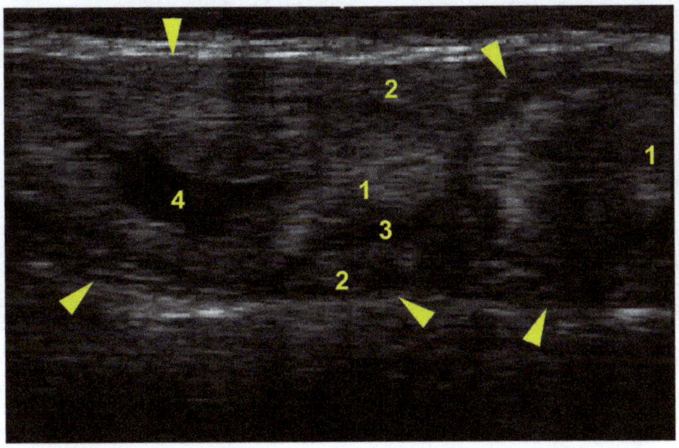

Figure 5.3. Ultrasonogram of two edges of a uterine horn in transverse section in a cow during estrus (probe 8 MHz; depth 4 cm). Note the considerable accumulation of endometrial mucus in the lumen of the uterus and the typical swollen appearance of the uterine wall in periestrus. 1: Endometrium; 2: Myometrium; 3: Vascular portion of the uterus; 4: Lumen of the uterus containing mucus; Arrowheads: Edge of the uterus.

ultrasound appearance of the uterine horns during diestrus. Compare these to Figures 5.4 and 5.5, which show images of the bovine uterus during periestrus.

Ultrasound appearance of the normal postpartum bovine uterus

Ultrasound examination of the postpartum uterus has allowed us to study the rate of involution according to parity and in the presence of any pathological conditions. In normal conditions with no complications (retained placenta, metritis, endometritis, and ovarian cysts), the bovine uterus completes its involution on average at day 23 in primiparous cows and day 27 in pluriparous cows[5] and at the latest at day 42 after parturition[17,22].

Figures 5.8–5.10 show the uterus during involution. Note the ultrasound appearance of the images obtained with a 5 to 7.5 MHz linear probe. In the first days after parturition, the caruncles can be seen (hyperechogenic), along with liquid in the uterine lumen and thickened uterine horns with a swollen and very nonuniform echogenic appearance.

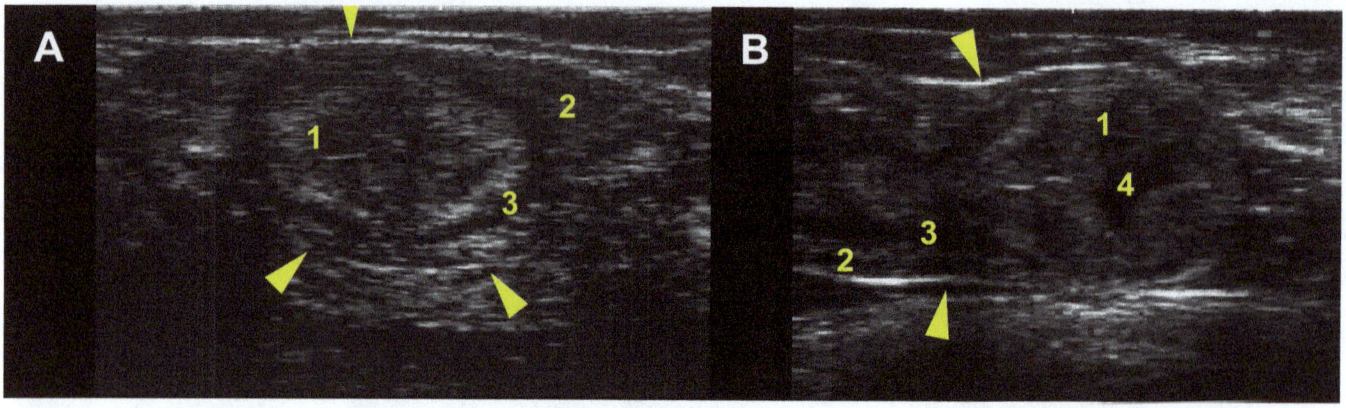

Figure 5.4. Sonograms of transverse (A) and longitudinal (B) sections of a uterine horn in a cow during proestrus (A: probe 10 MHz, depth 3 cm; B: probe 8 MHz, depth 4 cm). Note the thickness of the myometrium and its uniform ultrasound appearance, the swollen appearance of the endometrium and the slight accumulation of endometrial mucus in the uterine lumen in the longitudinal section. 1: Endometrium; 2: Myometrium; 3: Vascular portion of the uterus; 4: Uterine lumen containing mucus; Arrowheads: Edge of the uterus.

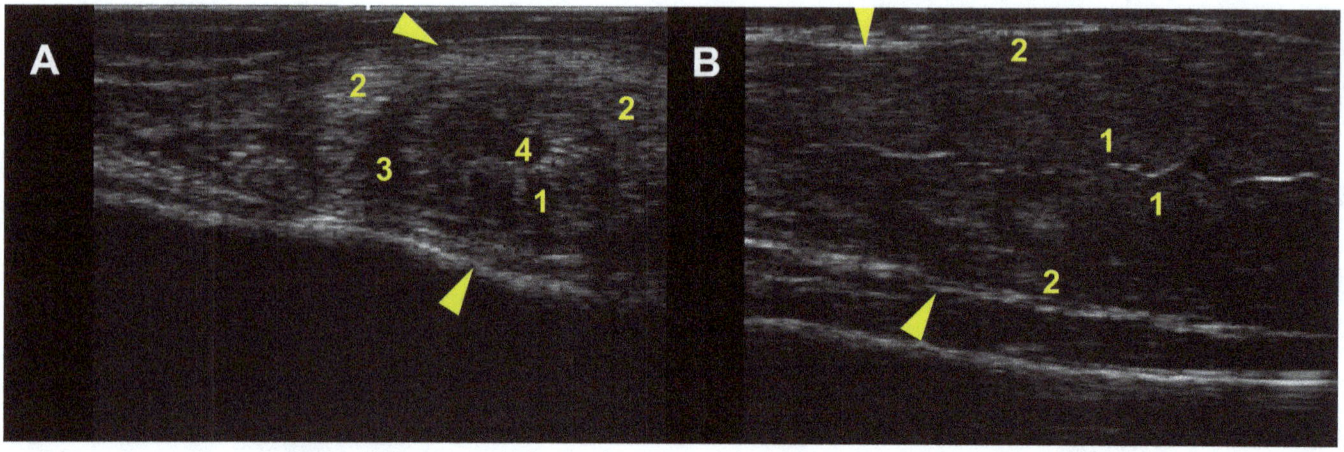

Figure 5.5. Sonograms of transverse (A) and longitudinal (B) sections of a uterine horn in a cow during estrus (probe 10 MHz; depth 4 cm). Note the thickness of the endometrium, the swollen appearance of the uterus, the hyperechogenicity of the endometrial mucosa, and the greater accumulation of endometrial mucus in the lumen in the transverse section. 1: Highly echogenic endometrium; 2: Myometrium; 3: Vascular portion of the uterus; 4: Lumen of the uterus containing mucus; Arrowheads: edge of the uterus.

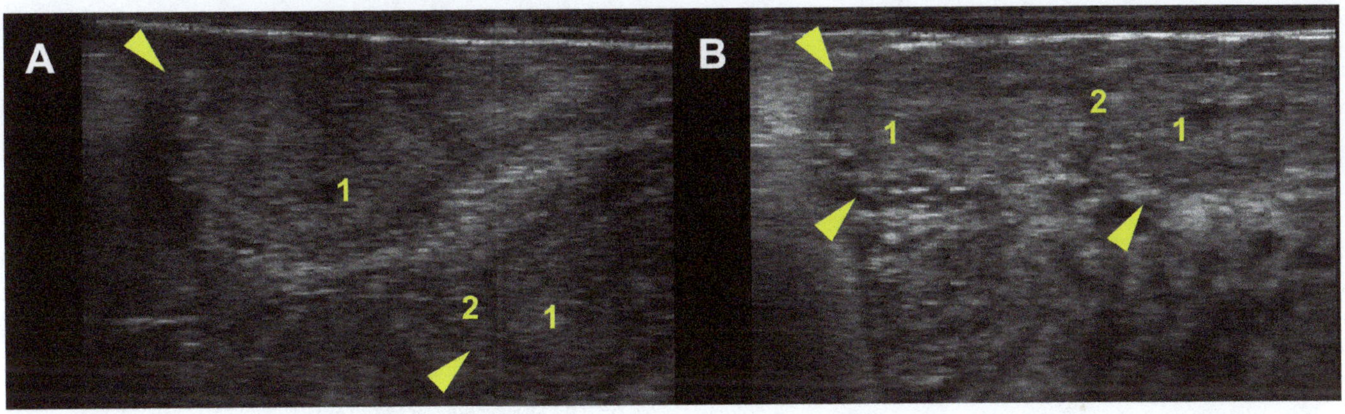

Figure 5.6. Sonograms of transverse sections of uterine horns during diestrus at day 8 (A) and day 15 (B) of the estrous cycle (probe 8 MHz; depth 4.5 cm). Note the decreased thickness of the uterus and the reduced distinction between the endometrium and the myometrium due to more uniform echogenicity and the absence of liquid in the lumen. 1: Endometrium; 2: Myometrium; Arrowheads: Edge of the uterus.

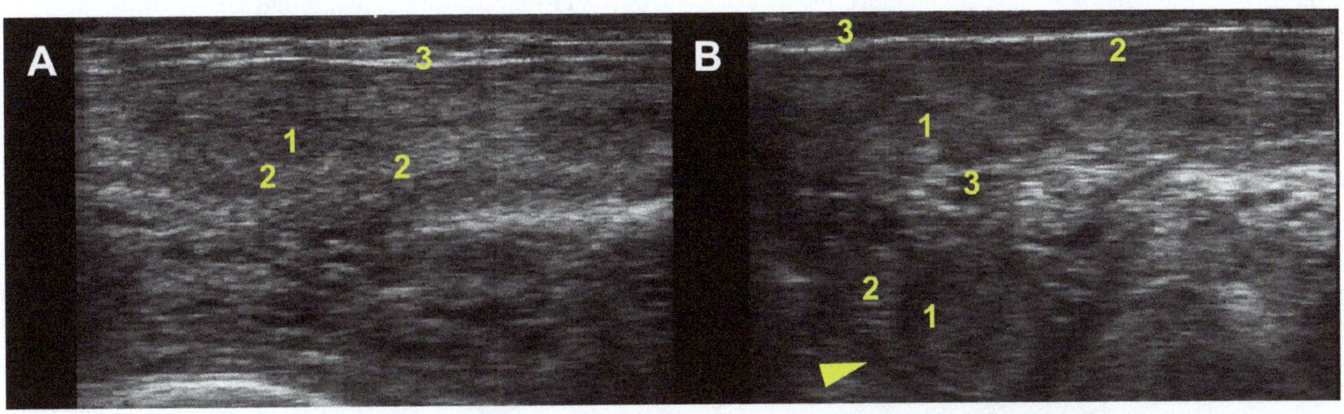

Figure 5.7. Sonograms of longitudinal sections of uterine horns during diestrus at day 8 (A) and day 11 (B) of the estrous cycle (probe 8 MHz; depth 4.5 cm). Note the reduced distinction between the endometrium and the myometrium in diestrus compared to periestrus in Figures 5.4B and 5.5B. B: In this ultrasonogram a transverse cut of a portion of the uterine horn (arrowhead) can also be visualized under the longitudinal section of the uterus. 1: Endometrium; 2: Myometrium; 3: Edge of the uterus; Arrowhead: Transverse section of the uterus.

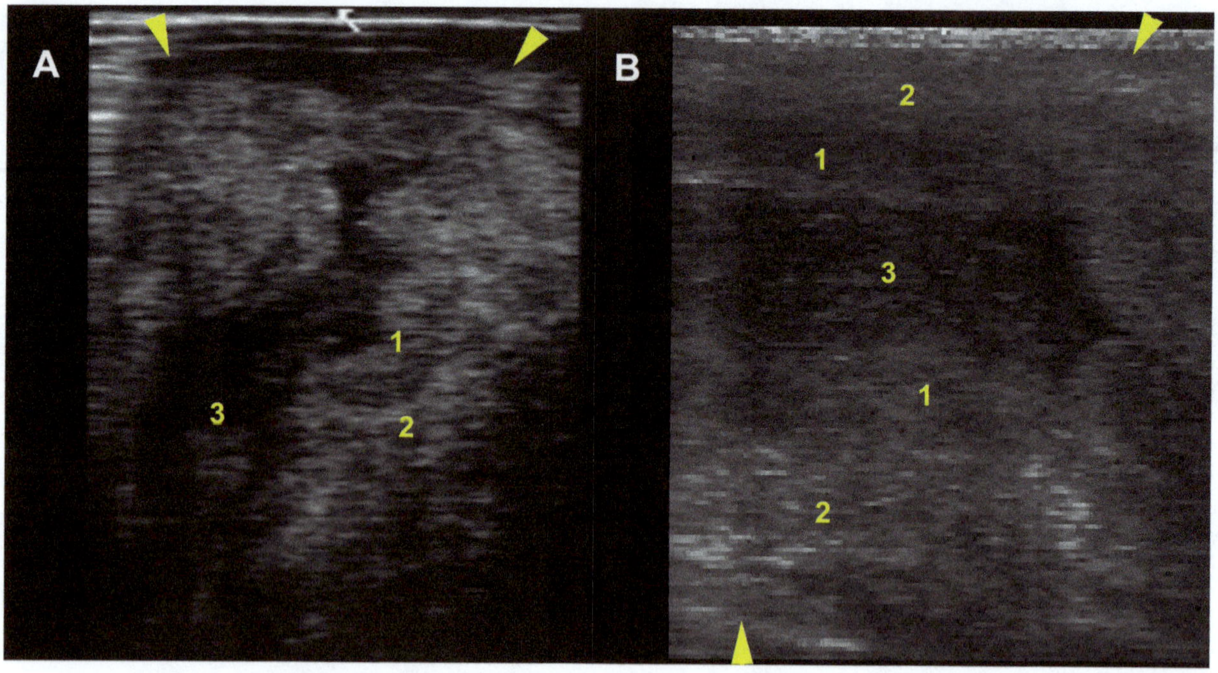

Figure 5.8. Ultrasonograms of normal uterine involution between 7 and 10 days postpartum. Note that the diameter of the uterine horn between the edges of the uterus is approximately 7 cm. A: probe 7.5 MHz, depth 8 cm; B: probe 5 MHz, depth 8 cm; 1: Thickened endometrium; 2: Thickened highly echogenic myometrium; 3: Normal liquid (lochia); Arrowheads: Edge of the uterus.

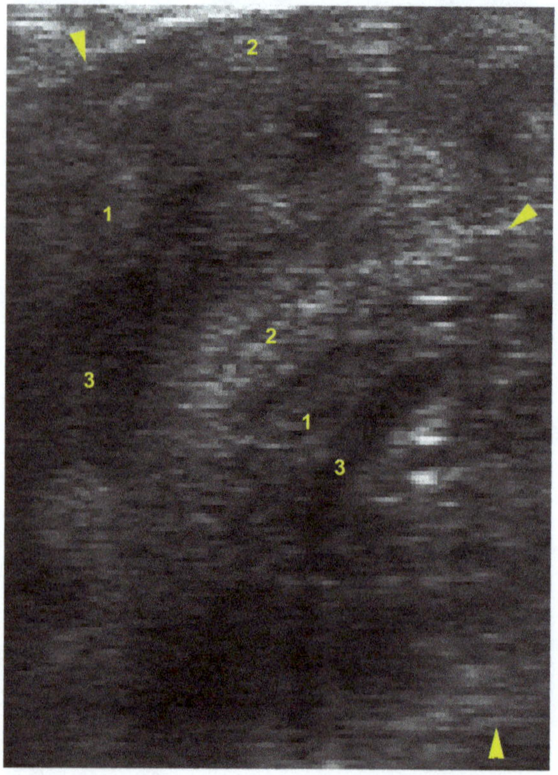

Figure 5.9. Ultrasonogram of a normal uterine involution in longitudinal view at 15 days postpartum (probe 5 MHz; depth 10 cm). Note the presence of liquid in the uterine lumen, a thickened uterine horn (especially the endometrium and to a lesser extent the myometrium). The diameter of the uterine horn is 5 cm at the level of the great curvature. 1: Endometrium; 2: Highly echogenic myometrium; 3: Normal liquid (lochia); Arrowheads: Edge of the uterus.

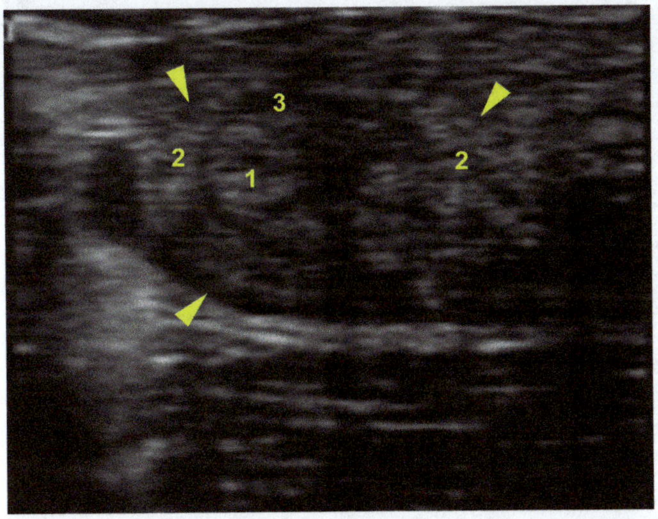

Figure 5.10. Ultrasonogram of a normal uterine horn in transverse view between 20 and 25 days postpartum (probe 7.5 MHz; depth 5 cm). Note that the appearance of this uterus resembles the one of a cow in periestrus (Figures 5.4A and 5.5A). The diameter of the uterine horn is 3 cm and the macroscopic involution seems to be completed. 1: Endometrium; 2: Myometrium; 3: Vascular portion of the uterus; Arrowheads: Edge of the uterus.

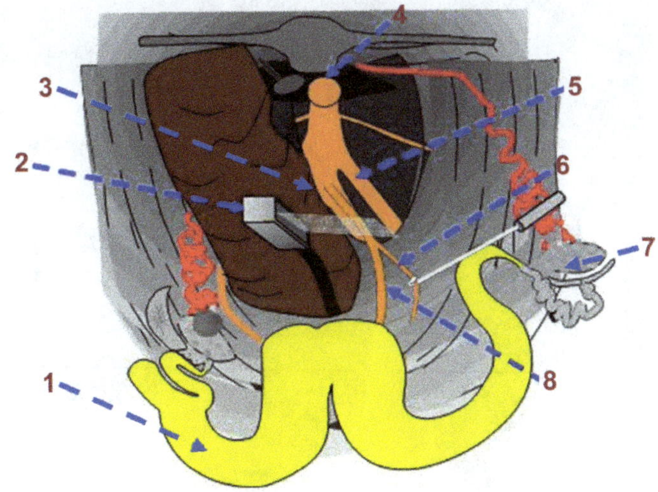

Figure 5.11. Schematic representation of the pelvic area of a cow and the position of the ultrasound transducer during Doppler sonographic examination of the left uterine artery. From Herzog and Bollwein (2007)[15], Blackwell Publishing. The uterine arteries can be found by following a systematic technique. With the ultrasound transducer oriented transversely and the face dorsally, the aorta can be easily found and followed caudally. At the level of the branching of the aorta, the external iliac artery can be identified coursing caudoventrally next to the body of the ilium. Proceeding caudally, the artery (A.) iliaca interna is observed. A common stem for the A. umbilicalis and the A. uterina is detectable about 4 cm caudal to the origin of the A. iliaca interna from its ventral wall. Because the A. umbilicalis is canalized only in its proximal 5 cm, the A. uterina is the functional continuation of the A. umbilicalis. The umbilical artery gives rise to a small vessel supplying the ureter[29]. The A. uterina represents the main supply of the uterus and shows a diameter of 2.8 to 5.0 mm in nulliparous, nonpregnant animals[5,22]. During pregnancy the diameter of the A. uterina can reach 10 to 12 mm. The A. uterina can be found within the mesometrium as a movable arterial vessel. Near its origin from the umbilical artery, the A. uterina can be visualized with the color Doppler technique. 1: Uterus; 2: Ultrasound probe; 3: A. iliaca interna; 4: Aorta; 5: Left external iliac artery; 6: Left umbilical artery; 7: Ovary; 8: Left uterine artery.

Color Doppler Sonography of the Uterine Blood Flow

Localization of uterine arteries

Uterine blood circulation can be studied by transrectal color Doppler sonography of both uterine arteries (Figure 5.11)[2,15].

Equipment, adjustments, and terminology

Transrectal pulsed Doppler ultrasound examinations of both uterine arteries take about 30 minutes for each cow. The Doppler measurements (Figure 5.12) can be performed using a Doppler ultrasound device equipped with a 7 MHz microconvex probe.

Adjustments of the equipment and terminology[15]

The size of the Doppler gate, which determines the location and area from which Doppler information is processed and displayed, should be adjusted to the diameter of the uterine artery (A. uterina). All blood flow velocity waveforms should be obtained at an interrogation angle between Doppler ultrasound beam and flow direction from 20 to 60 degrees. The analysis is based on the envelope of the Doppler shift spectrum (Figure 5.13).

Terminology and parameters[2,20]

The following parameters are suitable for measurements of uterine blood flow in cycling cows: the time averaged maximum velocity (TAMV), the Doppler

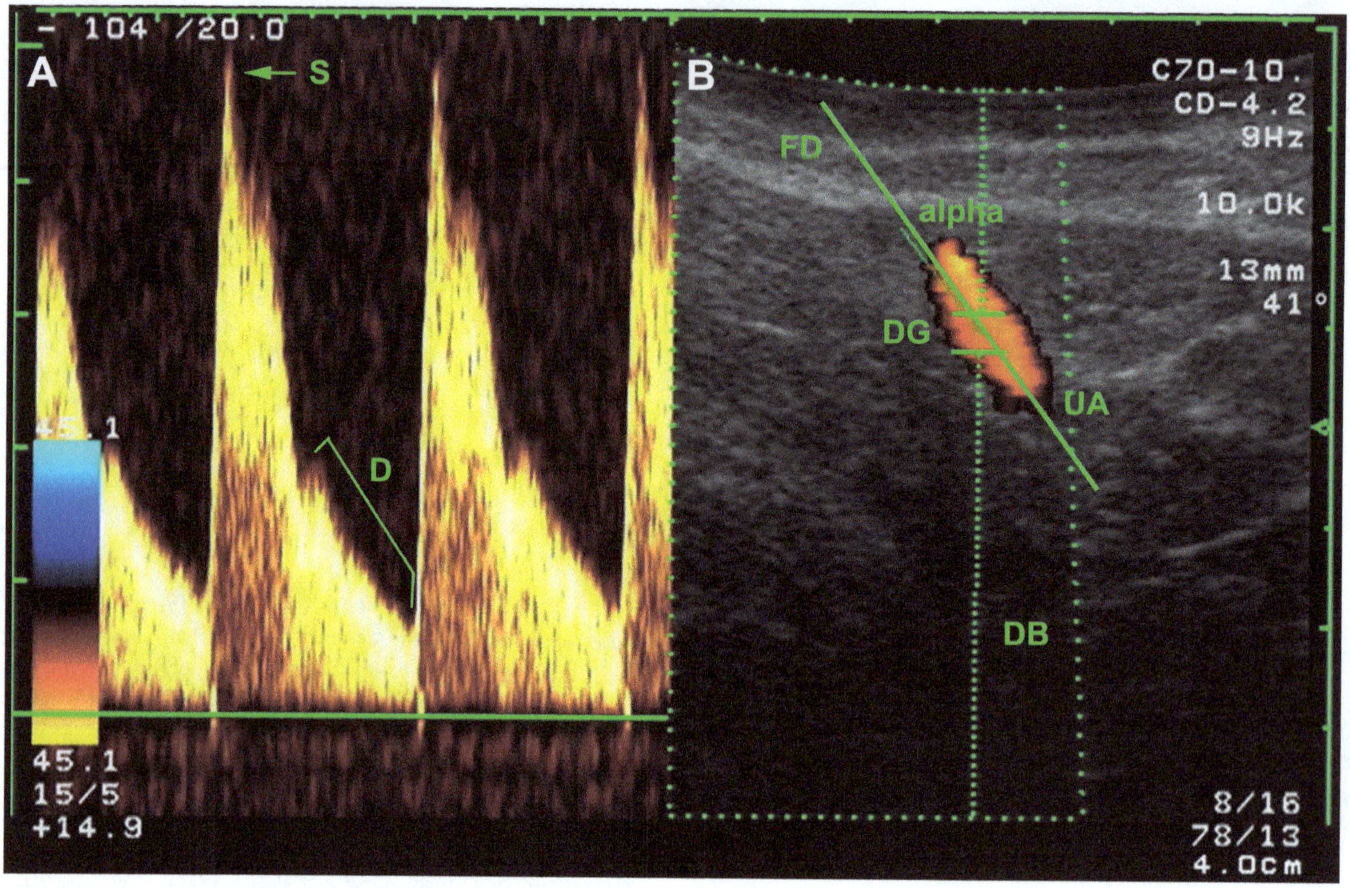

Figure 5.12. Doppler sonography of the right uterine artery (UA) in a cow 7 days after insemination. From Herzog and Bollwein (2007)[15], Blackwell Publishing. A: Uterine artery systolic peak frequency shift (S) and diastolic frequency shift (D); B: Uterine artery (UA) with Doppler gate (DG) and interrogation angle (α = alpha) between Doppler beam (DB) and flow direction (FD).

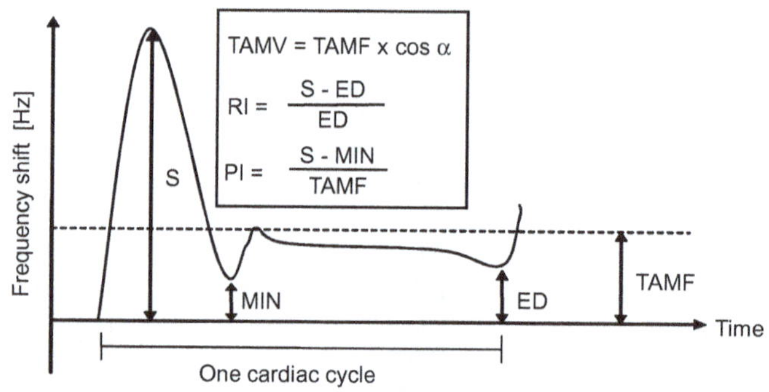

Figure 5.13. Schematic view of a Doppler wave with maximum systolic (S), minimum diastolic (MIN), end-diastolic (ED), and time averaged maximum frequency shift (TAMF) during one cardiac cycle and formulas for determination of time averaged maximum velocity (TAMV); alpha (α) = interrogation angle between Doppler beam and blood flow direction, Doppler indices resistance index (RI), and pulsatility index (PI). From Herzog and Bollwein (2007)[15], Blackwell Publishing.

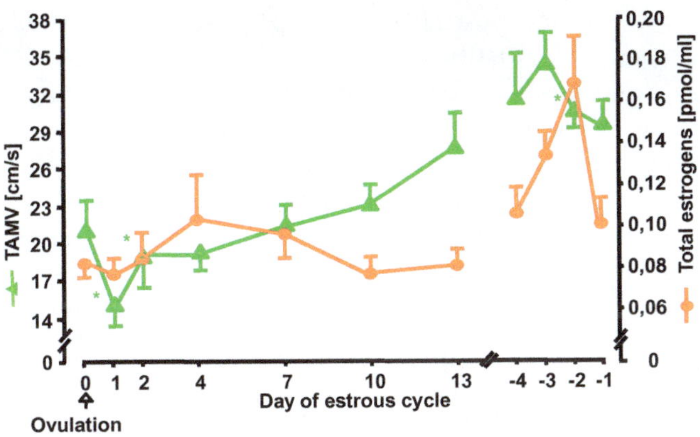

Figure 5.14. Variation of the uterine blood flow during the course of the estrous cycle in cows. From Herzog and Bollwein (2007)[15], Blackwell Publishing. Changes of time averaged maximum velocity (TAMV) from the uterine arteries and of total estrogens. Values are means ± SEM of 4 cows and 2 estrous cycles. Values with asterisks differ from those of the previous measurements ($P < 0.05$).

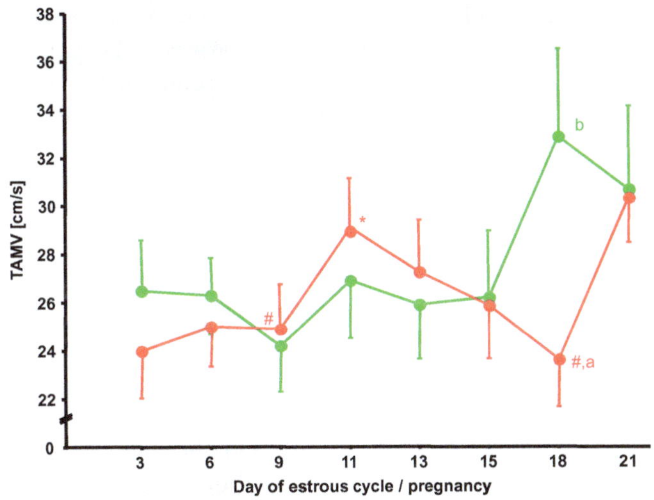

Figure 5.15. Changes of time averaged maximum velocity (TAMV) from the uterine artery ipsilateral to the corpus luteum in cycling (green line) and pregnant cows (red line). From Herzog and Bollwein (2007)[15], Blackwell Publishing. Values are means ± SD of 14 cycling cows and 18 pregnant cows. Values with different symbols (#,*) and letters (a,b) differ ($P < 0.05$).

indices resistance index (RI) and pulsatility index (PI). Due to the limited size of the uterine arteries, a reliable measurement of vessel area is not possible; therefore, the uterine blood volume flow can not be established accurately in cycling cows.

Blood flow is typically evaluated semiquantitatively using the so-called "Doppler indices." These indices are not a direct measure of blood flow, but describe the resistance to blood flow in vessels peripheral to the vessel being examined. As the values increase, so does blood flow resistance and vice versa[6]. The Doppler indices are relative quantities obtained from the maximum systolic (S), minimum diastolic (Min), end-diastolic (ED) or mean frequency shift (Mean) during one cardiac cycle[16]. This means that knowledge of the angle α, which is required for determination of blood flow velocity, is not required.

Uterine blood flow changes during estrous cycle and early pregnancy in cows

Estrous cycle

A study of cows that were examined during the estrous cycle showed that uterine blood flow had a characteristic pattern (Figure 5.14) with the highest TAMV values during proestrus and estrus and lowest values on day 1 (ovulation = day 0). TAMV stayed at a fairly constant level during early diestrus and mid-diestrus and had started to increase already at the end of diestrus. In this study, the cycle-associated changes in uterine blood flow velocity correlated with the plasma concentration of total estrogens, although the correlation was only moderate.

Early pregnancy

In pregnant cows, changes in uterine blood supply can be observed during the first 3 weeks after insemination compared to cycling cows (Figure 5.15). There is an initial short-term rise in uterine blood supply on day 11, which is followed by a decline until day 18. The reasons for these phenomena are unclear. Because no relationship could be observed with peripheral sexual steroid hormone levels, the alterations in uterine perfusion seem to be caused by local embryo-maternal interactions.

Previous studies have suggested that older animals are less fertile because of a low uterine perfusion[7]. In human medicine, the resistance to uterine artery blood flow is used to predict a hostile uterine environment prior to embryo transfer[27]. Goswamy and Steptoe (1988) treated women with a high resistance to uterine blood flow with estrogens and noticed an improvement in uterine perfusion and a trend toward higher pregnancy rates[13].

Due to the relatively high interindividual variability of TAMV and PI values both during estrous cycle and early pregnancy, the use of color Doppler sonography is not clinically helpful for an early pregnancy detection in cows.

Ultrasound of the Postpartum Abnormal Uterus and Vagina

The principal pathologic conditions of the uterus are infectious. Acute puerperal metritis, endometritis, pyometra, and abscesses are the most frequent infectious problems of the uterus. Other noninfectious pathologic conditions of the uterus that can be diagnosed with ultrasound are mucometra and pneumouterus. Gestational abnormalities may also be encountered, such as death of the embryo or a mummified fetus (see Chapter 6). Lymphosarcoma may infiltrate the uterine wall and create a thickened uterus with multiple masses.

The main vaginal abnormalities that can be viewed with ultrasound are urovagina, pneumovagina, hematoma, abscesses, and vaginitis. Some of these abnormalities do not need ultrasonographic examinations to confirm their diagnosis because transrectal and vaginal examinations are generally adequate. The ultrasonographic examination may help to differentiate between a hematoma and a vaginal abscess when the history of the cow is not readily available to the practitioner. It can also assist in the differentiation of vaginitis and clinical endometritis or metritis when vaginal discharge is present.

Routine evaluation of the postpartum uterus

The value of routine postpartum evaluation of the reproductive tract is controversial. In well-managed, healthy herds such examinations may cost more than the small benefit they would provide. In such herds good record systems flag problem cows and PreSynch protocols are often used. In these herds perhaps only cows with a history of dystocia, retained fetal membranes, puerperal metritis, and metabolic problems must be examined for uterine health prior to breeding.

However, most veterinarians work with herds that do not achieve this standard of excellence. In these herds routine postpartum and prebreeding examinations may be justified.

There are also regional differences in the management of reproductive programs. In North America there is a tendency to manage the entire herd as a single unit. In some European countries individual cow management is more common. Animal welfare regulations in some countries also make individual cow management more acceptable and expected by producers.

In any case, research has indicated that palpation does not have economic benefits for these examinations. Ultrasound provides a much more accurate and objective evaluation of the postpartum reproductive tract than palpation.

Ultrasound uterine evaluation during the first 10 days after parturition

Based on our experience, the ultrasound appearance of the uterus within the first week after calving is not obviously different in the normal and pathological uterus. Thus, the practitioner should use other more obvious clinical signs (cow off-feed, fever, malodorous vaginal discharge, etc.) to establish the final diagnosis of an acute puerperal metritis (Figure 5.16).

Ultrasound uterine evaluation between 10 and 21 days after parturition

Ultrasound evaluation is the best cow-side diagnostic tool to evaluate the physiopathological conditions of uterus and ovary in the early postpartum period. Table 5.1 presents the diagnostic sensitivity of different examination methods available to bovine practitioners to detect infectious pathological conditions of the early postpartum uterus[9,10,12,21,25,26].

When a uterine infection is diagnosed it is important to establish whether the cow has metritis or endometritis. In a case of metritis, the inflammatory process involves both the endometrium and the myometrium (Figure 5.17A). In cases of endometritis the inflammation is limited to the endometrium (Figure 5.17B). The correct diagnosis helps to select therapy and to propose reevaluation plans of the affected cow.

In some cows, the ovarian cycle starts as early as day 12. This first heat is generally silent in most cows but it is a very good indicator for the prognosis of the pathologic uterus because uterine health generally improves after estrus.

Starting at around 15 days after parturition, the ultrasound evaluation of the ovary may detect the

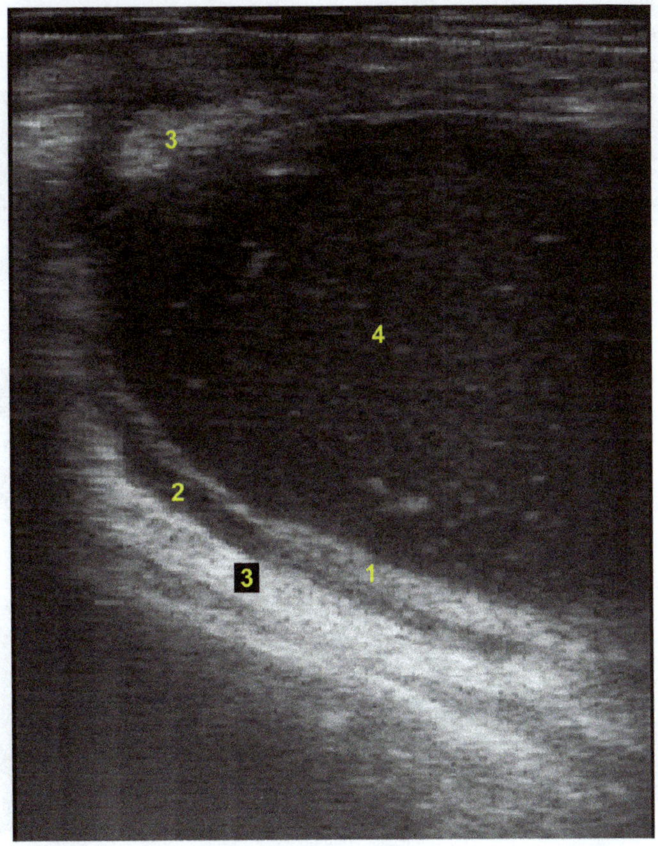

Figure 5.16. Ultrasonographic image of an acute puerperal metritis in a dairy cow 8 days after calving (probe 6 MHz; depth 8 cm). Acute puerperal metritis produces infected lochia in the uterine cavity and delayed uterine involution. Ultrasonograms of this pathological condition of the uterus may show a thickened, highly vascular uterine wall with no caruncles, and grayish liquid containing hyperechogenic particles. If the expulsion of fetal membranes did not take place the overall image is abnormally large, showing considerable delay in uterine involution. Clinical symptoms and vaginal examination should be included to support the diagnosis. 1: Endometrium; 2: Highly vascular portion of the uterus; 3: Thickened hyperechogenic myometrium; 4: Lumen contents with hyperechogenic particles.

Table 5.1.

Diagnostic sensitivity (Se) of different examination methods to detect infectious pathological conditions of the uterus in the early postpartum period in cows (adapted from Miller et al. 1980; Gilbert 1992, 2005, 2006; Ginther 1998; Sheldon et al. 2002; Riddle 2004)

Examination Methods	Se	Comments
Transrectal examination	22%	Quick but not accurate method. The sensitivity of this method is too low to make an adequate clinical assessment of the uterus.
Vaginal speculum	60–80%	Accurate method but impractical because the reusable speculum needs to be disinfected between cows. It is possible to use a disposable cardboard speculum but this increases the cost to the producer. Hygienic preparation required prior to the exam is another limiting factor.
Vaginal evaluation with a gloved hand	60–80%	Accurate method but the compliance to hygienic conditions during the execution of the exam makes this method impractical. False negatives occur when there is no liquid in the vestibule.
Metricheck	60–80%	Accurate method but false negatives occur when there is no liquid in the vestibule. It also requires disinfection of the instrument between cows.
Cytology	95%	Accurate method but not a cow-side test. Data are not in real time, making this method impractical for day-to-day use.
Ultrasonography	94%	Accurate method with very high sensitivity and specificity. Quick diagnosis in real time. Changing the sleeve and disinfecting the probe between exams to prevent leukosis transmission is very fast.

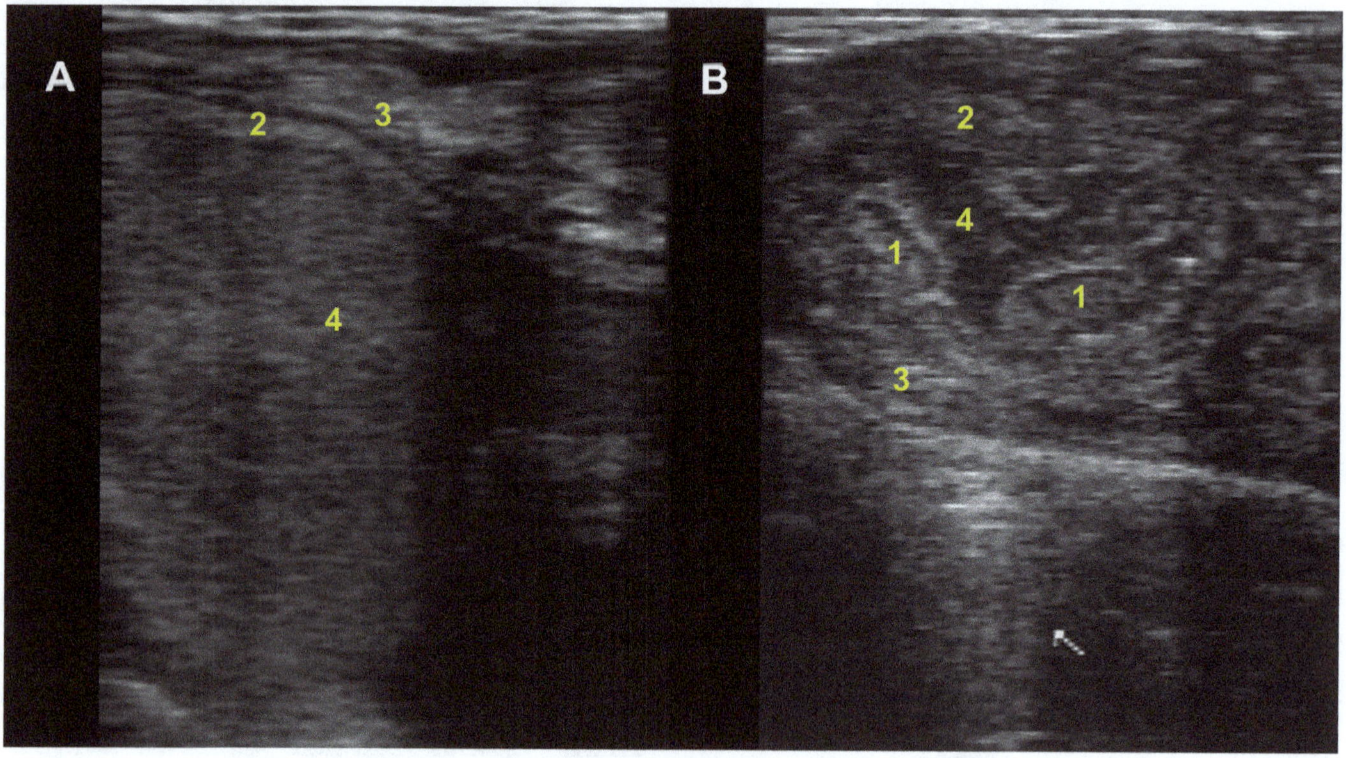

Figure 5.17. Metritis (A) and endometritis (B) ultrasonograms in cows 12 and 19 days respectively after parturition (probe 7.5 MHz; depth 8 cm). A: There is abundant thick liquid inside the uterus: lochia, blood, pus, fibrin, and polymorphonuclear cells. The image looks like a snowstorm. The endometrium and myometrium are thickened. B: There is thick liquid inside the uterus, delay in involution of the uterus, and a thickening of the endometrium. The caruncles are still evident due to a delay in uterine involution. 1: Caruncle; 2: Endometrium; 3: Myometrium; 4: Uterine content.

presence of corpus luteum (CL). When a CL is present the use of prostaglandins to treat metritis/endometritis may be more effective[19] (Figure 5.18).

Ultrasound uterine evaluation between 21 days and the end of the voluntary waiting period (VWP)

Ultrasound examination of the uterus during the voluntary waiting period (VWP) period allows the veterinarian to assess the presence/absence of endometritis (Figures 5.19, 5.20). This examination must also include the evaluation of the ovaries for the presence/absence of a CL. In cases of endometritis with the presence of a CL, a PreSynch program will likely induce three heats in 35–38 days. The heats induced by this protocol stimulate the uterine immune system and assist in evacuation of purulent material. Manual determination of a CL has a low specificity, which causes many diagnostic errors. The use of an accurate ultrasonographic examination of the ovaries is highly recommended in order to improve the efficiency of reproductive synchronization programs (see Chapter 4 for more details).

Ultrasound uterine evaluation past the VWP

Beyond the VWP ultrasound examinations, it is essential to recognize the presence of a CL and/or the presence of a chronic subclinical endometritis (Figure 5.21), pyometra (Figure 5.22), or mucometra (Figures 5.23, 5.25). Manual examination is nearly useless for diagnosing subclinical metritis and is unable to distinguish pyometra from mucometra. The ultrasound examination helps to establish which therapeutic strategy should be adopted. The presence of a CL after the VWP allows the veterinarian to direct the cow toward one of the following reproduction synchronization programs: PreSynch, OvSynch,

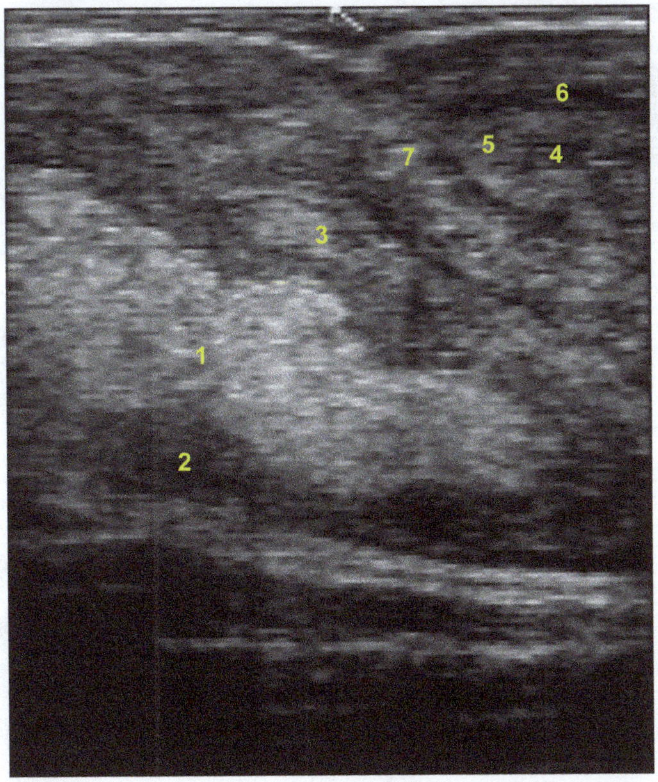

Figure 5.18. Endometritis ultrasonogram at 21 days after parturition (probe 7.5 MHz; depth 7 cm). Note the differences between the infected uterine horn on the left longitudinal view and the normal one on the right in transverse section. 1: Dense and hyperechoic pus in the lumen of the left uterine horn; 2: Endometrium; 3: Myometrium; 4: Lumen of the normal right uterine horn; 5: Endometrium of the normal horn; 6: Vascular portion of the right horn; 7: Myometrium of the normal horn.

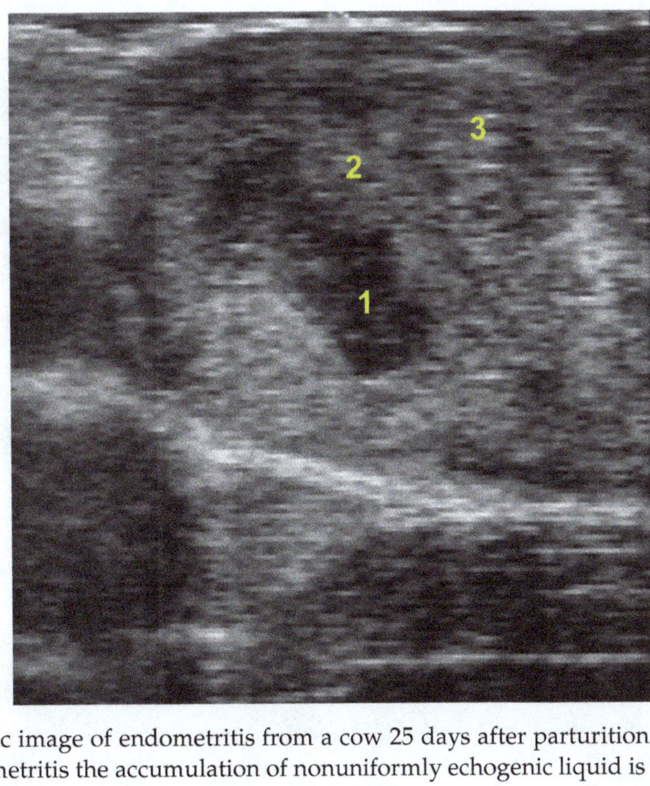

Figure 5.19. Ultrasonographic image of endometritis from a cow 25 days after parturition (probe 7.5 MHz; depth 6 cm). On this less extreme form of endometritis the accumulation of nonuniformly echogenic liquid is usually visible only in the cranial and lower segment of the uterine horns (see also Figure 5.20A). Without an ultrasound examination this may give the veterinarian the impression of early gestation, resulting in diagnostic error. 1: Purulent uterine content; 2: Endometrium; 3: Myometrium.

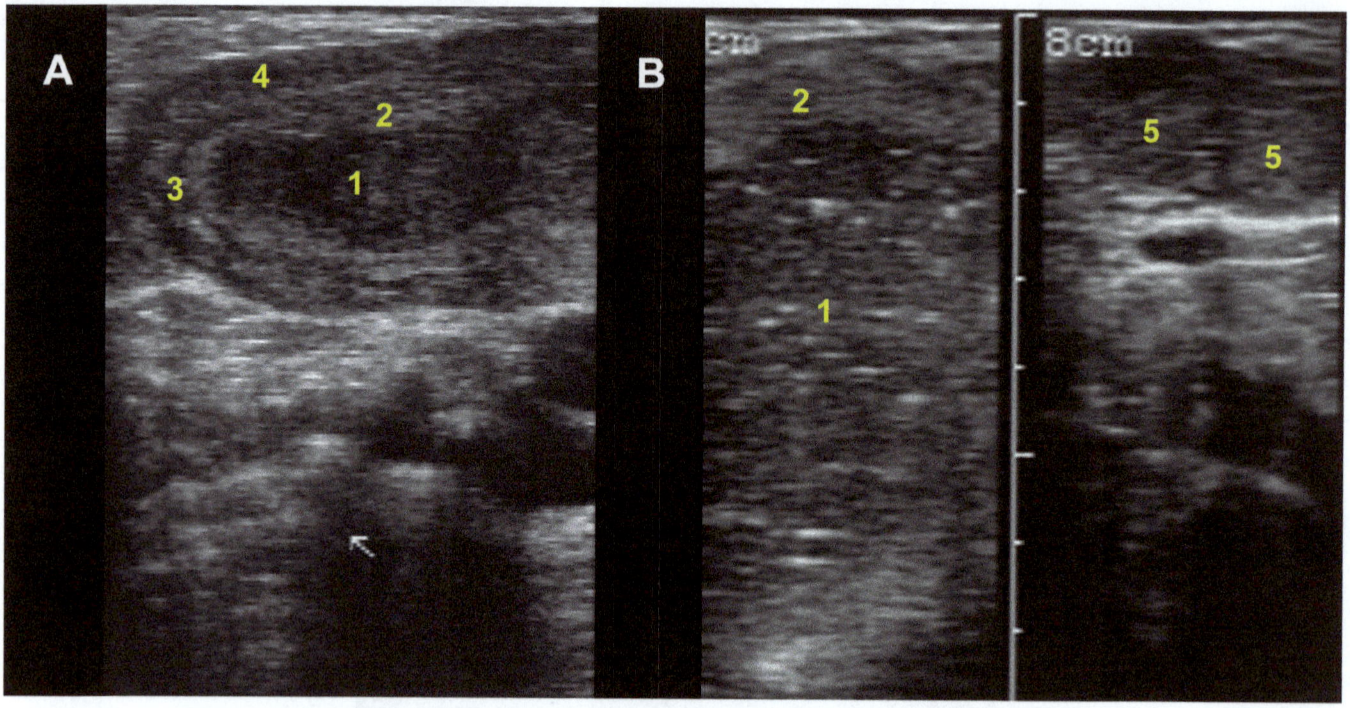

Figure 5.20. Ultrasonograms of endometritis in cows between 25 and 30 days after parturition (probe 7.5 MHz; depth 8 cm). A: Note the clear delimitation between the endometrium and the myometrium; B: Split image ultrasonogram in BB-mode. On the left side one can see the "snowstorm" uterine content with multiple hyperechoic particles. On the right side there are two corpora lutea (CL). This is a good case in which to apply a PreSynch protocol. 1: Purulent content of the uterus; 2: Endometrium; 3: Vascular portion; 4: Myometrium; 5: CL.

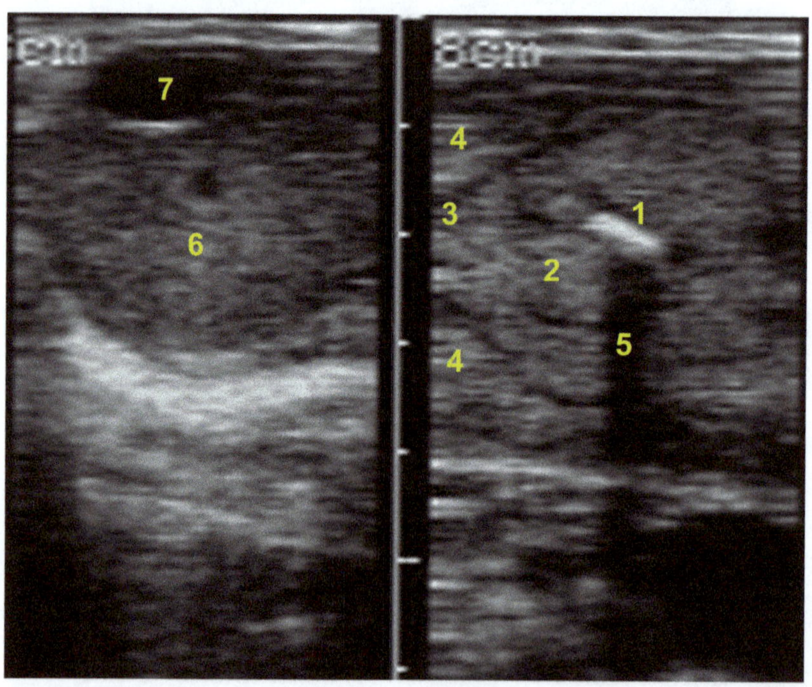

Figure 5.21. Ultrasonogram in BB-mode of a chronic endometritis from a cow at 55 days after parturition (probe 7.5 MHz; depth 6 cm). Note the presence of a CL and of a follicle on the left side of the image. In the less extreme forms of chronic endometritis the accumulation of nonuniformly echogenic liquid is usually visible in the cranial and lower segment of the uterine horns. The more echogenic portion (1) of the accumulated fluid contains fibrins, pus, and mucus. 1: Hyperechogenic content of the uterus; 2: Endometrium; 3: Vascular portion of the uterus; 4: Myometrium; 5: Shadow artifact; 6: CL; 7: Follicle.

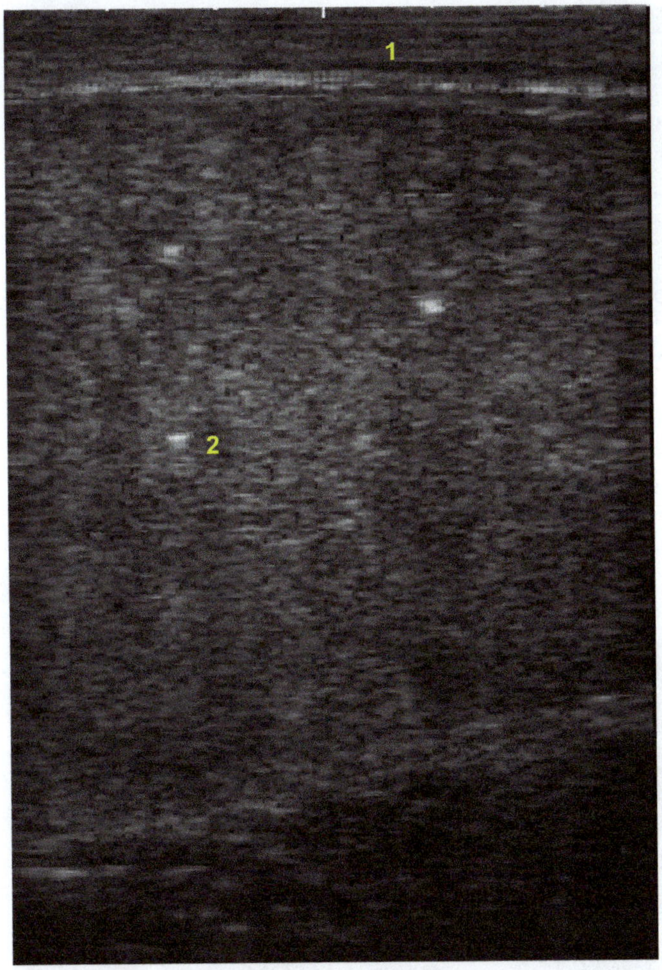

Figure 5.22. Ultrasonogram of a pyometra from a cow at 62 days postpartum (probe 8MHz; depth 9cm). In the ultimate form of endometritis, pyometra, ultrasound also shows the accumulation of a large quantity of a heterogenous echogenic liquid and a thickened uterine wall. The liquid is visible throughout the uterus. By balloting the uterus a few times the suspended hyperechogenic particles will be sent into movement within the uterine liquid, creating a snowflake effect. The diameter of the uterine cavity in pyometra is generally between 5cm and 20cm, but a uterine size similar to that of late gestation can also be observed[1]. 1: Uterine wall; 2: Lumen contents with highly echogenic particles.

CoSynch, or Target Breeding. In the absence of a CL, the use of a slow-release progesterone device can be an alternative to combine with an OvSynch protocol.

Even with ultrasound examination the resolution of the equipment does not always allow the demonstration of nonuniform echogenicity in a cavity that is less than 5mm in diameter (Figure 5.23). In this case it is not always possible to differentiate between the presence of uterine anechogenic liquid due to estrus (Figure 5.24), pregnancy (Figure 5.25B), follicular cyst, or mucometra (Figure 5.25A) and nonuniform echogenic liquid indicating endometritis[17] or early embryonic death (see Chapter 6). Scanning the ovaries and checking the breeding records will be helpful in these cases to guide the practitioner toward a probable diagnosis and plan of action.

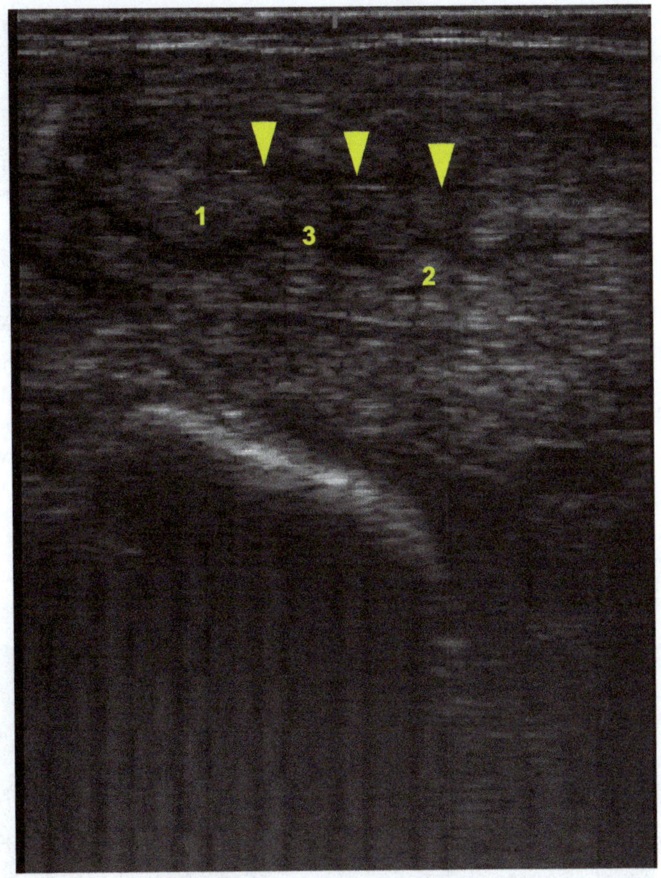

Figure 5.23. Longitudinal section of a uterus from a cow with vaginal mucopurulent material (probe 6MHz; depth 6cm). The diagnosis of this cow is uncertain. Is it endometritis or an accumulation of endometrial liquid during estrus? It is difficult to establish a definitive diagnosis without other additional examinations. Note that the appearance of the uterus is similar to that of a cow in estrus (see Figures 5.3 to 5.5 and 5.24B). 1: Endometrium; 2: Myometrium; 3: Vascular portion of the uterus; Arrowheads: Accumulation line of clear uterine content.

Differential diagnosis of endometritis

Figures 5.24 and 5.25 present ultrasonograms that must be evaluated carefully in order to differentiate nonuniform echogenic liquid in the uterus of cows.

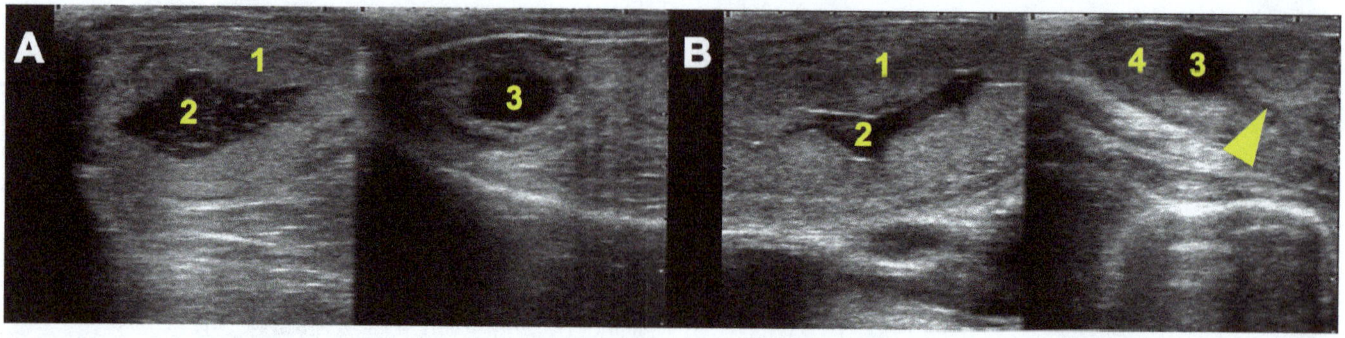

Figure 5.24. Split sonograms of endometritis (A) and of normal uterus during estrus (B) (probe 5 MHz; depth 5 cm). The difference between endometritis and uterus of a cow in heat is obvious in these ultrasonograms when viewed side by side. In both of these cases one can visualize the presence of a dominant follicle. Another possible differential diagnosis of this case of endometritis is the early embryonic death if the cow was bred 25 to 40 days prior to the ultrasound examination (see Chapter 6 for more details). 1: Uterus; 2: Accumulation of content (pus or mucus); 3: Follicle; 4: Old CL; Arrowhead: Tip of uterine horn in transverse view.

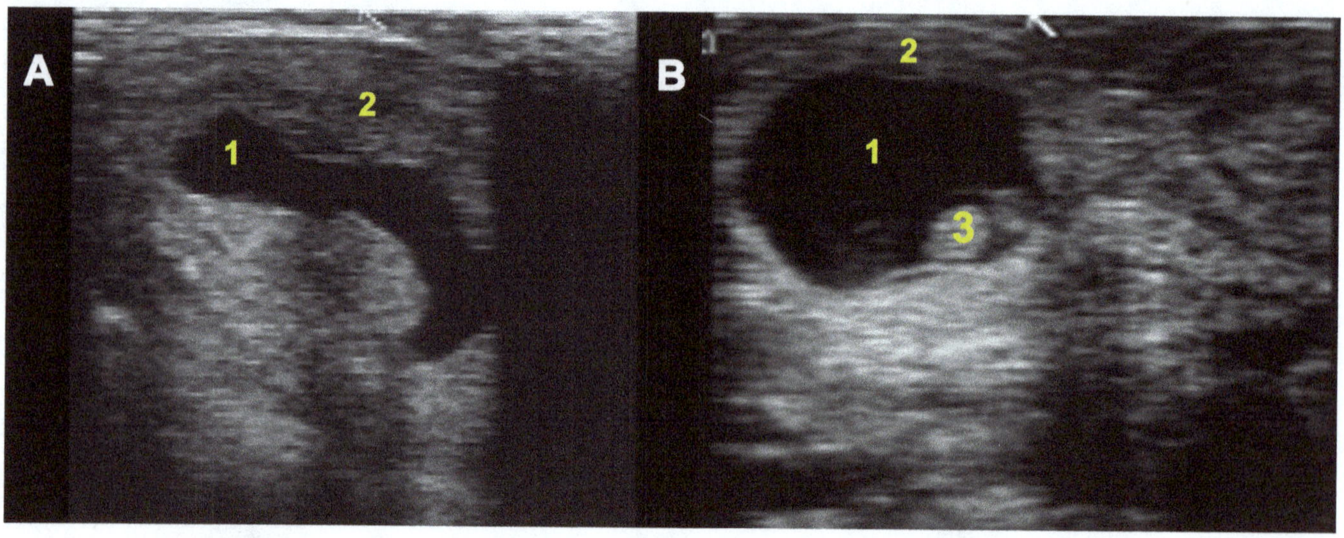

Figure 5.25. Differential diagnosis of mucometra (A) and early pregnancy (B) (probe 7.5 MHz; depth 5 cm). Mucometra is an accumulation of nonpurulent, noninfectious fluid in the uterine lumen. The fluid may be completely clear or contain very small echogenic flecks, as opposed to the more echogenic fluid in endometritis and to the very anechogenic fluid in normal early pregnancy. The uterine wall tends to be thin and the uterus flaccid, in contrast to the uterus of a cow in estrus. Often, but not always, mucometra is associated with the presence of a follicular cyst. A false positive diagnosis of pregnancy must be avoided by carefully examining the uterus for the definitive signs of pregnancy described in Chapter 6. Please note the difference between the thickness of the uterine wall in these two situations. 1: Accumulation of clear anechogenic content; 2: Uterine wall; 3: Embryo.

Other uterine abnormalities

Although rare, it is possible to view an abscess in the uterine wall or in the broad ligament in cows with a perforated uterus due to obstetrical manipulation, artificial insemination, or embryo transfer manipulation, or following intrauterine administration of antibiotics or uterine flushing (Figure 5.26). Figure 5.27 presents the ultrasonographic appearance of a pneumouterus.

Urovagina

Figure 5.28 shows an ultrasonographic image of the urovagina.

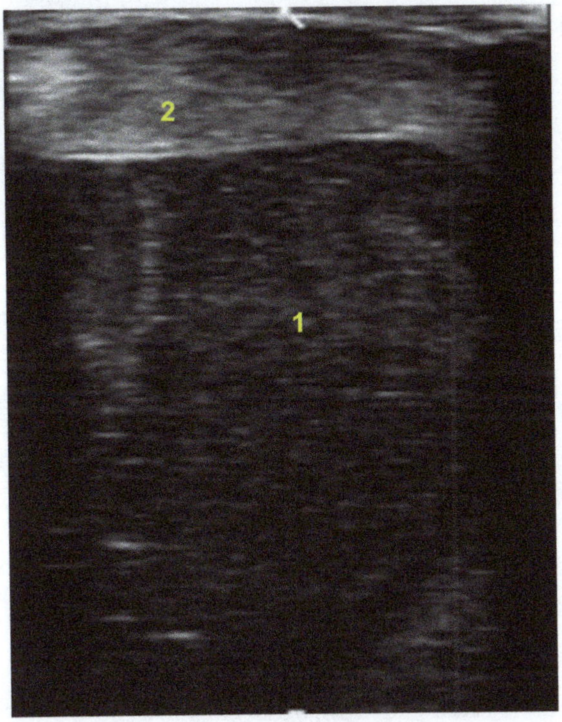

Figure 5.26. Ultrasound image of an abscess in the broad ligament of a dairy cow (probe 7.5 MHz; depth 8 cm). Note the typical ultrasound appearance of the abscess with the accumulation of a large quantity of nonuniformly echogenic liquid and many hyperechogenic particles. 1: Accumulation of nonuniform purulent liquid; 2: Edge of the abscess.

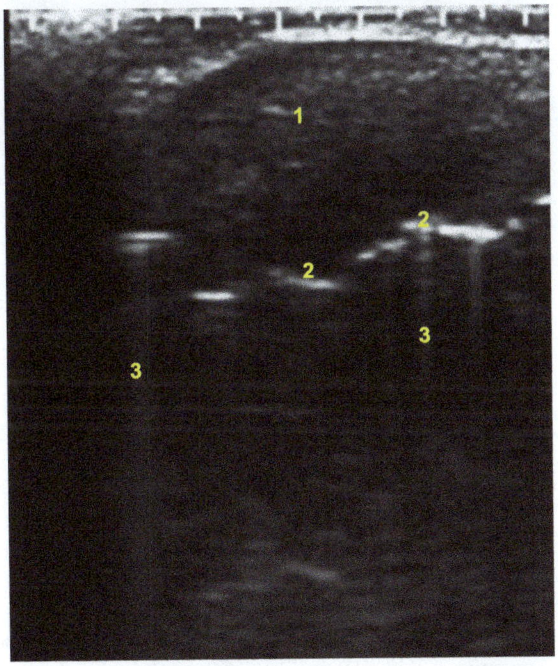

Figure 5.27. Ultrasonogram of a pneumouterus in a dairy cow (probe 5 MHz; depth 8 cm). Pneumouterus also occurs rarely and presents as a series of air pockets in the uterus producing hyperechogenic images under which a shadow cone is formed (reflected ultrasound waves). 1: Uterus; 2: Air pocket; 3: Shadow cones.

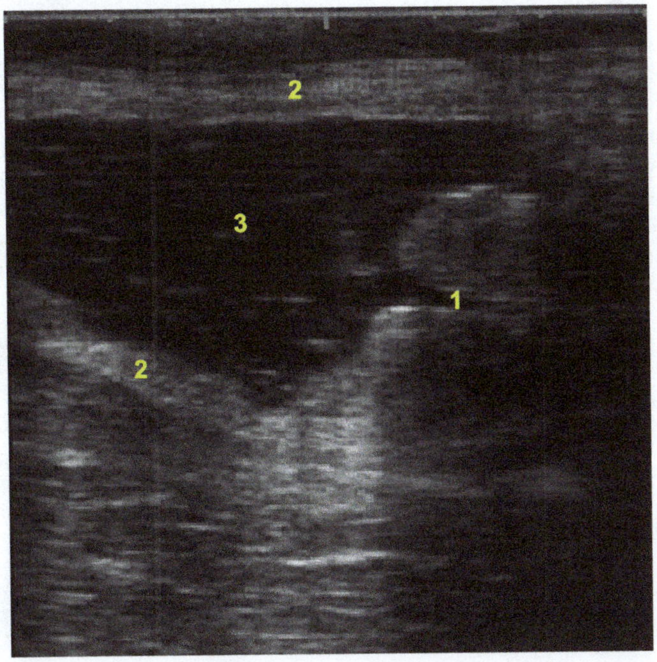

Figure 5.28. Ultrasonographic image of an urovagina (probe 6 MHz; depth 6 cm). In the same image one can see the caudal portion of the cervix. The anechogenic image is the urovagina. The vaginal wall is irregular and the urine contains large, hyperechogenic particles in suspension. 1: Cervix; 2: Vagina wall; 3: Accumulated urine.

REFERENCES

1. Barlund CS, Carruthers TD, Waldner CL, Palmer CW (2008). A comparison of diagnostic techniques for post-partum endometritis in dairy cattle. Theriogenology 69(6): 714–723.
2. Bollwein H, Meyer HH, Maierl J, Weber F, Baumgartner U, Stolla R (2000). Transrectal Doppler sonography of uterine blood flow. Theriogenology 53: 1541–1552.
3. Bonafos LD, Kot K, Ginther OJ (1995). Physical characteristics of the uterus during the bovine estrous cycle and early pregnancy. Theriogenology 43: 713–721.
4. Carrière P, DesCôteaux L, Durocher J (2005). Ultrasonography of the reproductive system of the cow. [CD-ROM]. Faculté de médecine vétérinaire, Université de Montréal, St-Hyacinthe, Québec.
5. De Lahunta A, Habel RE (1986). Ovary and uterus. In: De Lahunta A, Habel RE (Eds.), Applied Veterinary Anatomy. WB Saunders Co., Philadelphia, pp. 258–260.
6. Dickey RP (1997). Doppler ultrasound investigation of uterine and ovarian blood flow in infertility and early pregnancy. Hum Reprod Update 3: 467–503.
7. Finch CE, Gosden RG (1986). Animal models for the human menopause. In: Mastroianni LJ, Paulsen CA (Eds.), Aging Reproduction and the Climacteric. Plenum Press, New York, pp. 3–34.
8. Fissore RA, Edmonson AJ, Pashen RL, Bondurant RH (1986). The use of ultrasonography for the study of the bovine reproductive tract II. Non-pregnant, pregnant and pathological conditions of the uterus. Anim Repro Sci 12: 167–177.
9. Gilbert RO (1992). Bovine endometritis: the burden of proof. Cornell Vet 82: 11–14.
10. Gilbert RO, Shin ST, Guard CL, Erb HN, Frayblat M (2005). Prevalence of endometritis and its effects on reproductive performance of dairy cows. Theriogenology 64(9): 1879–1888.
11. Gilbert RO (2006). Personal communication.
12. Ginther OJ (1998). Ultrasonic Imaging and Animal Reproduction: Cattle. Equiservices Publishing. Wisconsin, 304 pages.
13. Goswamy RK, Steptoe PC (1988). Doppler ultrasound studies of the uterine artery in spontaneous ovarian cycles. Hum Reprod: 721–726.
14. Hajurka J, Macak V, Hura V (2005). Influence of health status of reproductive organs on uterine involution in dairy cows. Bull Vet Inst Pulawy 49: 53–58.
15. Herzog K, Bollwein H (2007). Application of Doppler ultrasonography in cattle reproduction. In: Reproduction in Domestic Animals. Blackwell Publishing, Ames, IA, Volume 42, pp. 51–58.
16. Honnens A, Voss C, Herzog K, Niemann H, Rath D, Bollwein H (2008). Uterine blood flow during the first 3 weeks of pregnancy in dairy cows. Theriogenology (in press).
17. Kähn W (1994). Atlas de diagnostics échographiques. Éditions Maloine, Paris, 255 pages.
18. Kamimura S, Ohgi T, Takahashi M, Tsukamoto T (1993). Postpartum resumption of ovarian activity and uterine involution monitored by ultrasonography in Holstein cows. J Vet Med Sci 55: 643–647.
19. LeBlanc SJ, Duffield TF, Leslie KE, Bateman KG, Keefe GP, Walton JS, Johnson WH (2002). The effect of treatment of clinical endometritis on reproductive performance in dairy cows. J Dairy Sci 85: 2237–2249.
20. Maulik D (1997). Spectral Doppler: Basic principles and instrumentation. In: Maulik, D (Ed.), Doppler Ultrasound in Obstetrics and Gynecology. Springer, New York, pp. 21–42.
21. Miller HV, Kimsey PB, Kendrick JW, Darien B, Doering L, Franti C, Horton J (1980). Endometritis of dairy cattle: diagnosis, treatment and fertility. Bov Pract 15: 13–23.
22. Okano A, Tomizuka T (1996). Post partum uterine involution in the cow. Japan Agri Res Quart 30: 113–121.
23. Pierson RA, Ginther OJ (1987). Ultrasonographic appearance of the bovine uterus during the estrous cycle. J Am Vet Med Assoc 190: 995–1001.
24. Ribadu AY, Nakao T (1999). Bovine reproductive ultrasonography: A review. J Repro Dev 45: 13–28.
25. Riddle G (2004). Metricheck a new way of diagnosis. World Buiatric Congress. Intervet Symposium. Québec City, Québec, Canada.
26. Sheldon IM, Noakes DE, Rycroft AN, Dobson H (2002). Effect of postpartum manual examination of the vagina on uterine bacterial contamination in cows. Vet Rec 151: 531–534.
27. Steer CV, Tan SL, Dillon D, Mason BA, Campbell S (1995). Vaginal color Doppler assessment of uterine artery impedance correlates with immunohistochemical markers of endometrial receptivity required for the implantation of an embryo. Fertil Steril: 101–108.
28. Stroud BK (1994). Clinical applications of bovine reproductive ultrasonography. Comp Cont Educ 16(8): 1085–1097.
29. Zietzschmann O (1943). Die arterien. In: Ellenberger W, Baum H (Eds.), Handbuch der Vergleichenden Anatomie der Haustiere. Springer Verlag, Berlin, pp. 627–717.

Points to Remember

- During periestrus ultrasound images of the uterus translate into less uniform gray tones. There is a swollen or swirled appearance of the uterine wall and a greater area of the uterus showing dark, anechogenic zones that denote areas of edema and increased vascularity under the endometrium.
- During the periestrous period it is also possible to view a small quantity of mucus in the uterine lumen.
- During estrus the endometrial mucosa becomes especially echogenic, the limit between the endometrium and the myometrium is more obvious, and the uterine lumen may show a greater accumulation of mucus over a longer segment of the uterine horns.
- In normal conditions with no complications, the bovine uterus completes its involution on average at day 23 in primiparous cows and day 27 in pluriparous cows.
- Ultrasound evaluation is the best cow-side diagnostic tool to evaluate the physiopathological conditions of uterus and ovary during the early postpartum period.
- The use of an accurate ultrasonographic examination of the ovaries and of the uterus is highly recommended in order to improve the efficiency of reproductive synchronization programs.
- During the estrous cycle the uterine blood flow has a characteristic pattern with the highest time averaged maximum velocity (TAMV) values during proestrus and estrus.
- During diestrus blood flow velocity remains at a fairly constant low level.
- Due to the relatively high interindividual variability of TAMV and pulsatility index values, the use of color Doppler sonography is not clinically helpful for early pregnancy detection in cows.
- The typical pyometra sonogram shows the accumulation of a large quantity of a heteregenous echogenic liquid and a thickened uterine wall. By balloting the uterus the suspended hyperechogenic particles will be sent into movement within the uterine liquid.

Summary Questions

1. A small quantity of nonechogenic fluid may be found in a nongravid uterus in one or more of those situations. Please select all possible choices.
   a. Uterus in heat
   b. Pyometra
   c. Mucometra
   d. Follicular cyst

2. Color Doppler ultrasonography is useful to detect any changes in the uterine artery blood flow. The increased blood flow in the uterine artery from day 16 after insemination is a valuable parameter to confirm early pregnancies in bovine species. True or False?
   a. True
   b. False

3. The following is an ultrasonographic image from the uterus of a cow that was taken 23 days after calving (probe 7.5 MHz; depth 7 cm). What is your diagnosis?
   a. Acute puerperal metritis
   b. Normal involution of the uterus
   c. Mucometra
   d. Endometritis

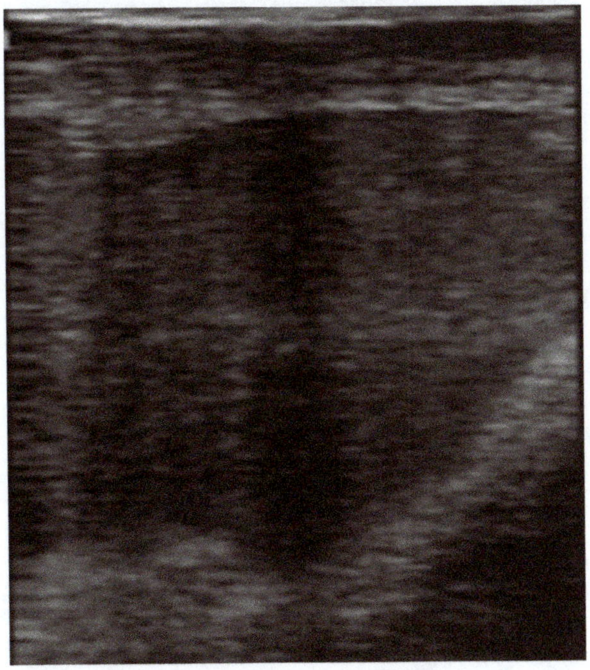

4. The following is an ultrasonographic image from the uterus of a cow that was taken 42 days after insemination (probe 7.5 MHz; depth 7 cm). What is your diagnosis?
   a. Uterus in heat
   b. Pyometra
   c. Gravid uterus
   d. Endometritis

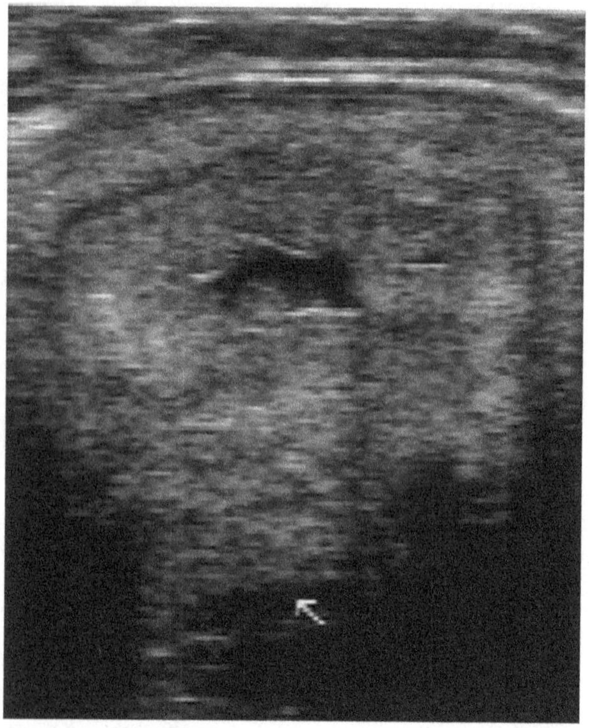

5. The following is an ultrasonographic image from the uterus of a cow that was taken 56 days after calving (probe 7.5 MHz; depth 6 cm). This cow demonstrated signs of nymphomania since a week before the ultrasonographic examination. What is your diagnosis?
   a. Uterus in heat
   b. Gravid uterus
   c. Mucometra
   d. Endometritis

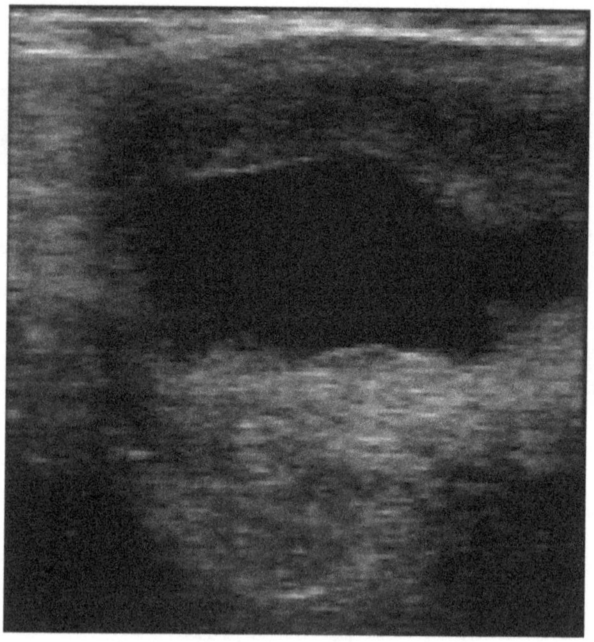

ANSWERS

1. a, c, and d
2. b
3. d
4. a
5. c

CHAPTER SIX

BOVINE PREGNANCY

Luc DesCôteaux, Jill Colloton, Véronique Gayrard, and Nicole Picard-Hagen

INTRODUCTION

Early pregnancy diagnosis in cows via ultrasound has been an integral part of dairy herd health programs since the mid-1990s. This rapid, accurate, and secure transrectal diagnostic procedure is considered to be essential and economical for dairy producers who want to improve the reproductive performance of their herd[4,7,8,9,22].

Linear probes with frequencies between 5 and 8 MHz are generally preferred for early pregnancy diagnosis in bovines[11].

This chapter presents the important stages of morphologic embryonic and fetal development up to day 55 of gestation to help the practitioner recognize the necessary ultrasound criteria for early diagnosis of gestation. This comes prior to providing a definitive diagnosis of fetal sex, the topic to be developed in the next chapter. The principal signs essential to the diagnosis of a normal gestation will be reviewed before presenting some ultrasound images of embryonic and fetal death. The initial signs along with the characteristics of ultrasound images of twin gestations also will be explained.

MORPHOLOGIC EMBRYONIC AND FETAL DEVELOPMENT UP TO DAY 55

The embryonic period is traditionally defined as the period between fertilization and the end of organogenesis on the 42nd day of gestation.

The beginning of the embryonic period can be described as a series of cell divisions and the first differentiations leading to the blastocyst stage, 6 days after fertilization. The zona pellucida disappears on day 9. The blastocyst changes in shape from spherical (0.2 mm in diameter) to oblong (1.5 to 3.3 mm by 0.9 to 1.7 mm) on day 12 or 13 of gestation[2].

Extraembryonic tissues

As early as the 12th day of gestation the extraembryonic tissues lengthen considerably, and the blastocyst becomes filamentous. During the entire period preceding implantation the conceptus grows within the uterine lumen and eventually occupies the entire ipsilateral horn with the corpus luteum on approximately day 17, when it reaches approximately 40 cm in length. The length of the embryonic vesicle nevertheless shows significant individual variations, measuring anywhere between 7 and 24 cm on day 16 of gestation[3,30]. Its diameter, however, remains constant at 2 mm from day 10 to day 18 of gestation (Figure 6.1). One end of the vesicle reaches the utero-tubular junction of the other horn on day 20–24[18]. At that time it resembles a long, hollow cord over 1 meter in length. The amnion appears as an oval-shaped fluid swelling 3–4 mm in diameter in the center. Fluid accumulation increases considerably at approximately day 25, when the embryo detaches from the uterine wall and is easier to detect by ultrasound.

The amniotic folds develop by about day 12, covering the embryo by approximately day 23 when a cavity is formed (Figure 6.2). The allantois can be seen on day 18, in the shape of a two-lobed bud that extends rapidly toward the ends of the conceptus until around day 24, when it resembles a tube. From about day 18 to day 35 the tips of the chorion degenerate, leading to a rapid

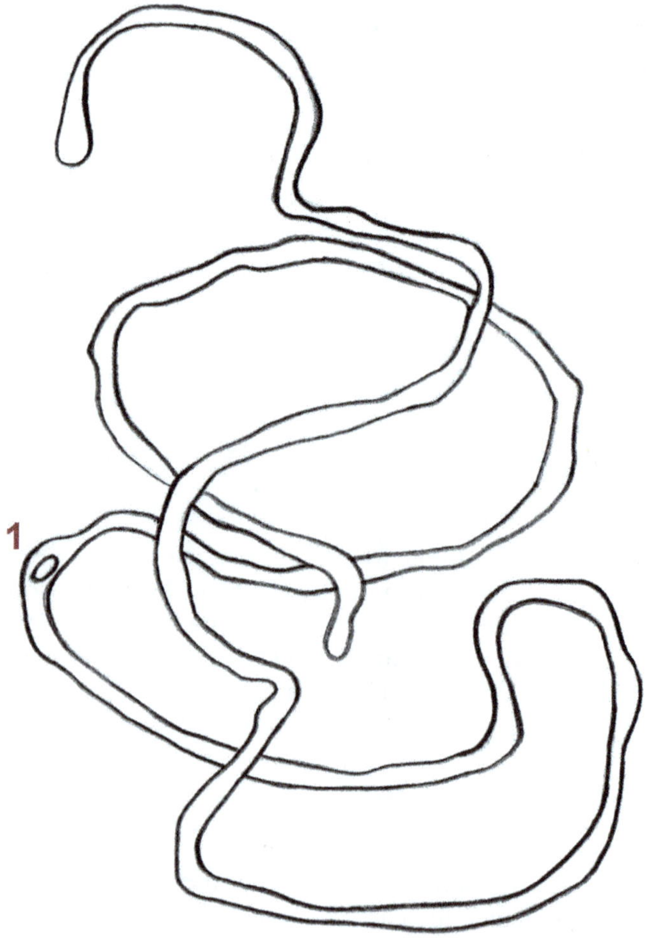

Figure 6.1. Blastocyst at day 18 measuring 40 cm in length (adapted from Barone 1990). 1: Developing amnion.

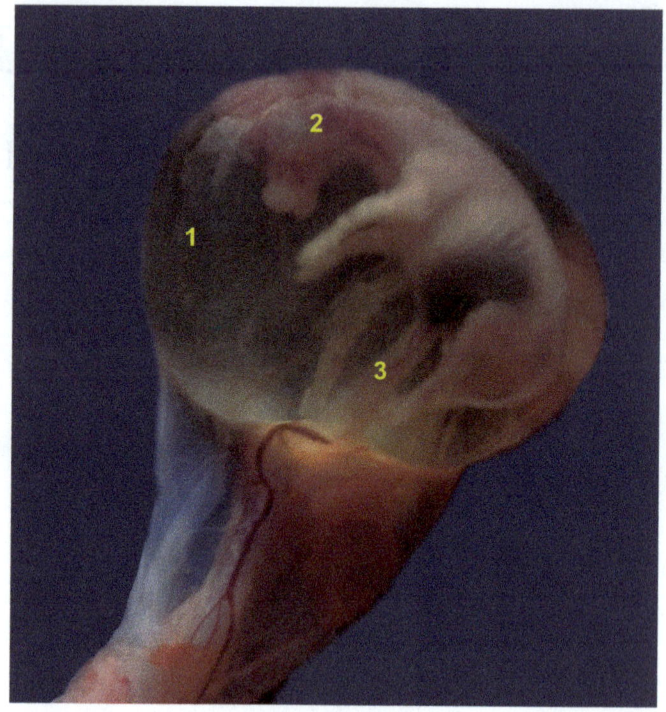

Figure 6.2. Amniotic cavity and 55-day-old bovine fetus. At this stage, the amniotic cavity resembles a bean-shaped swelling. 1: Amnion; 2: Fetus; 3: Umbilical cord.

shortening of the conceptus at the allantoic extremities (Figure 6.3). The conceptus thus acquires its definitive appearance, measuring 30 cm in length, although the maximum width does not exceed 3 cm[23].

Implantation of the conceptus in the uterus begins on day 19 of gestation, and on the 20th day the first placental villi develop. Toward day 27 bunches of villi located across from the uterine caruncles form the first cotyledons[2,19] (Figure 6.4). The placentomes initially develop close to the embryo, followed by 100 to 120 convex placentomes that arrange in four to six parallel rows over the whole surface of the chorion[24].

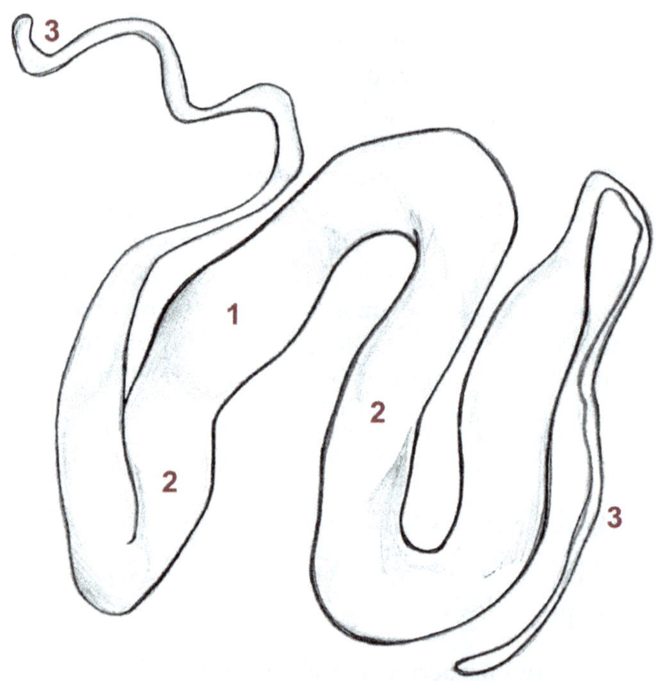

Figure 6.3. 30-day-old conceptus measuring 60 cm in length (adapted from Barone 1990). 1: Amnion; 2: Allantois covered by the chorion; 3: Degenerated chorionic extremity.

Morphogenesis and organogenesis of the bovine embryo

The embryo is well demarcated by approximately day 18, with a highly accentuated curve in its anterior-posterior axis. The first somites are formed around day

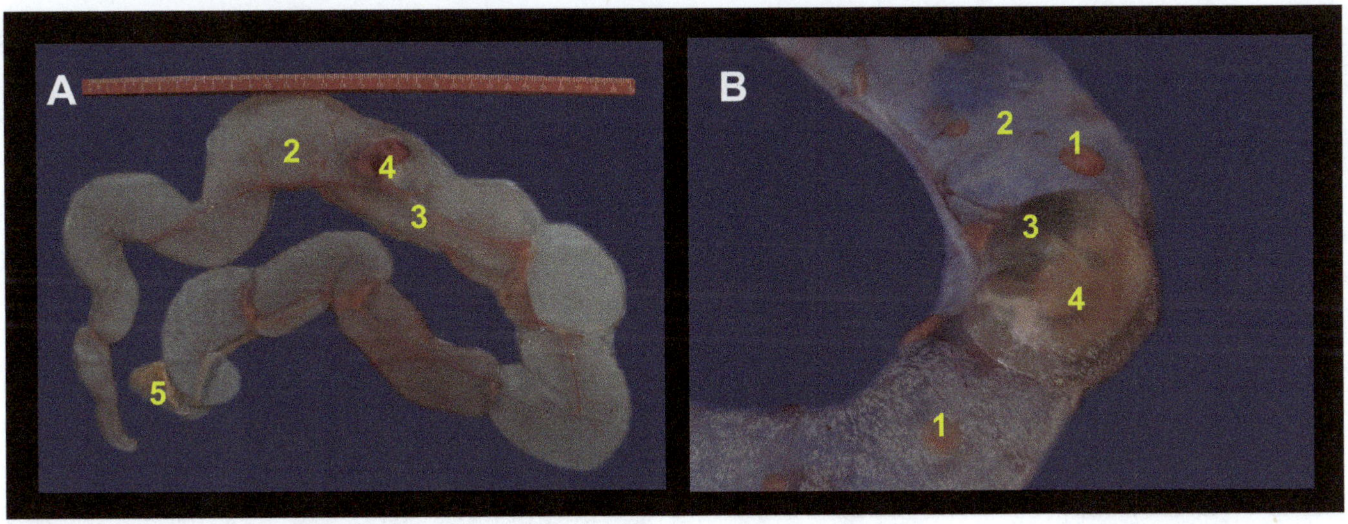

Figure 6.4. Fetus and fetal tissues on day 45 (A) and on day 55 (B) of gestation. The cotyledons are visible on the surface of the allantochorion. 1: Cotyledon; 2: Allantochorion; 3: Amnion; 4: Fetus; 5: Degenerated chorionic extremity.

Table 6.1.
Development of the bovine embryo and fetus up to day 55 of gestation (according to Barone 1990; Ginther 1998)

Stage of Gestation (Days)	Transverse Diameter of the Embryonic Vesicle (mm)	CRL* (mm)	Observations
20	2–3	3	Heartbeats
22	3–5	4–5	Optic vesicles
25	10	5–7	Limb buds
30	18–20	8–12	Optic primordium (no eyelids)
35	20–25	13–17	Folds around eyes
			Neck is developed
			Digits recognizable on all four limbs
40	30–35	17–24	Genital tubercle (undifferentiated stage)
			Embryonic movement
45	35–40	23–26	Rudimentary eyelids
			Rudimentary ear pinnae
			Mammary primordium
			Tactile hair follicles (lips, eyelids)
50	40–45	35–45	Migration of the genital tubercle in both sexes
			Atrophy of labial tubercle
55	45–55	45–60	Fusion of the urogenital folds and the genital tubercle

*CRL: Crown-rump length.

19. At that time the embryo is 3–4 mm long, the neural tube is beginning to close, and the prominent cardiac primordium begins to beat[10].

Table 6.1 presents the stages of bovine embryonic and fetal development. On day 22 the optical vesicles are formed, as well as the hepatic primordium and the mesonephros. On day 25 the anterior limb buds appear in the form of elongated swellings, and the next day, the posterior buds appear. On day 26 the embryo curves in upon itself and measures 7–8 mm long. Starting from the moment it becomes visible, and up to day 50 of gestation, it grows by an average of 1.1 mm/day[23] (Table 6.1). Toward day 30 the optic buds are prominent but the eyelids are not formed.

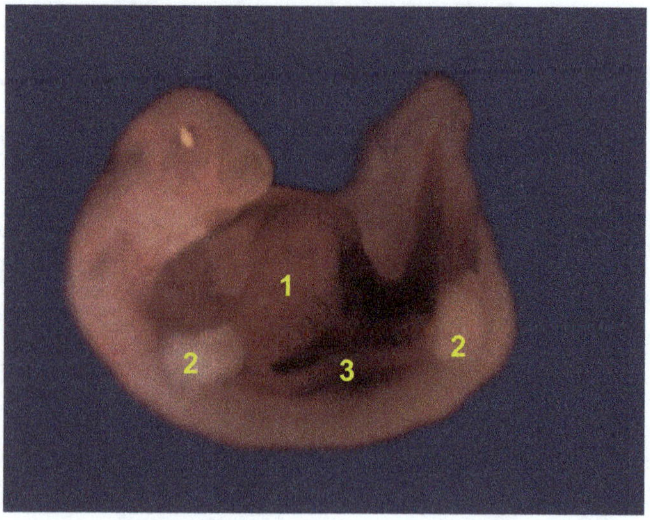

Figure 6.5. 35-day-old embryo. The crown-rump length (CRL) is 1.5 cm. The embryo is C-shaped. The head is distinguishable. The heart cavity is prominent. 1: Heart cavity; 2: Limb buds; 3: Hepatic primordium.

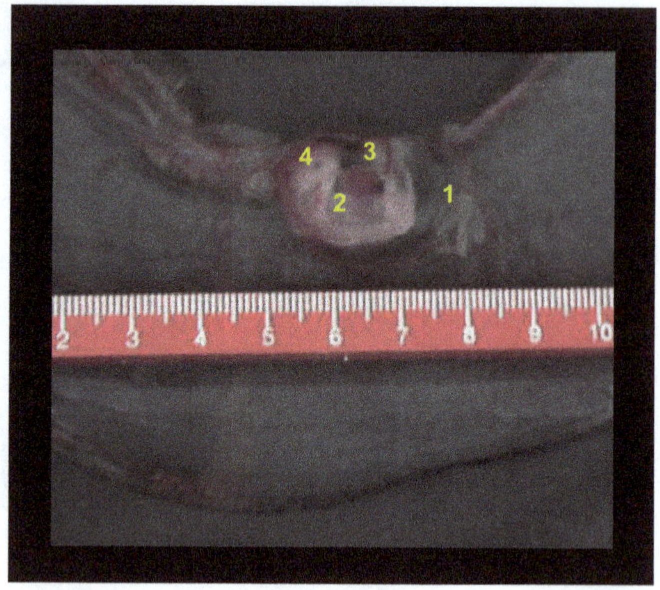

Figure 6.6. 40-day-old embryo. The crown-rump length (CRL) is 2.0 cm. The embryo is L-shaped in the amniotic cavity. The head is distinct. The eyes are prominent. 1: Amnion; 2: Embryo; 3: Umbilical cord; 4: Eye.

Toward day 35 the embryo assumes an "L" shape; the eyes are bordered by thin folds or rudimentary eyelids (Figure 6.5); the neck is clearly developed and the digits are recognizable on all four limbs.

On day 40 of gestation the genital tubercle is prominently located on the median line between the posterior limbs (Figure 6.6). It becomes the embryonic penis in the male and the clitoris in the female. Urogenital folds, which are the embryonic prepuce in males and vulvar lips in females, are visible caudal to the genital tubercle. The labio-scrotal folds, which form the scrotum in males, are visible between the umbilicus and the genital tubercle, beside the median line (see Figure 6.8A). At this stage there is no macroscopic difference in the genital tubercle between the two sexes, but the presence of the urogenital orifice and the anogenital raphe indicate that the embryo is male[16].

At approximately day 45 of gestation the fetus loses its rudimentary embryonic shape, and its face, neck, limbs, and tail have lengthened and become more defined. The mammary primordium is recognizable in both sexes and the digits can be distinguished separately (Figure 6.7).

Migration of the genital tubercle and determination of fetal sex

At approximately day 47 of gestation in the male fetus the genital tubercle begins to migrate toward the umbilicus. This migration results in a relative increase in the distance separating the genital tubercle from the fetus' tail and is usually completed by day 56 to 58 after insemination (Figures 6.8, 6.9). The urogenital folds fuse with the genital tubercle on day 55 of gestation[14].

In females the genital tubercle migrates toward the anus starting at day 48–49 to reach its final position at approximately 53 days postinsemination (Figure 6.10). The labio-scrotal fold progressively atrophies starting on day 50, eventually disappearing completely.

Ultrasound of the conceptus before day 55

During the early development of the embryo before day 30 the development of the embryonic tissues and the different organs take place earlier (Table 6.1) than they can be viewed using ultrasound (Table 6.2). This delay is mainly related to the size of the structures compared to the probe's accuracy of resolution. The typical ultrasound appearance of the bovine conceptus and the gravid uterus up to day 55 will be presented in the following section.

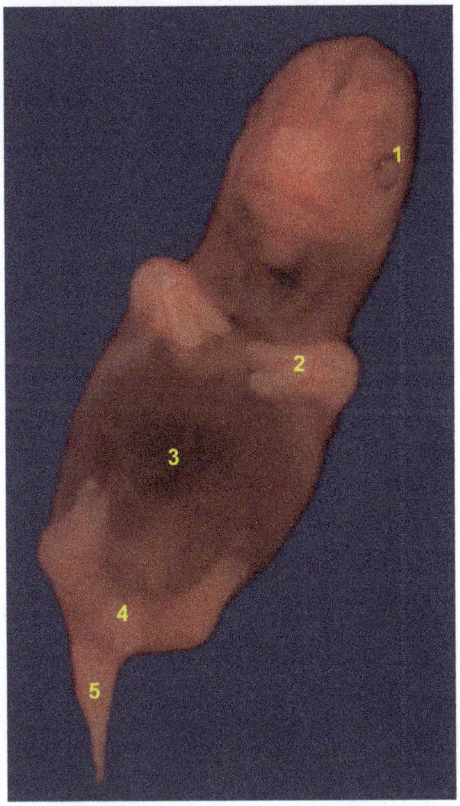

Figure 6.7. Fetus of undifferentiated sex at day 45 of gestation. The crown-rump length (CRL) is 3.1 cm. The genital tubercle is located between the two posterior limbs. 1: Eye; 2: Limbs and digits; 3: Hepatic primordium; 4: Genital tubercle; 5: Tail.

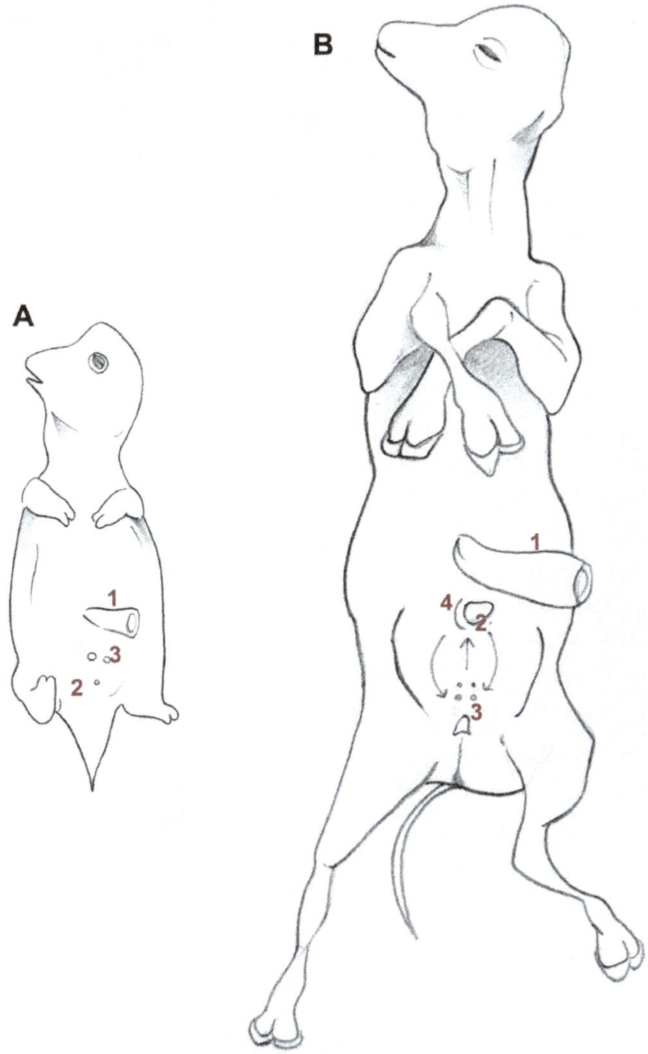

Figure 6.8. Anatomy of the external genital organs of the male fetus between days 40 (A) and 55 (B) of gestation. 1: Umbilicus; 2: Genital tubercle; 3: Labio-scrotal fold (scrotum); 4: Urogenital folds.

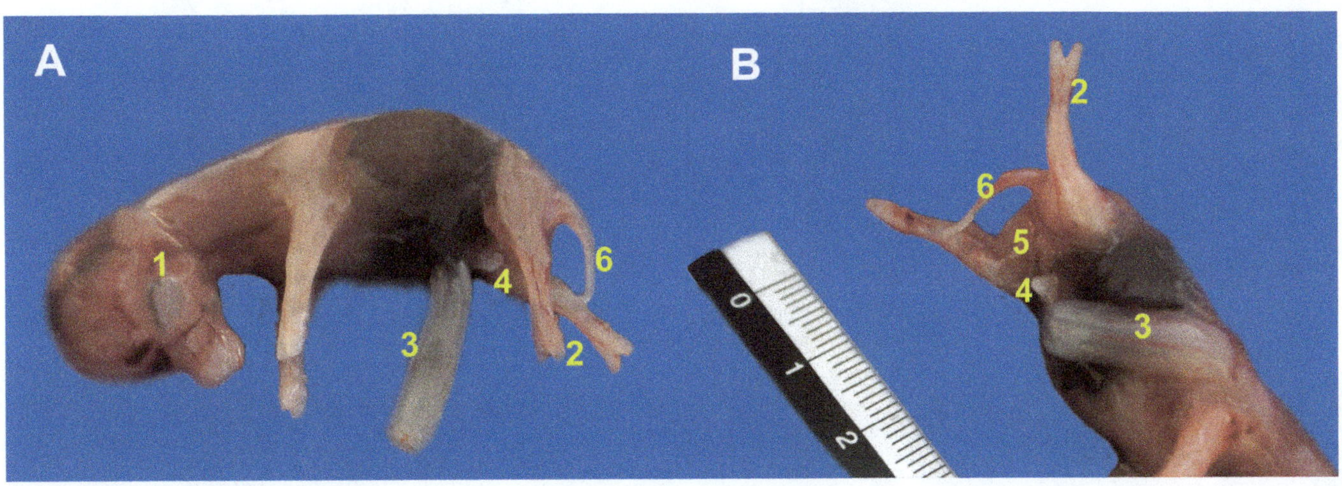

Figure 6.9. 55-day-old male fetus. The crown-rump length (CRL) is 6.0 cm. The genital tubercle has migrated caudal to the umbilical cord. 1: Eye; 2: Limbs and digits; 3: Umbilical cord; 4: Genital tubercle caudal to the umbilical cord; 5: Labio-scrotal folds (scrotum); 6: Tail.

Table 6.2.
Summary of embryonic and fetal measurements, principal characteristics of the conceptus, and their moment of apparition in ultrasound examinations (+) between days 25 and 55 of gestation (adapted from Curran et al. 1986; Ginther 1998; Kolour et al. 2005)

	Day 25	Day 30	Day 35	Day 40	Day 45	Day 50	Day 55
CRL* (cm)	0.5–0.7	0.8–1.2	1.3–1.7	1.7–2.4	2.3–2.6	3.5–4.5	4.5–6.0
Embryonic shape	C	C	L	L	L	L	L
Cardiac frequency (b/min)	140–150	160–180	170–190	170–190	170–190	180–200	180–200
Allantois	+	+	+	+	+	+	+
Amnion		+	+	+	+	+	+
Spinal column		+	+	+	+	+	+
Anterior limbs		+	+	+	+	+	+
Posterior limbs			+	+	+	+	+
Trunk diameter (cm)			0.6	0.9	1.2	1.5	1.7
Placentome (cm)			0.3	0.5	0.6	0.8	1.0
Claws					+	+	+
Movements					+	+	+
Eye diameter (cm)						0.3	0.4
Ribs						+	+

*Crown-rump length measurement of the embryo/fetus.

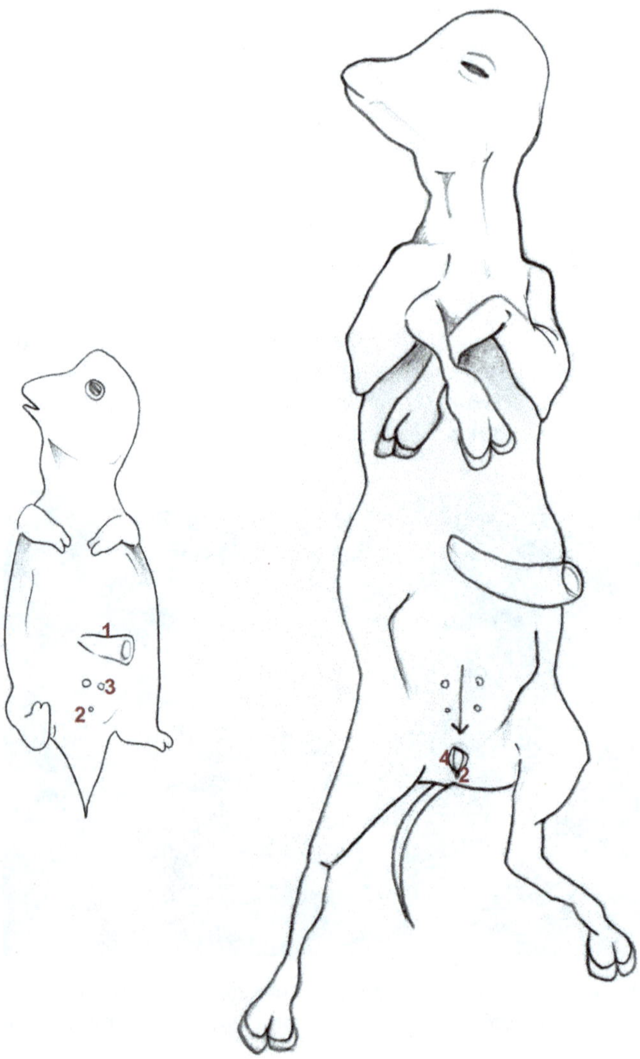

Figure 6.10. Anatomy of the external genital organs in the female fetus between days 40 (A) and 55 (B) of gestation. 1: Umbilicus; 2: Genital tubercle; 3: Labio-scrotal fold; 4: Urogenital folds.

Ultrasound Landmarks of Standard Early Pregnancy Diagnosis

Ultrasound diagnosis of bovine gestation can be carried out beginning at day 25–26 after insemination[11,15,27]. This diagnostic method has excellent sensitivity, indicating the ability to detect gestation when the animal is truly pregnant. Sensitivity is superior to 95% as early as day 26 after insemination, and close to 100% after day 29[11]. This excellent diagnostic capability allows bovine practitioners to propose reproduction synchronization programs for nonpregnant cows with the goal of successful insemination in the best possible time frame (see Chapter 4)[9].

The principal landmarks that are essential to early diagnosis of normal gestation are reviewed in the following section.

Normal appearance of the gravid uterus and the bovine conceptus between days 25 and 55 of gestation

Early ultrasound diagnosis of gestation reveals a uterine lumen containing a variable quantity of anechogenic fluid produced by the conceptus[26]. Fluid accumulation and uterine distension depend largely on the stage of gestation (Table 6.1) and the age of the cow[4,26]. There is normally too little fluid inside the uterus prior to day 27 of gestation to be able to confirm a diagnosis, which explains the better reported diagnostic value of ultrasound examinations carried out after this date. As well, fluid accumulation during estrus in nonpregnant cows can be confused with the anechogenic image of the conceptus and cause potential diagnostic error by less experienced users[4,11,26].

It is sometimes difficult to locate the embryo in the slight quantity of amniotic and allantoic fluid before day 30 of gestation[11,26] because the young embryo is often lodged close to the uterine wall and may even be concealed by an endometrial fold[4]. Careful examination in the zone of anechogenic fluid generally reveals the presence of the embryo close to the uterine folds. Starting on day 30 it is also possible to view the echogenic amniotic membrane that produces specular reflections due to its round shape[4,18] (Figures 6.11, 6.12).

The placentomes can be identified starting on day 35 of gestation and are visible close to the young embryo. Table 6.2 provides the approximate dimensions of the placentomes according to the age of the conceptus. On

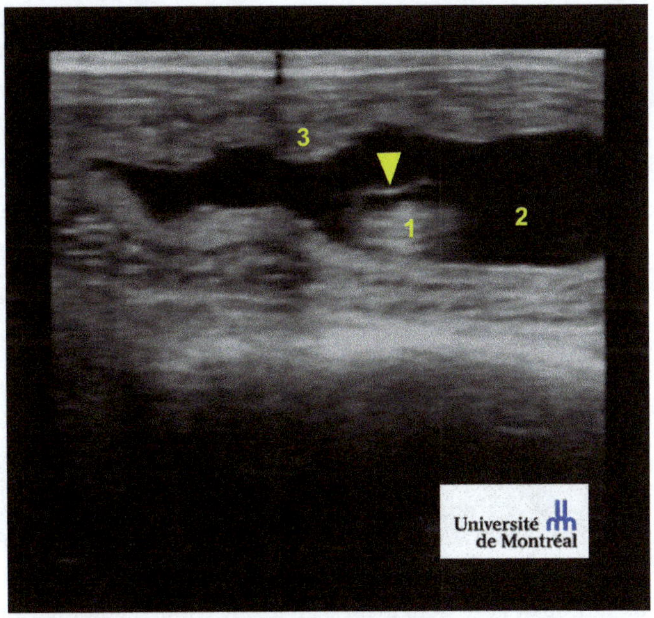

Figure 6.11. A 30-day-old embryo measuring 12 mm is located close to some uterine folds that are the same size as the embryo (7.5 MHz probe; depth 6 cm). Courtesy of the Université de Montréal. There is a smaller quantity of amniotic fluid compared to the allantoic fluid. 1: Embryo; 2: Allantoic fluid; 3: Uterine fold; Arrowhead: amnion.

Figure 6.12A we can distinguish a 0.5 cm placentome near the 40-day-old embryo.

Other important signs of normal embryonic and fetal development are the appearance of the umbilical cord attachment to the uterus of the cow starting at day 40 of gestation (Figure 6.13) and a view of the ossified ribs in the fetus starting at day 50 (Figure 6.14).

Other ultrasound landmarks of normal fetal development before day 55

Measurements used to determine embryonic or fetal age

A growth curve helps determine the age of the embryo according to its size. The rate of fetal growth increases after day 50 of gestation compared to that of the preceding period[18]. Several different ultrasound machines come with a program allowing the veterinarian to estimate the age of the bovine embryo or fetus using specific measurements. Among these are the distance between the top of the head (the crown) and the rump (crown-rump length or CRL) and the diameters of the head and trunk; these are the easiest measurements to obtain and are also the best predictors of gestational

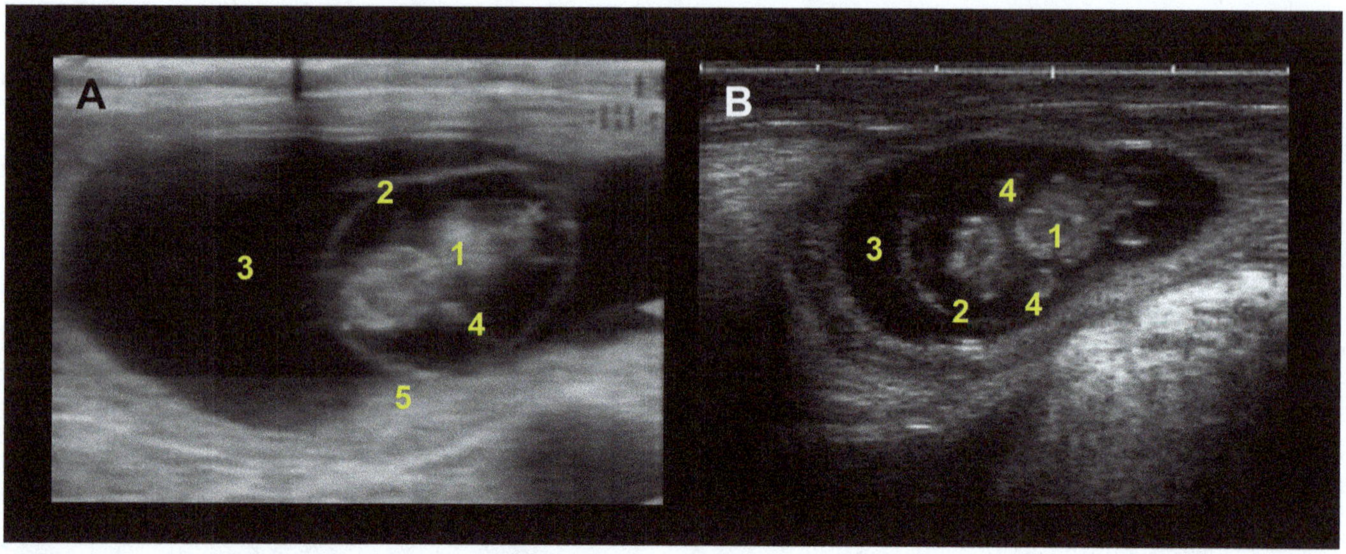

Figure 6.12. 40-day-old embryo measuring 21 mm (A: probe 7.5 MHz, depth 4.5 cm; B: probe 10 MHz, depth 4 cm). Starting on day 30 of gestation, there is generally enough amniotic and allantoic fluid in the uterus to be able to position and view the bovine embryo in the center of the zone of accumulated fluid. On these ultrasonograms, the head, the anterior and posterior limb buds, and a 0.5 cm placentome are visible. 1: Embryo; 2: Amnion; 3: Allantoic fluid; 4: Limbs; 5: Placentome.

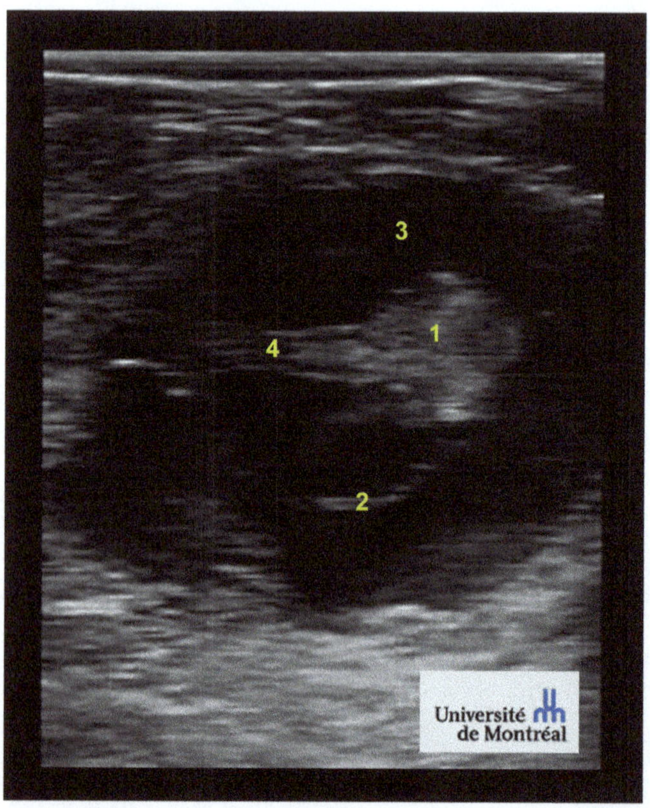

Figure 6.13. Fetus on day 47 with the umbilical cord. Courtesy of the Université de Montréal. 1: Fetus; 2: Amnion; 3: Allantoic fluid; 4: Umbilical cord.

age[17,29,31] (Figure 6.15). According to the experience of users, the CRL measurement is the easiest and most precise in estimating gestational age before days 50 to 55; the other two measurements are more practical after day 55 due to the fact that most ultrasound probes cannot provide a view of the entire length of the fetus at this stage. Tables 6.1 and 6.2 of this chapter provide a good summary of CRL measurements and also give the principal landmarks to evaluate normal embryonic and fetal development up to day 55. The following chapter includes a table with practical landmarks for the more mature fetuses.

Fetal heartbeat and movement and appearance of the fluid

During pregnancy diagnosis it is also important to evaluate the embryo's viability by paying special attention to the heartbeat. The heartbeats are generally visible starting on day 25 of gestation and appear at the center of the embryo in the form of a scintillating light with variable frequency depending on the age[4] (Table 6.2).

Starting on day 45 one can also observe the first movements of the fetus[18]. The fetus moves slightly within the amniotic vesicle between days 45 and 55. According to the observations carried out between the

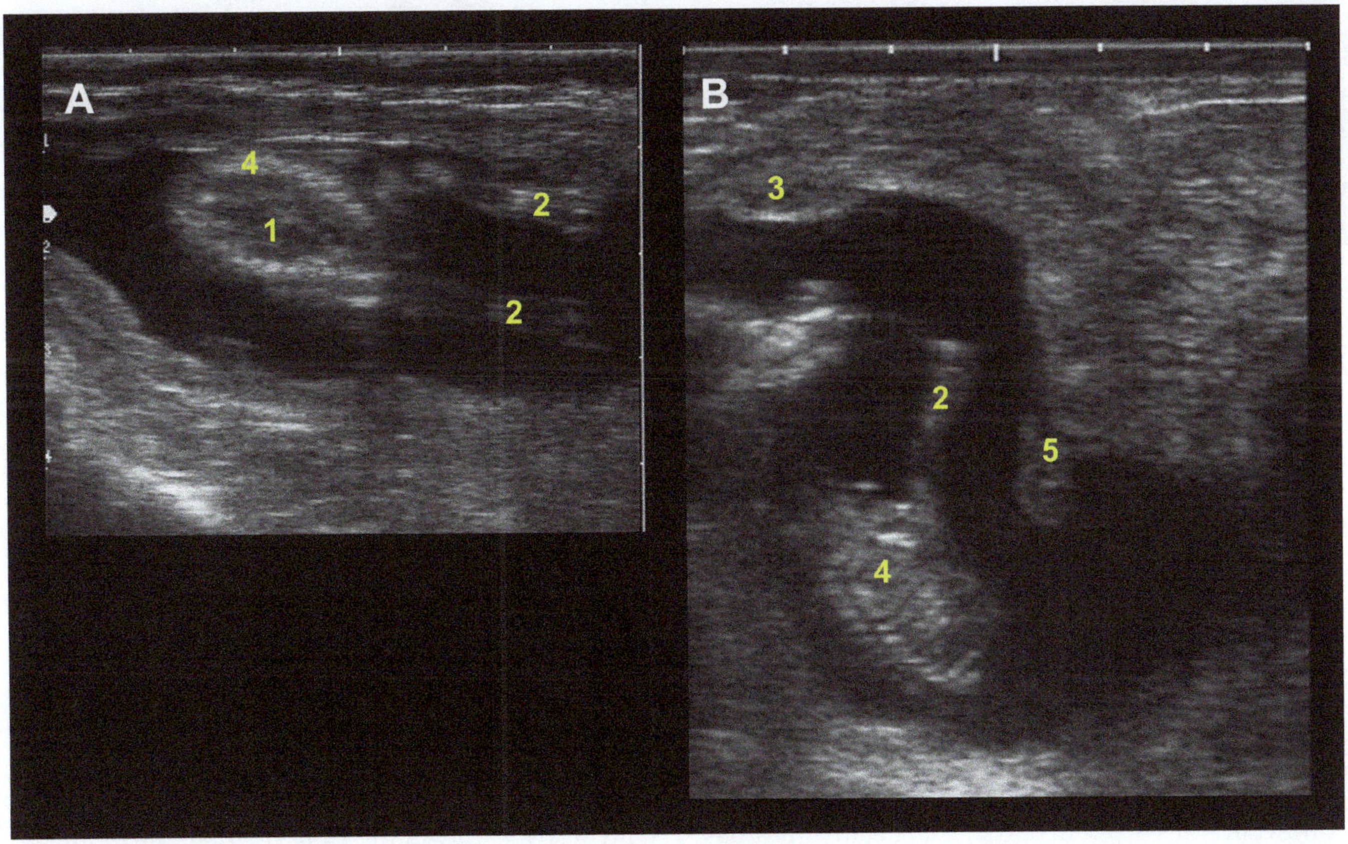

Figure 6.14. Fetus on day 59 with the first view of the ribs. A: transverse section of the fetus at the level of the anterior portion of the thorax (probe 10 MHz; depth 5 cm); B: longitudinal section (probe 8 MHz; depth 7 cm). 1: Fetus; 2: Anterior limb; 3: Placentome; 4: Ribs; 5: Umbilical cord.

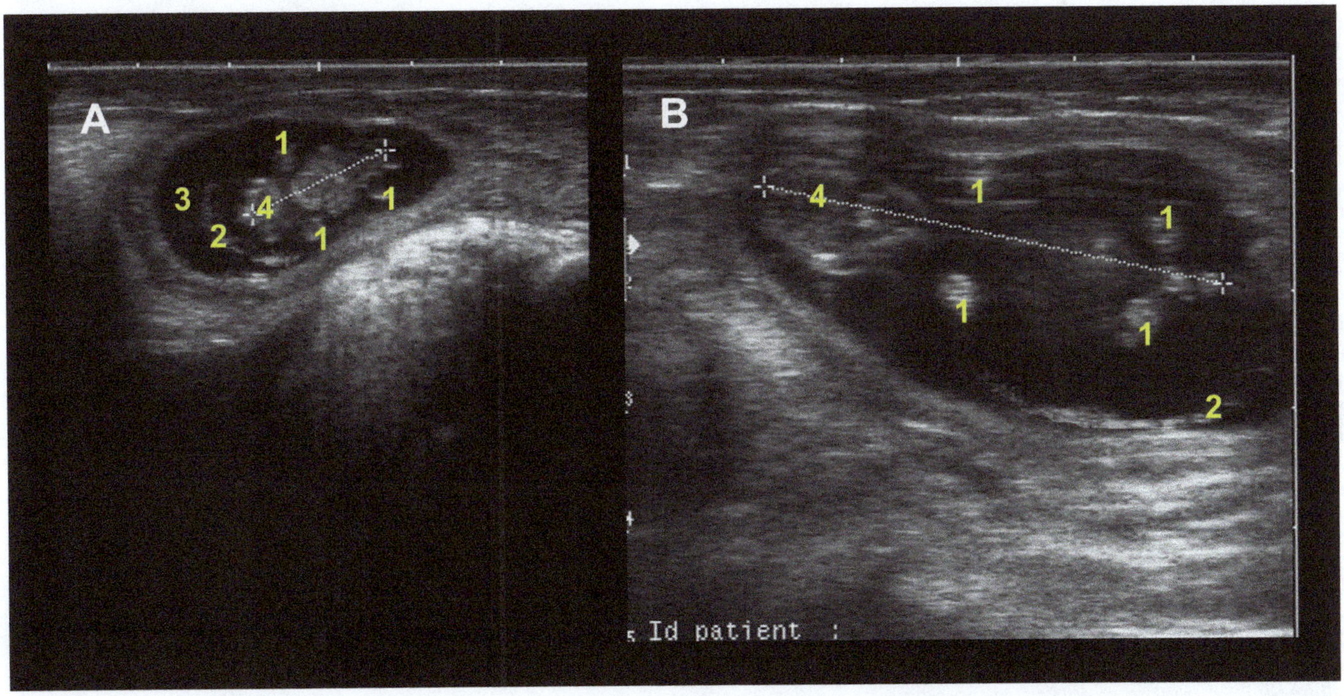

Figure 6.15. Evaluation of gestational stage by measuring the crown-rump length (CRL) of a 40-day-old embryo (A) and a 53-day-old fetus (B) with respective measurements of 1.63 cm and 3.97 cm (10 MHz linear probe; depth 5 cm). 1: Limbs; 2: Amnion; 3: Allantoic fluid; 4: Head.

second and third month of gestation the most significant fetal movements as it floats in the allantoic fluid cause changes in presentation, position, and posture[14]. During fetal observation periods that lasted for 5 minutes the authors reported a percentage of normal fetal activity of approximately 3 minutes, or 60% of the observation period, which remained essentially the same between days 65 and 175 of gestation[14]. In the absence of fetal movement a reevaluation of the gestation is recommended to ensure fetal viability.

Finally, it is important to observe the presence of clear (anechogenic) fluid in adequate quantities around the embryo or fetus to confirm that the conceptus is developing normally (Figures 6.11 to 6.15).

Early Embryonic and Fetal Death

Embryonic death is defined by the loss of an embryo between the time of fertilization and the end of organogenesis at approximately day 42. After this period loss of the conceptus is referred to as fetal death or mortality[1]. Even though the majority of embryonic deaths occur before day 25 of gestation, the period between days 25 and 42 is critical to the proper attachment of the embryonic membranes to the uterine epithelium. Embryonic death between days 28 and 42 has been reported to range from 10 to 15%[11,14], whereas fetal deaths were reported at 6.3% and 3.4%, respectively, for the periods between days 42 and 56, and days 56 and 98[14]. Fetal and embryonic loss varies considerably with climate, general health of the herd, and biosecurity procedures applied.

Ultrasound observations

When the veterinarian observes cloudy (echogenic) debris in the amniotic and allantoic fluids, or poorly defined fetal structures, mortality should be suspected and the ultrasound examination of the conceptus must be carried out even more thoroughly. In this situation, it is important to review the different signs of embryonic and fetal viability with the goal of obtaining a precise diagnosis.

Spontaneous embryonic and fetal mortality, contrary to therapeutic abortion induced by prostaglandin $F_{2\alpha}$, often has a characteristic ultrasound appearance with a more obvious degeneration of the bovine conceptus[14] (Table 6.3).

Figures 6.16 through 6.19 illustrate the principal ultrasound signs observed in embryonic or fetal mortality. The majority of these observations are too subtle to be detected by transrectal palpation, which delays veterinary interventions in problem cows.

Fetal mummification most often reveals poorly defined ultrasound images, a mass of hyperechogenic intrauterine tissue with no fluid, hyperechogenic bone matter with shadow cones, and sometimes a thickened uterine wall[12].

Table 6.3.
Summary of the principal differences in the ultrasound examination of a gravid uterus in a cow having undergone therapeutic abortion with prostaglandin $F_{2\alpha}$ compared to spontaneous embryonic or fetal death in the first trimester of gestation (adapted from Ginther 1998)

Signs	Therapeutic Abortion by Prostaglandin $F_{2\alpha}$ Injection	Spontaneous Embryonic or Fetal Death
Expulsion of the embryo or fetus	Less than 5 days	Several days to several weeks
Embryonic or fetal degeneration	None to minimal	Minimal to significant
Ultrasound observations		
✓ Embryo often intact	Frequently	Rarely
✓ Irregular contours of the embryo or fetus	+	++ to +++*
✓ Debris on the surface of various structures	+	++ to +++
✓ Debris in the amniotic or allantoic fluid	Rarely	++ to +++
✓ Break in the amniotic membrane	Rarely	++
✓ Reduction in the quantity of amniotic and allantoic fluid prior to expulsion of the embryo or fetus	Rarely	++

*+: often; ++: very often; +++: most of the time.

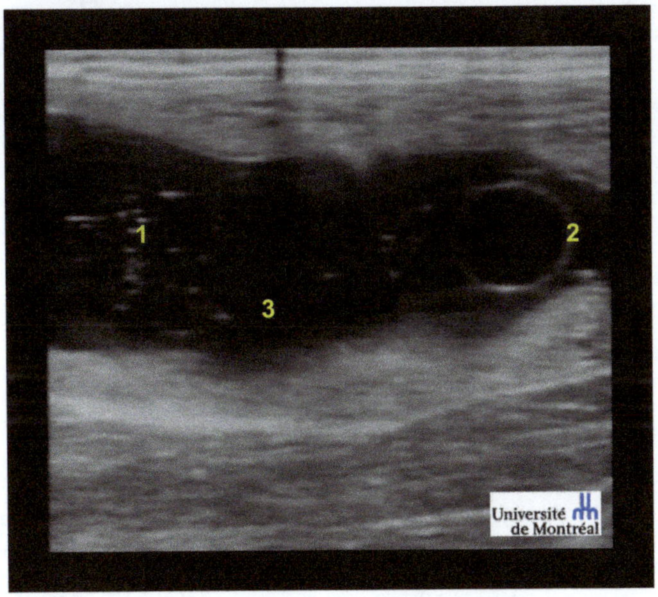

Figure 6.16. Ultrasound image of embryonic mortality observed at day 30 (7.5 MHz linear probe; depth 5 cm). Courtesy of the Université de Montréal. Debris from the dead embryo has been released outside the amniotic cavity. 1: Embryonic debris; 2: Amnion; 3: Allantoic fluid.

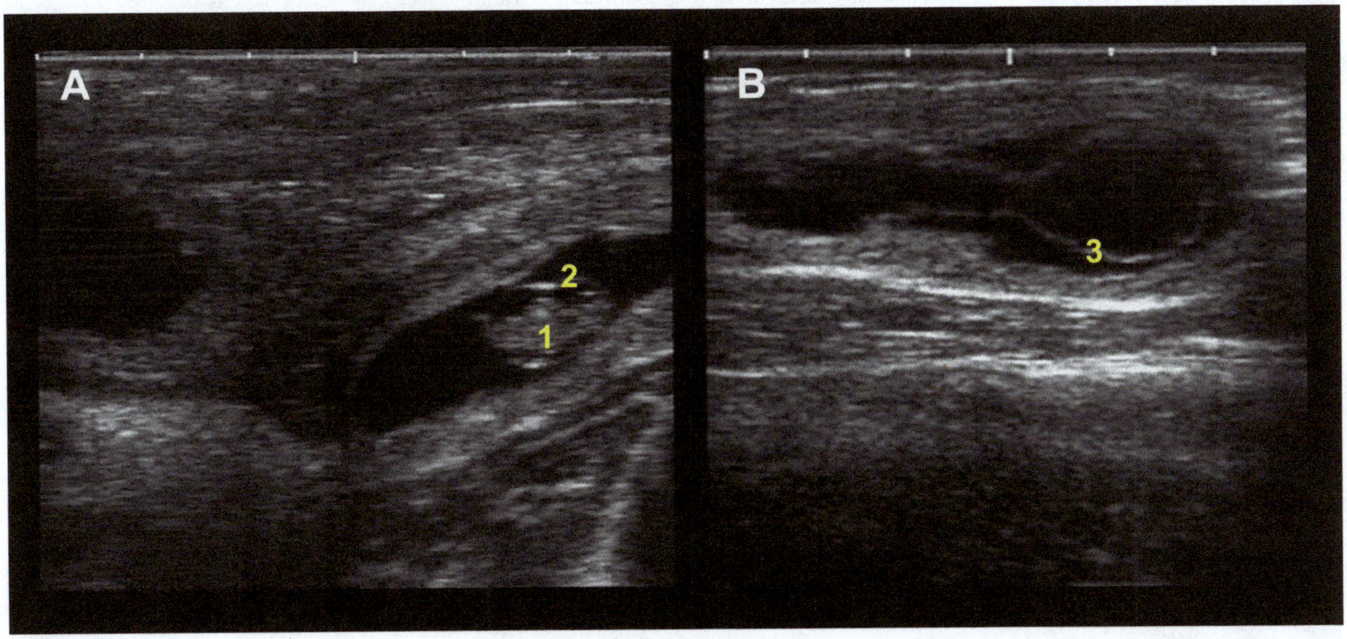

Figure 6.17. Ultrasound images of embryonic death identified on day 32 of gestation including an embryo with poorly defined contours and irregular, hyperechogenic amniotic and chorioallantoic membranes (8 MHz linear probe; depth 5 cm). 1: Embryo; 2: Amnion; 3: Allantois.

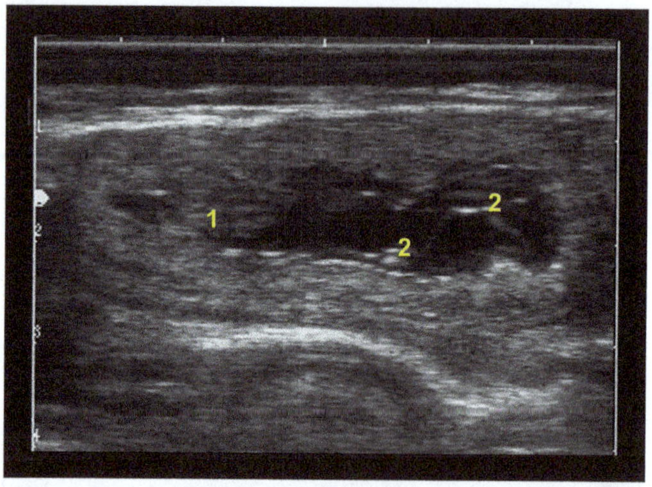

Figure 6.18. Ultrasound image of the same bovine uterus as in the preceding figure on day 45, 13 days after diagnosis of embryonic death (10 MHz linear probe; depth 4 cm). The allantoic fluid remains cloudy. The debris from the conceptus was completely expelled on day 50. 1: Embryonic debris; 2: Irregular chorioallantoic membrane.

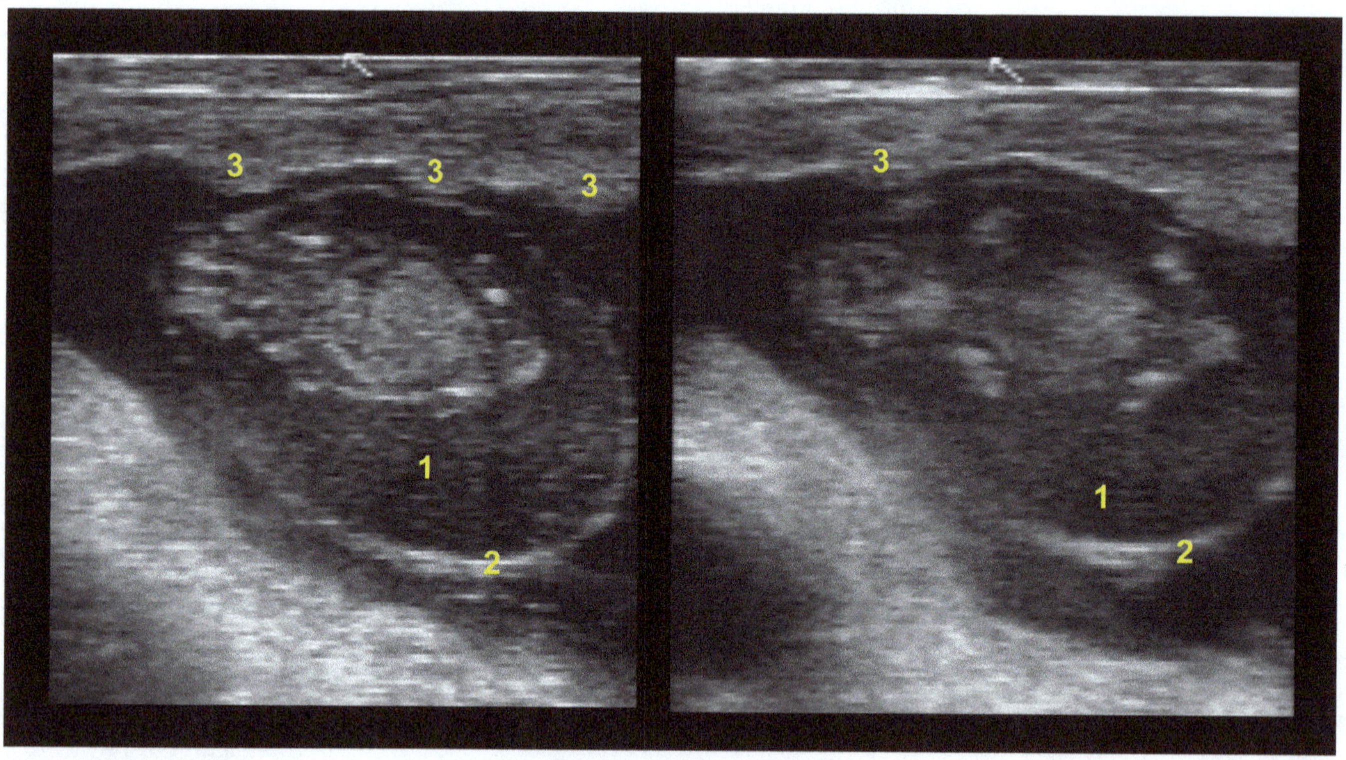

Figure 6.19. Ultrasound images of fetal death estimated on day 48 (CRL: 3 cm) on which one can see the beginning of fetal degeneration with significant accumulation of hyperechogenic debris in the amniotic fluid (7.5 MHz linear probe; depth 6 cm). Observe the irregular, hyperechogenic appearance of the amniotic membrane and placentomes above the dead fetus. 1: Fetal debris; 2: Amniotic membrane; 3: Placentomes 0.6 cm in diameter.

Finally, it is important to remember that the embryo, the fetus, and the fetal debris are generally expelled via the cervix rather than being reabsorbed by the uterus[4,18].

Twins

The rate of twinning in lactating dairy cattle is increasing. In one study of historical data the rate has increased from 4.54% in 1959 to 6.86% in 1997[6]. Today, many practitioners work for herds with twinning rates over 10%. There appears to be a direct positive correlation between twinning rate and milk production although the mechanism is uncertain at this time[6,13]. Twinning rates in beef cattle are significantly lower.

Cows carrying twins are more prone to abortion, dystocia, and postpartum problems such as metritis, displaced abomasum, ketosis, and fatty liver[28]. When a cow is known to be carrying twins, management changes can be made to monitor her more closely before, during, and after parturition. It is generally not recommended that twins be intentionally aborted due to the difficulty of getting dairy cows pregnant. Furthermore, high-producing cows are likely to continue to double ovulate in subsequent cycles, thus increasing the risk of conceiving twins again.

Ultrasonographic examination method and imaging

Systematic examination procedure of the reproductive tract

A thorough examination of the entire reproductive tract is critical to identify twins. The authors prefer to begin with an examination of the ovaries. Fifty percent of pregnant cows with two corpora lutea will have twins (Figure 6.20). Monozygous twins comprise less than 5% of bovine twins[25]. Fortunately, monozygous twins are usually close together in the same uterine horn (Figure 6.21), so they will often be identified even though examination of the ovaries reveals only one corpus luteum.

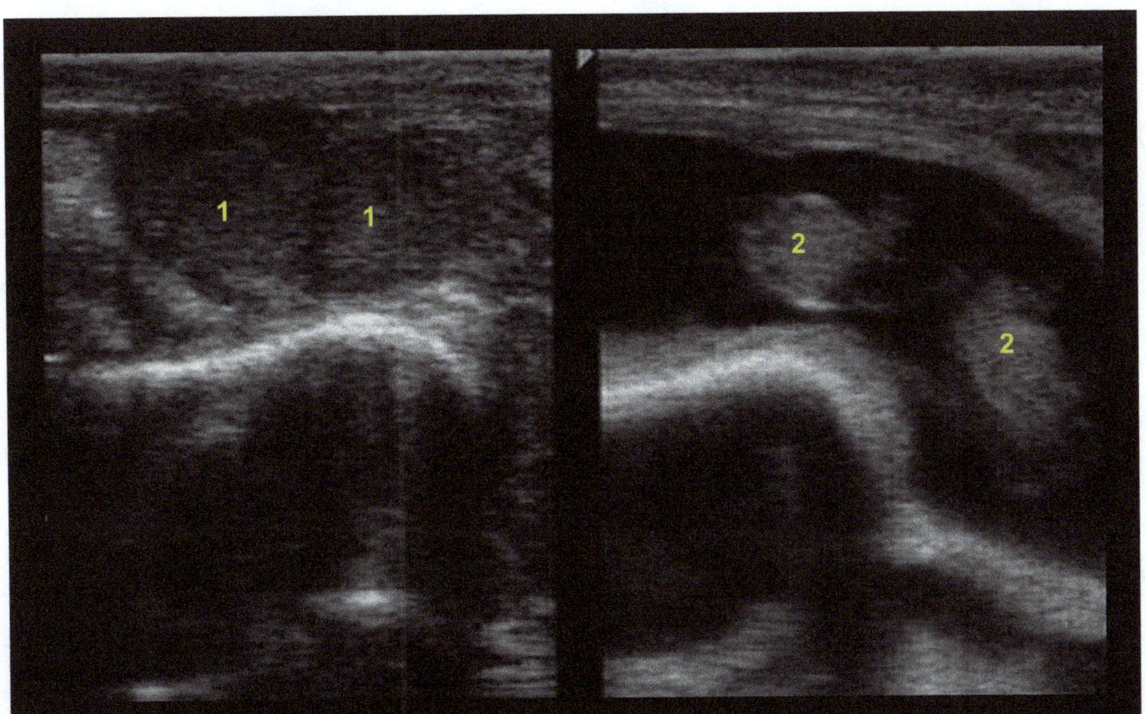

Figure 6.20. Ultrasound image of dizygous twins (BB-mode; probe 5 MHz; depth 7 cm). Note the presence of two corpora lutea on the ovary (left) and twins in the same uterine horn (right). Dizygous twins may be in one or both uterine horns. In this case they are ipsilateral. 1: Corpus luteum; 2: Embryos.

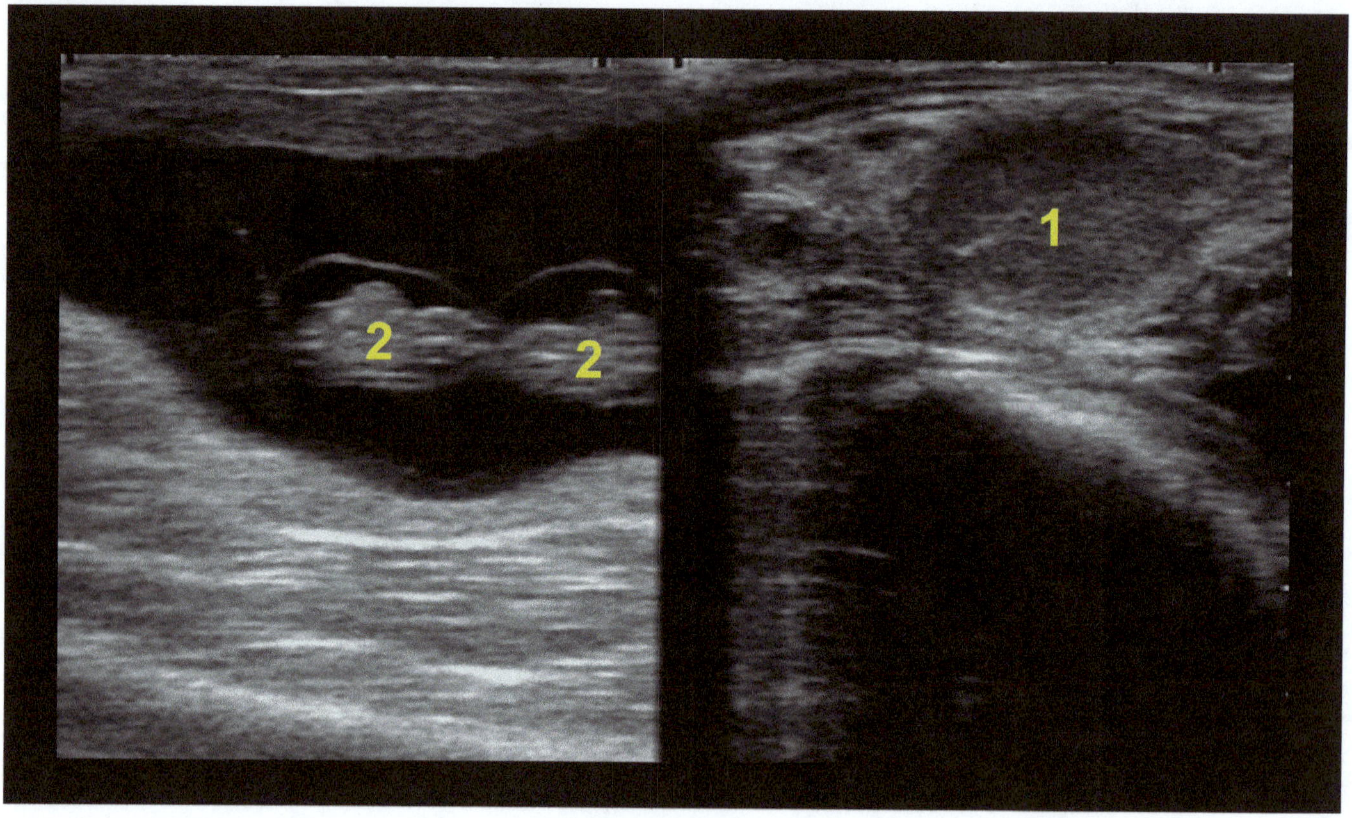

Figure 6.21. Ultrasonogram of monozygous twins (BB-mode; probe 5 MHz; depth 7 cm). Monozygous twins are almost always in the same uterine horn and tend to be close together. Note the presence of only one corpus luteum (right). 1: Corpus luteum; 2: Embryos.

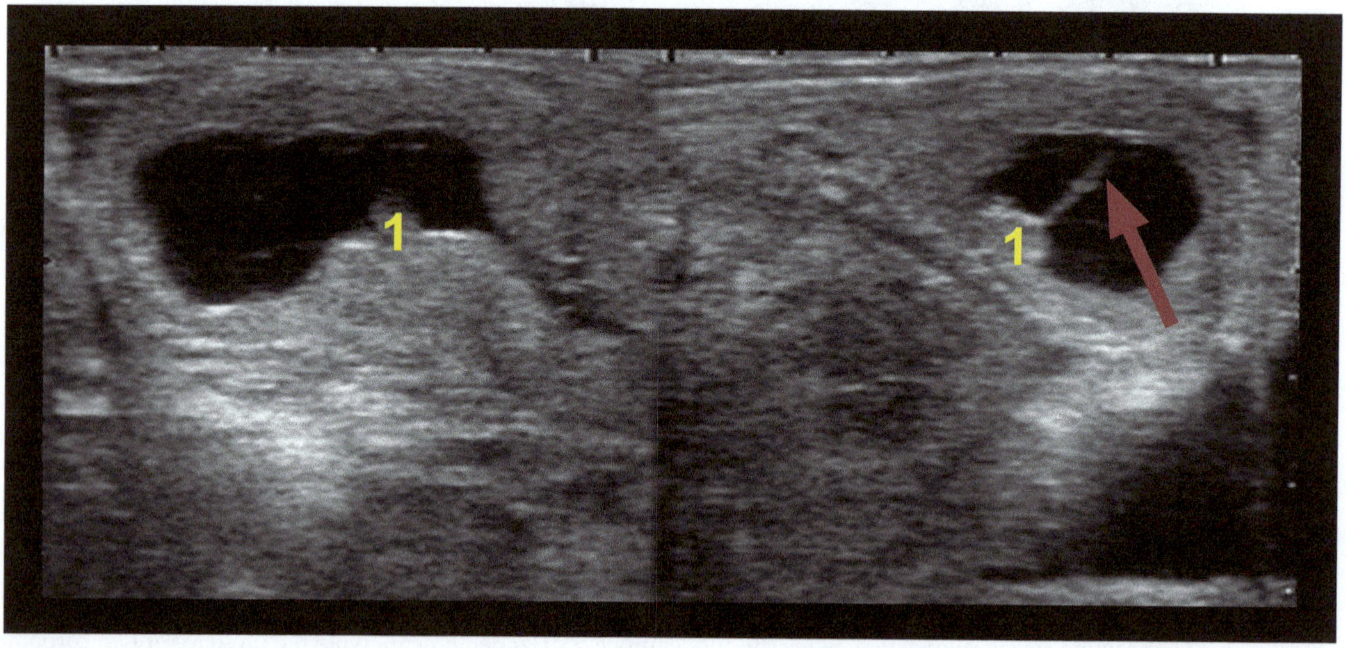

Figure 6.22. Ultrasonographic appearance of the twin line in a 26-day twin pregnancy (BB-mode; probe 5 MHz; depth 5 cm). 1: Embryo; Red arrow: Twin line.

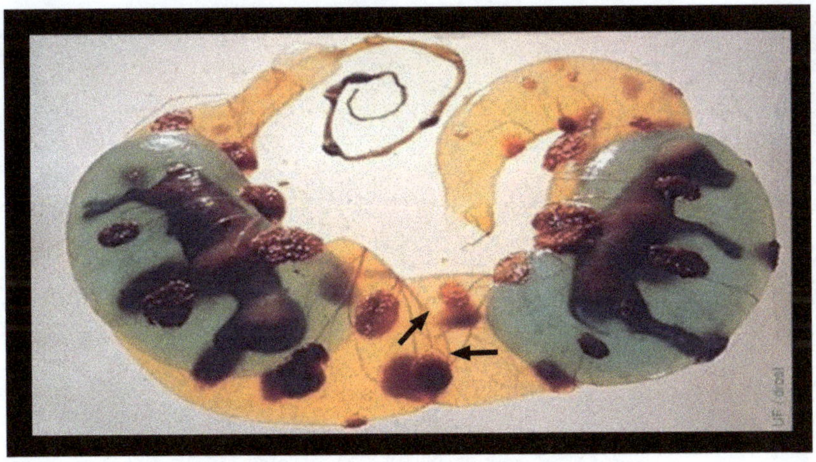

Figure 6.23. Twin line/chorioallantoic membrane. Courtesy of the Drost Project (http://drostproject.vetmed.ufl.edu/drost_bovine_contents.html). Distinguish the amniotic vesicles (in blue) from the allantoic vesicles (in yellow) and the shared chorioallantoic membrane (black arrows).

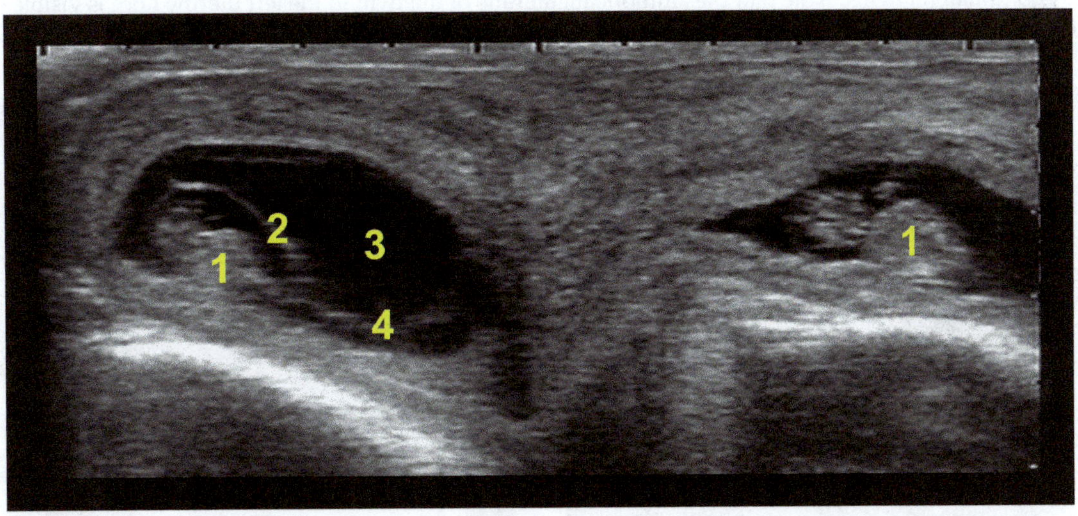

Figure 6.24. Ultrasonogram of a 39-day twin pregnancy (BB-mode; probe 5 MHz; depth 5 cm). This split-screen image shows twins in contralateral uterine horns. Both are normal. 1: Embryo; 2: Amnion; 3: Allantoic fluid; 4: Twin line.

Ultrasound appearance

Examination of the uterus may reveal more fluid than expected for the stage of pregnancy, more amniotic membrane than expected for a single pregnancy, or a "twin line." The twin line is the shared chorioallantoic membrane between the fetuses (Figures 6.22, 6.23). It appears to move away from one or both fetuses, so it will not be confused with the amniotic membrane that appears as a circle around each fetus. It is not always seen, but when it is, a thorough examination for twins is indicated. Figures 6.24 and 6.25 are ultrasonograms of a 39-day twin pregnancy and a 43-day twin pregnancy, respectively.

Embryonic and fetal death risk of twins

Recheck examinations after 60 days of pregnancy are even more critical for twins than for single pregnancies. In one study the rate of loss of contralateral twins from first examination at 36–42 days to recheck at 90 days was 8%[21]. In the same time period the rate of loss of ipsilateral twins was 32%.

In the same study one of the twin fetuses was lost in 6.2% of twin cases, and the second fetus survived (Figure 6.26). If the surviving twin is a heifer and the lost twin was a bull there is a possibility of freemartinism, particularly if the bull twin was lost after the embryonic period (past 42 days). Figure 6.27 is an ultrasonogram of 54-day dead twins.

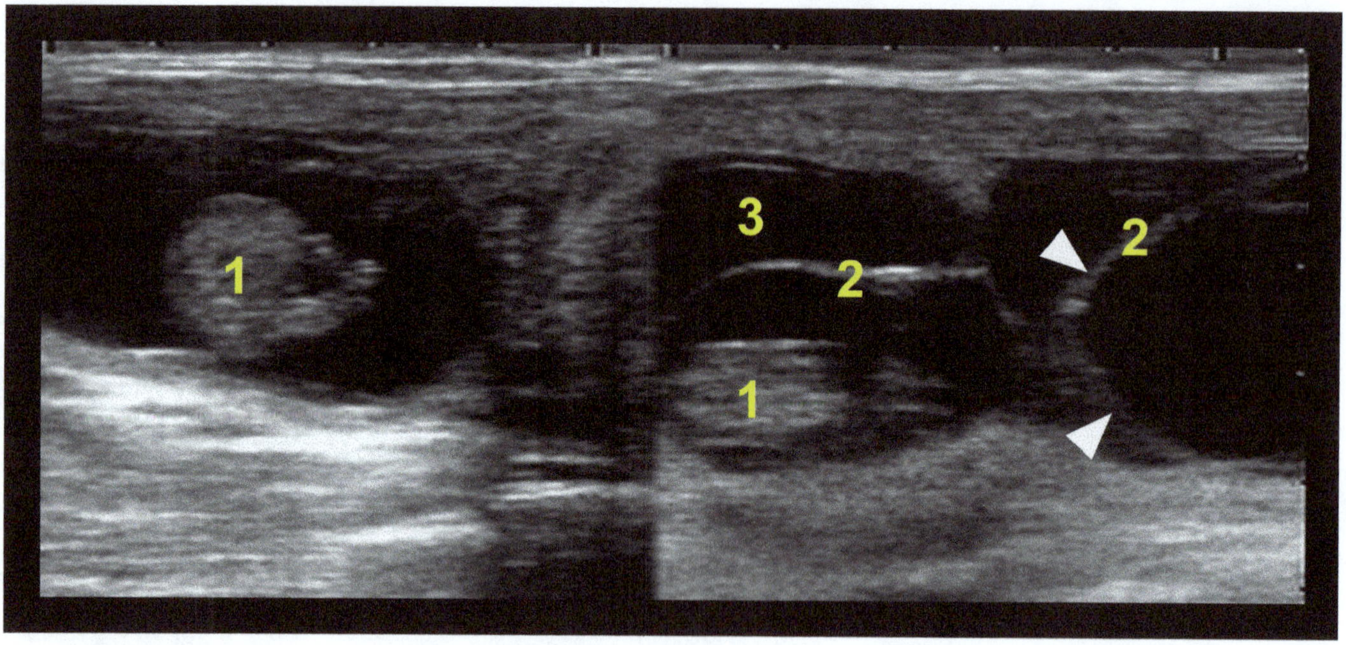

Figure 6.25. Ultrasonogram of a 43-day twin pregnancy (BB-mode; probe 5 MHz; depth 5 cm). The split image presents normal 43-day contralateral twins. Note that the amniotic membrane of the twin in the left uterine horn is visible on the image of the twin in the right uterine horn (white arrowheads). 1: Embryo; 2: Amnion; 3: Allantoic fluid.

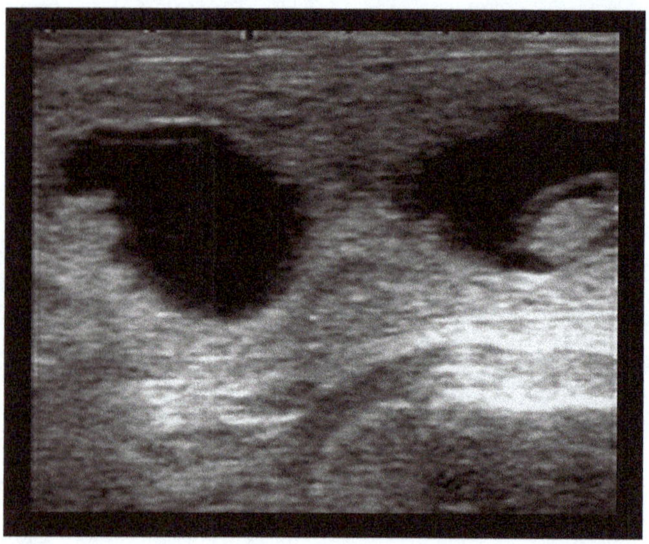

Figure 6.26. Ultrasonographic image of 30-day twins in which one embryo is alive and the other one is dead (probe 5 MHz; depth 5 cm). The fetus to the right is normal. The fetus to the left is degraded and dead. This is a high-risk pregnancy and the cow should be rechecked at the next herd visit.

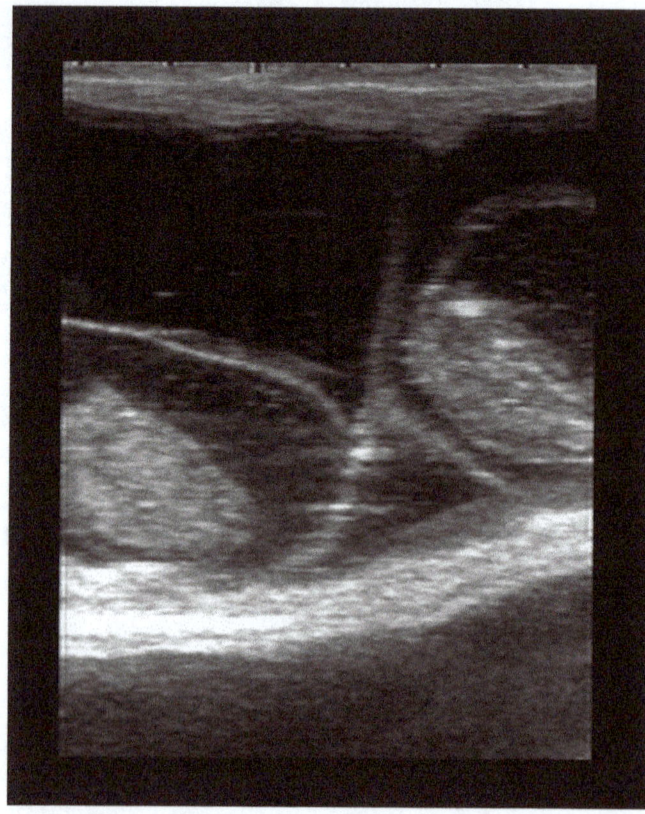

Figure 6.27. Ultrasonogram of 54-day dead twins (probe 5 MHz; depth 8 cm). Both twins in this 54-day recheck examination were dead. Note the cloudy amniotic fluid (more obvious around the embryo on the left) and the lack of fetal definition. At this stage of pregnancy a normal fetus will have clear limbs, head, and movement. This pregnancy felt completely normal on palpation.

References

1. Ayalon N (1978). A review of embryonic mortality in cattle. J Reprod Fert 54: 483–493.
2. Barone R (1990). Anatomie comparée des mammifères domestiques. Tome 4. Splanchnologie II, Appareil urogénital, foetus et ses annexes, péritoine et topographie abdominale, Vigot Ed., pp. 506–674.
3. Betteridge KJ, Eaglesome MD, Randall GCB, Mitchell D (1980). Collection, description and transfer of embryos from cattle 10–16 days after estrus. J Reprod Fertil 59: 205–216.
4. Carrière P, DesCôteaux L, Durocher J (2005). Ultrasonography of the reproductive system of the cow. [CD-ROM]. Faculté de médecine vétérinaire, Université de Montréal, St-Hyacinthe, Québec.
5. Curran S, Pierson RA, Ginther OJ (1986). Ultrasonographic appearance of the bovine conceptus from days 20 through 60. J Amer Vet Med Assoc 189: 1295–1302.
6. Day JD, Weaver LD, Franti CF (1997). Association of twin pregnancy diagnosis and parturition with days open, days pregnant at diagnosis, parity, and milk production in dairy cattle. Bov Pract No. 31. 2: 25–28.
7. DesCôteaux L, Fetrow J (1998). Economic evaluation of the use of ultrasound in early pregnancy diagnosis in dairy cows: A decision analysis approach. Proceedings of the 50th annual convention of the Canadian Veterinary Medical Association. Toronto, Ontario, pp. 367–371.
8. DesCôteaux L, Fetrow J (1998). Does it pay to use an ultrasound machine for early pregnancy diagnosis in dairy cows? Proceedings of the annual convention of the American Association of Bovine Practitioners 31: 172–174.
9. DesCôteaux L (1997). Est-il rentable d'utiliser l'appareil échographique pour le diagnostic de gestation précoce chez la vache laitière? Compte-rendu du 56e congrés de l'Ordre des médecins vétérinaires du Québec, pp. 9–16.
10. Evans HE, Sacks WO (1973). Prenatal development of domestic and laboratory mammals: growth curves, external features and selected references. Anat Histol Embryol 2: 11–45.
11. Filteau V, DesCôteaux L (1998). Valeur prédictive de l'utilisation de l'appareil échographique pour le diagnostic précoce de la gestation chez la vache laitière. Méd Vét Québec 28: 81–85.
12. Fissore RA, Edmonson AJ, Pashen RL, Bondurant RH (1986). The use of ultrasonography for the study of the bovine reproductive tract II. Non-pregnant, pregnant and pathological conditions of the uterus. Anim Repro Sci 12: 167–177.
13. Fricke P, Wiltbank MC (1999). Effect of milk production on the incidence of double ovulation in dairy cows. Theriogenology 52: 1133–1143.
14. Ginther OJ (1998). Ultrasonic Imaging and Animal Reproduction: Cattle. Equiservices Publishing. Wisconsin, pp. 134–143.
15. Hanzen C, Delsaux B (1987). Use of transrectal B-mode ultrasound in early pregnancy in cattle. Vet Rec 121: 201–202.
16. Inomata T, Eguchi Y, Yamamoto M, Asari M, Kano Y, Mochizuki K (1982). Development of the external genitalia in bovine fetuses. Jpn J Vet Sci 44: 489–496.
17. Kahn W (1989). Sonographic fetometry in the bovine. Theriogenology 31: 1105–1121.
18. Kastelic JP, Curran S, Pierson RA, Ginther OJ (1988). Ultrasonic evaluation of the bovine conceptus. Theriogenology 29: 39–54.
19. King GJ, Atkinson BA, Robertson HA (1980). Development of the bovine placentome from days 20 to 29 of gestation. J Reprod Fert 59: 95–100.
20. Kolour AK, Batavani RA, Ardabili FF (2005). Preliminary observations on the effect of parity on first day ultrasonic detection of embryo and its organs in bovine. J Vet Med A 52: 74–77.
21. Lopez-Gatius H, Hunter R (2005). Spontaneous reduction of advanced twin embryos: its occurrence and clinical relevance in dairy cattle. Theriogenology 63: 118–125.
22. Oltenacu PA, Ferguson JD, Lednor AJ (1990). Economic evaluation of pregnancy diagnosis in dairy cattle: A decision analysis approach. J Dairy Sci 73: 2826–2831.
23. Pierson RA, Ginther OJ (1984). Ultrasonography for detection of pregnancy and study of embryonic development in heifers. Theriogenology 22: 225–233.
24. Schlafer DH, Fisher PJ, Davies CJ (2000). The bovine placenta before and after birth: placental development and function in health and disease. Anim Reprod Sci 64: 13–20.
25. Silva del Rio N, Kirkpatrick BW, Fricke PM (2006). Observed frequency of monozygotic twinning in Holstein dairy cattle. Theriogenology 66: 1292–1299.
26. Stroud BK (1994). Clinical applications of bovine reproductive ultrasonography. Comp Cont Educ 16(8): 1085–1097.
27. Taverne MAM, Szency O, Szetag J, Piros A (1985). Pregnancy diagnosis in cows with linear-array real-time ultrasound scanning: a preliminary. Vet Quarterly 7(4): 264–270.
28. Van Saun RJ (2001). Comparison of pre- and postpartum performance of Holstein dairy cows having either a single or twin pregnancy. Proceedings of the annual convention of the American Association of Bovine Practitioners 34, p. 204.
29. White IR, Russel AJF, Wright IA, Whyte TK (1985). Real-time ultrasonic scanning in the diagnosis of pregnancy and the estimation of gestational age in cattle. Vet Rec 117: 5–8.
30. Winters LM, Green WW, Comsock RE (1942). Prenatal development of the bovine. Minn Tech Bull 151: 1–50.

31. Wright IA, White IR, Russel AJF, Whyte TK, McBean AJ (1988). Prediction of calving date in beef cows by real-time ultrasonic scanning. Vet Rec 123: 228–229.

Points to Remember

- The embryonic period is traditionally defined as the period between fertilization and the end of organogenesis on the 42nd day of gestation.
- Before 30 days of gestation a careful examination in the zone of anechogenic fluid generally reveals the presence of the embryo close to the uterine folds.
- The placentomes can be identified starting on day 35 of gestation and are visible close to the embryo.
- Other important signs of normal embryonic and fetal development are the appearance of the umbilical cord attachment to the uterus of the cow starting at day 40 of gestation and a view of the ossified ribs in the fetus starting at day 50.
- Starting on day 45 one can also observe the first movements of the fetus.
- On day 40 of gestation the genital tubercle is prominently located on the median line between the posterior limbs. It becomes the embryonic penis in the male and the clitoris in the female.
- At approximately day 47 of gestation in the male fetus the genital tubercle begins to migrate toward the umbilicus and is usually completed by day 56 to 58 after insemination.
- In females the genital tubercle migrates toward the anus starting at day 48–49 to reach its final position at approximately 53 days postinsemination.
- The crown-rump length (CRL) measurement is the easiest and most precise in estimating gestational age before days 50 to 55.
- Embryonic death between days 28 and 42 is generally in the range of 10 to 15%, whereas fetal deaths are 6.3% and 3.4%, respectively, for the periods between days 42 and 56, and days 56 and 98.
- Embryonic or fetal mortalities should be suspected when the ultrasonographer observes cloudy (echogenic) debris in the amniotic and/or allantoic fluids or poorly defined fetal structures.
- The rate of twinning in lactating dairy cattle is increasing.
- Monozygous twins comprise less than 5% of bovine twins.
- Ultrasound examination of the uterus may reveal more fluid than expected for the stage of pregnancy, more amniotic membrane than expected for a single pregnancy, or a "twin line." Recheck examinations after 60 days of pregnancy are critical for twins because the rate of loss of contralateral twins from first examination to recheck at 90 days is 8% and the rate of loss of ipsilateral twins is 32%.

Summary Questions

1. On day 30 of gestation the maximum diameter of the embryonic vesicle is approximately
   a. 0.2 cm
   b. 2 cm
   c. 10 cm
   d. 25 cm

2. Which of the following statements is true regarding the genital tubercle (the fetal structure allowing early determination of fetal sex by ultrasound)?
   a. The genital tubercle corresponds to the testicles in the male.
   b. The genital tubercle corresponds to the development of the vulva in the female.
   c. At day 45 of gestation the genital tubercle is located between the posterior limbs in the male.
   d. At day 55 of gestation the genital tubercle begins its migration toward the tail in the female.

3. What is the name of the echogenic band (specular reflection) around the 40-day-old embryo?
   a. An artifact
   b. Chorioallantoic membrane
   c. Allantoic membrane
   d. Amniotic membrane

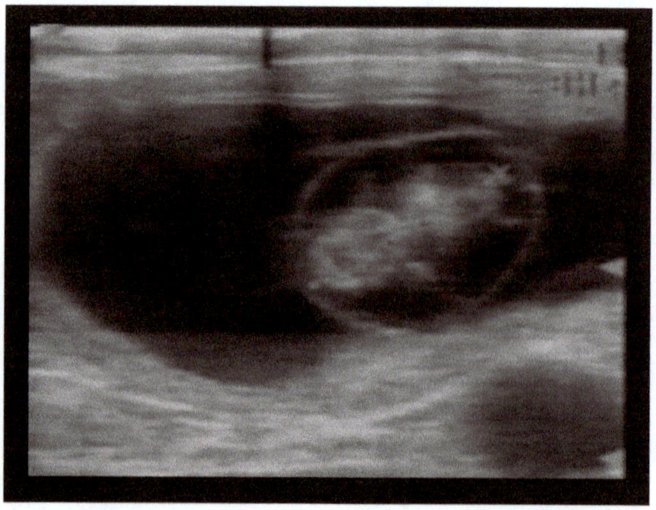

4. What is the youngest age of pregnancy at which it is possible to visualize the umbilical cord of the embryo?
   a. 25 days
   b. 30 days
   c. 40 days
   d. 60 days

5. What are the ultrasonographic signs that one can use in order to confirm that a 45-day fetus is normally developed and viable? Select all answers that apply.
   a. Movements of the fetus are obvious
   b. Presence of heart beats
   c. The fetus has a crown-rump length between 1 and 1.5 cm
   d. The fetus has a crown-rump length between 2.5 and 3 cm

6. Identify the twin line in the following image:
   a. 1
   b. 2
   c. 3
   d. 4

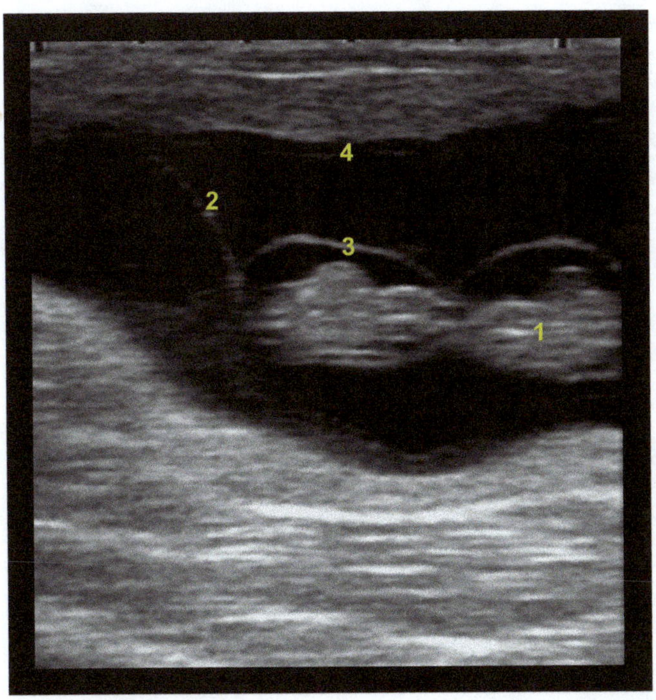

7. The approximate rate of loss for ipsilateral twins from about 38–90 days of gestation is
   a. 6%
   b. 17%
   c. 32%
   d. 60%

Answers

1. b
2. c
3. d
4. c
5. a, b, and d
6. b
7. c

CHAPTER SEVEN

Bovine Fetal Development after 55 Days, Fetal Sexing, Anomalies, and Well-Being

Luc DesCôteaux, Nicole Picard-Hagen,
Jean Durocher, Sébastien Buczinski, Jill Colloton,
Sylvie Chastant-Maillard, and Sandra Curran

Fetal Development after 55 Days

Following the organogenesis of the embryonic period, there is a long fetal period of 7.5 months during which the fetus grows considerably in size[9]. Individual organs can be identified by ultrasound examination when their size exceeds the resolution power of the ultrasound probe, and if their echogenicity can be distinguished from that of adjacent organs and tissues.

Table 7.1 describes the principal macroscopic and ultrasound characteristics of the bovine fetus during its development. Estimation of fetal age is based on fetal mass, measurements of fetal size or body parts, and hair growth[1,19] (Tables 7.1 to 7.3). However, only fetal measurements can be evaluated by ultrasound (Tables 7.2 and 7.3).

Table 7.1.
Principal physical characteristics of the bovine fetus during its development, starting at day 60 of gestation (according to Maneely 1952; Evans and Sacks 1973; Barone 1990)

Stage of Gestation (Months)	CRL* (cm)	Macroscopic and Ultrasound Observations
2	6–7	Fusion of eyelids
		External genital organs (clitoris, scrotum)
		Claws on all 4 limbs
		Omasum and abomasum
		First centers of ossification in the skull and vertebrae
3	14–15	Differentiated stomach compartments
		Hair follicles near the eyes and lips
		Ossification of limbs and vertebrae
4	25	Teats (female)
		Claws cornified
		Dental development
5	40	Descent of testicles completed
6	46	Eyelashes, hair on ears and end of tail
7	60	Eyelids open
		Hair all over the body
8	60–80	Full coat of short hair
9	65–85	Hair tuft at end of tail

*CRL: crown-rump length.

Head

The first centers of ossification in the skull, which appears very echogenic on the ultrasound image, appear toward the end of the second month of gestation, especially in the mandibular and maxillary bones. Ossification of the skull is complete at day 100 of gestation[12].

The diameter of the eye increases during the first two trimesters of gestation[11] (Table 7.3, Figure 7.1). The head of the fetus is generally accessible to ultrasound examination during the entire gestation, allowing fetal age to be determined based on the diameter of the eye (Table 7.3). At 2 months of gestation, the eyelids cover the eyes and become fused together (Figure 7.2), to reopen at 6.5 months of gestation.

Table 7.2.
Summary of the principal fetal measurements from 60 to 140 days of gestation (adapted from Winters et al. 1942; White et al. 1985; Hughes and Davies 1989; Kähn 1989)

	60 Days	70 Days	80 Days	90 Days	100 Days	120 Days	140 Days
CRL* (cm)	6–7	9–13	12–13	13–17	19	22–32	33
Eye diameter (mm)	4	6	8	10	12	16	19
Trunk diameter (cm)	1.7–2.2	2.3–2.9	3.0–3.7	3.9–4.5	5.1–5.3	7.0–8.7	8.9–14.8
External skull diameter (cm)	1.6–1.8	2.0–2.3	2.5–2.8	3.2–3.3	3.8–4.0	4.9–6.2	5.9 9.6

*CRL: crown-rump length.

Table 7.3.
Changes in crown-rump length and eye diameter, heart rate and fetal presentation from months 2 to 9 of gestation (adapted from Winters et al. 1942; Scanlon 1974; Kähn 1989; Barone 1990; Ginther 1998)

	2 Mos	3 Mos	4 Mos	5 Mos	6 Mos	7 Mos	8 Mos	9 Mos
CRL* (cm)	6–7	14–15	25–27	37–40	46–54	60–70	60–82	65–88
Heart rate (beats/min)	160–195	150–180	145–165	140–155	135–155	135–145	125–135	120–125
Diameter of the eye (mm)	4	10	16	20	24	26	27	27
Fetal presentation (%) Anterior	50	43–50	43–50	50–65	50–70	70–80	85–95	95–98
Posterior	50	43–50	43–50	22–50	28–50	20–25	2–15	2–5

*CRL: crown-rump length.

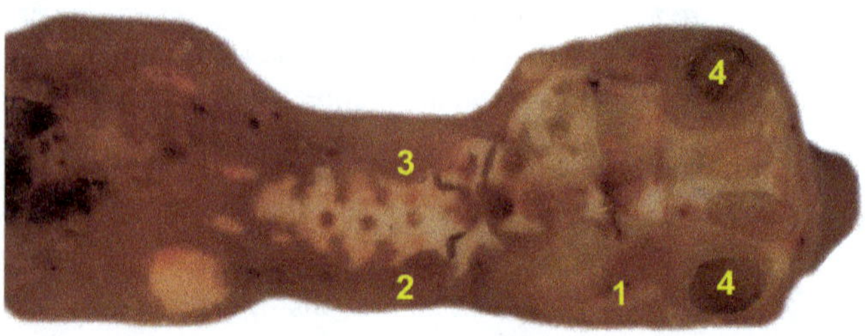

Figure 7.1. Frontal view of the head and neck of a bovine fetus at 4 months of gestation. The skull bones and vertebrae are ossified. The eyes are visible. 1: Head; 2: Neck; 3: Cervical vertebrae; 4: Eye.

Various signs of fetal viability can be observed on the head, such as eyelid movements, swallowing, and muzzle licking.

Spinal column

Cervical, thoracic, lumbar, and sacral vertebrae begin to ossify starting on days 61 to 65 of gestation, with the coccygeal vertebrae starting on day 86 of gestation[12].

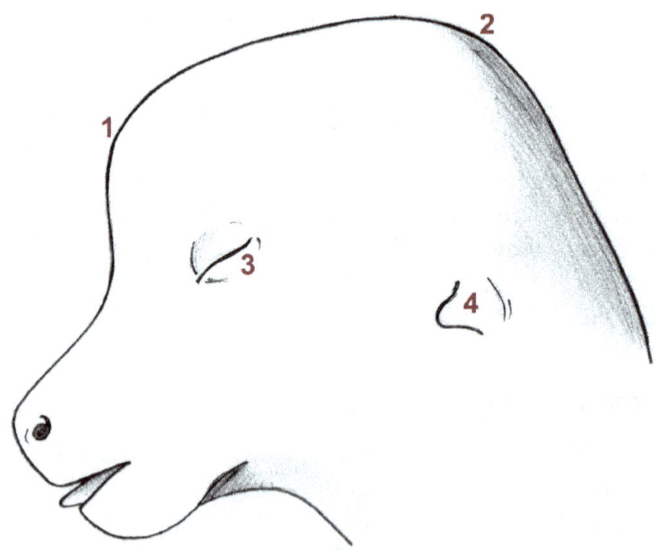

Figure 7.2. Head of a bovine fetus on day 58 of gestation (adapted from Barone 1990). The eyelids are fused together. 1: Fetal telencephalon; 2: Fetal metencephalon; 3: Fused eyelids; 4: Ear pinna.

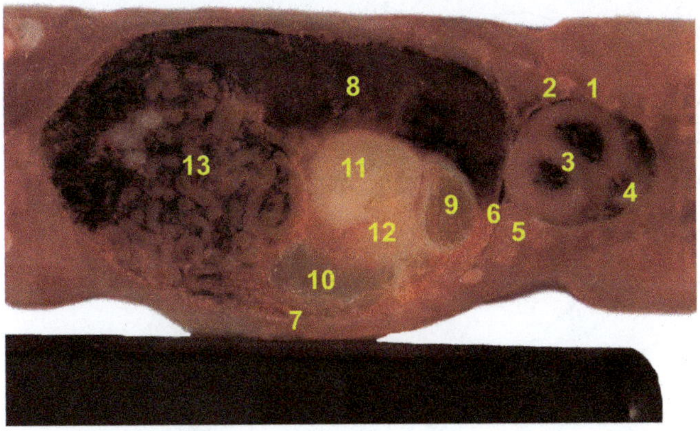

Figure 7.3. Frontal view of the thoracic and abdominal cavities of a bovine fetus at 4 months of gestation. The 10 cm linear probe is located on the left side of the fetus. 1: Thoracic cavity; 2: Ribs; 3: Heart (left and right ventricles); 4: Pulmonary trunk; 5: Lungs; 6: Diaphragm; 7: Abdominal cavity; 8: Liver; 9: Reticulum; 10: Rumen; 11: Omasum; 12: Abomasum; 13: Intestines.

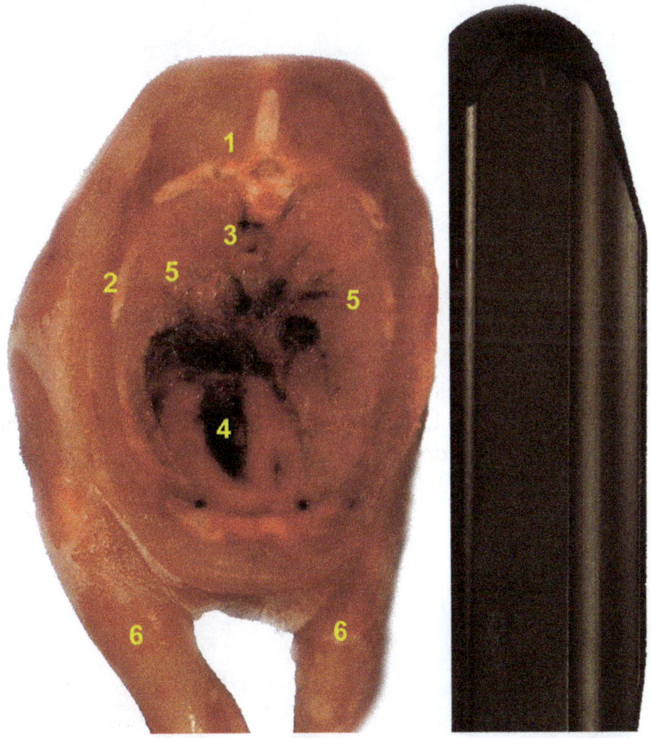

Figure 7.4. Transverse section view of the thoracic cavity of a bovine fetus at 100 days of gestation. The linear probe is located on the right side of the fetus. 1: Thoracic vertebra; 2: Rib; 3: Aorta; 4: Heart; 5: Lung; 6: Anterior limb.

Thorax

The ossification of the ribs occurs earlier, between days 55 and 60 of gestation, whereas the sternum begins to ossify between 81 and 85 days of gestation[12].

The cone-shaped cranial section of the thorax is occupied almost entirely by the heart. Its four chambers are separated by the septum and the valves (Figure 7.3). The heart is easy to visualize with ultrasound due to its obvious beating. The heart rate varies considerably, even at different times in the same individual, because it increases during phases of fetal activity[16]; it is also much faster than that of the mother (Table 7.3). The lungs fill the space around the heart, extending to the cranial surface of the diaphragm (Figure 7.4).

Abdomen

The embryonic abdominal cavity is occupied almost entirely by the liver and the mesonephros. On day 65 of gestation, the liver weighs one-tenth the total weight of the fetus and extends past the umbilicus caudally[1]. Its growth slows down during the second half of gestation, when it is displaced slightly to the right and caudal to the diaphragm, gradually ceding space to the other viscera[2] (Figure 7.3). The liver has a rich vascular network that can be visualized by ultrasound (Figure 7.28C).

At 2 months of gestation, the stomach is divided into its four compartments—the rumen and the reticulum are similar in size to the abomasum, whereas the omasum is clearly larger (Figures 7.5, 7.6). The abomasum and the omasum appear as hyperechogenic spots, whereas the rumen is the largest hypoechogenic region in the trunk[11,18]. Starting at 6 months, the abomasum grows considerably; at the time of birth, it is three times larger than the rumen[1].

The jejunum and ileum are differentiated as early as day 40 of gestation, but the differentiation of the large intestine and its proximal segments comes later, beginning at 4.5 months of gestation (Figures 7.7, 7.3).

During the embryonic period, the mesonephros occupies a large volume and extends over practically the entire lumbar region; it subsequently atrophies at approximately day 70 of gestation[1, 21]. The definitive kidneys emerge from the development of the metanephros starting at 30 days of gestation. The kidneys possess their definitive appearance and lobulation at approximately 3 months of gestation (Figures 7.8, 7.9).

In the fetal stage, the bladder can be viewed by ultrasound with a variable degree of filling.

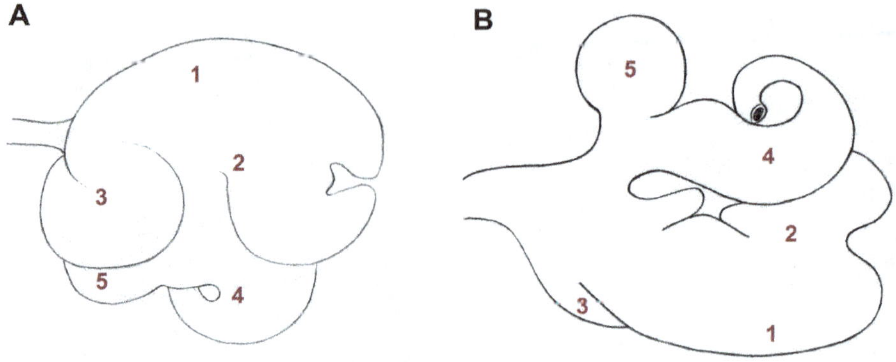

Figure 7.5. Development of the stomach compartments in the bovine fetus at day 70 of gestation (adapted from Noden and De Lahunta 1985). Lateral view (A) and dorsal view (B). The dorsal sac of the rumen has been displaced to the right in B. 1: Dorsal sac of the rumen; 2: Ventral sac of the rumen; 3: Reticulum; 4: Abomasum; 5: Omasum.

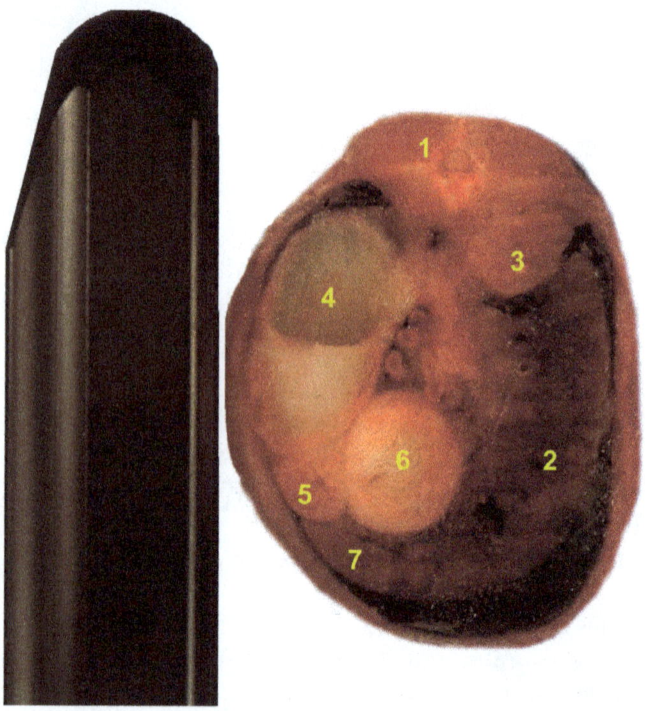

Figure 7.6. Ventral view from a transverse section of the abdomen of a bovine male fetus at 100 days of gestation. The linear probe is located on the left side of the fetus. 1: Lumbar vertebra; 2: liver; 3: Right kidney; 4: Rumen; 5: Abomasum; 6: Omasum; 7: Spleen.

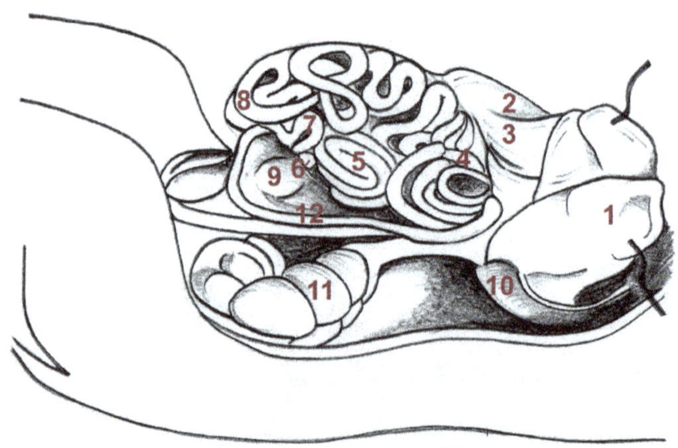

Figure 7.7. Abdominal organs in a bovine fetus at day 90 of gestation (adapted from Barone 1990). Left lateral view. The rumen and the greater omentum have been displaced to the left to display the intestines. 1: Rumen displaced cranially (dorsal sac, ventral sac); 2: Abomasum; 3: Greater omentum; 4: Proximal segment of the jejunum; 5: Ascending colon; 6: Cecum; 7: Descending segment of the duodenum; 8: Distal segment of the jejunum; 9: Right kidney (under the duodenum); 10: Spleen; 11: Left kidney; 12: Ascending segment of the duodenum.

Genital organs

After day 70 of gestation, the genital tubercle is covered by small labia or by the prepuce, which decreases its echogenicity. Therefore, beginning at this stage there is no longer a genital tubercle; the external genital organs have taken its place.

In the male fetus at 60 days of gestation, the scrotal folds fuse on the median line to form the scrotum. The width of the scrotum increases over the course of gestation, measuring 4, 10, and 33 mm, respectively, at 2, 3, and 7 months of gestation[18] (Figures 7.10, 7.11). The teats remain rudimentary. The testicles cross the inguinal space during the 4th month of gestation and reach their definitive position in the scrotal sac between the 3rd and 5th months[1,22]. Thus an empty scrotum, resem-

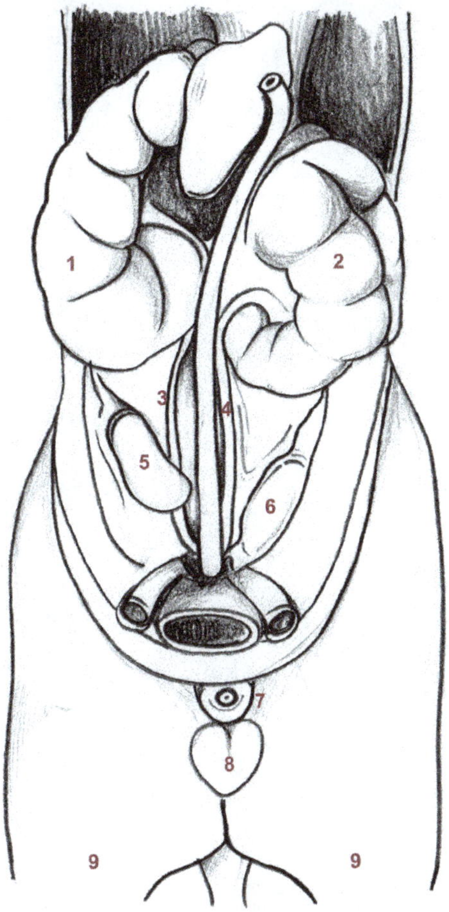

Figure 7.8 Urinary and genital organs in a bovine male fetus at 90 days of gestation (adapted from Barone 1990). The kidneys are well developed within the abdominal cavity. 1: Right kidney; 2: Left kidney; 3: Right ureter; 4: Left ureter; 5: Right testicle; 6: Left testicle; 7: Penis and prepuce; 8: Scrotum; 9: Section of posterior limbs.

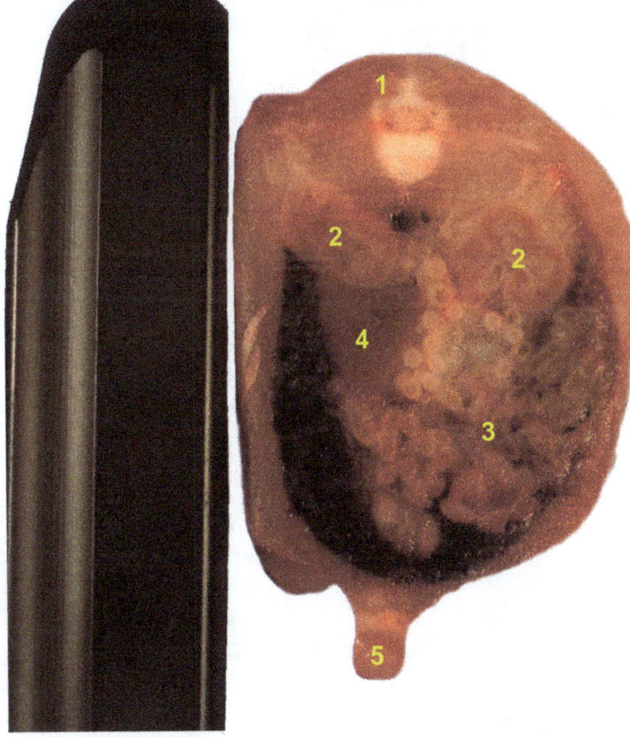

Figure 7.9 Transverse section view of the lower abdomen and penis of a bovine male fetus at 100 days of gestation. The linear probe is located on the right side of the fetus. 1: Lumbar vertebra; 2: Kidneys; 3: Intestines; 4: Liver; 5: Penis.

bling two white circles with black centers, is often observed until the end of the 3rd month of gestation.

In the female fetus, the labio-scrotal folds are smaller than in the male and they do not move from their position between the posterior limbs; however, they disappear completely by day 75 of gestation. The rudimentary teats are clearly visible by ultrasound, which reveals four hyperechogenic corners of a square or rhombus (Figures 7.12, 7.13). Even though they are present in the male fetus, these structures are usually not visible by ultrasound with field units. The urogenital folds lift and form two labia that completely surround the genital tubercle during the 5th month of gestation[15]. They are visible by ultrasound as an equals sign (=) immediately beneath the tail.

Pelvis and limbs

The scapula, ilium, and ischium become ossified at approximately 70 days of gestation[12].

During the 2nd month of gestation, the claws can be seen on the four limbs as small cone-shaped tubercles (Figure 7.14). A few cornified structures appear in the 4th month of gestation. The long bones of the limbs begin to ossify as early as days 61 to 65 of gestation, with ossification of the digits occurring later, between days 81 and 85 of gestation[12] (Figure 7.15). The anterior and posterior limbs of the fetus measure 2.1 and 1.2 cm, respectively, on day 60 of gestation. Exponential growth takes place after that and the diaphysis of the long bones of the limbs reaches a length between 5.5 and 6.5 cm around the 6th month of pregnancy[18].

Fetal mobility and position in the uterus

The fetus is active approximately 60% of the time. Its activity level remains stable between days 65 and 175

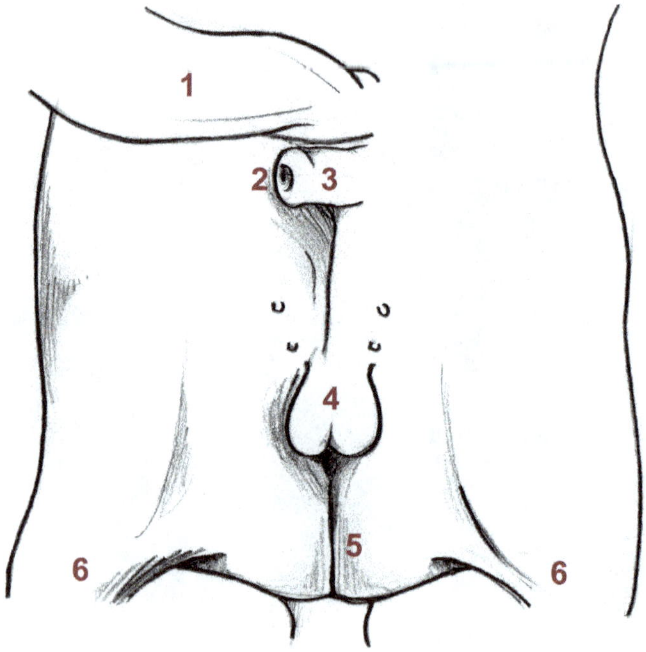

Figure 7.10. Development of the external genitalia in a bovine male fetus at 70 days of gestation (adapted from Barone 1990). 1: Umbilical cord; 2: Penis; 3: Prepuce; 4: Scrotum; 5: Perineal raphe; 6: Posterior limbs.

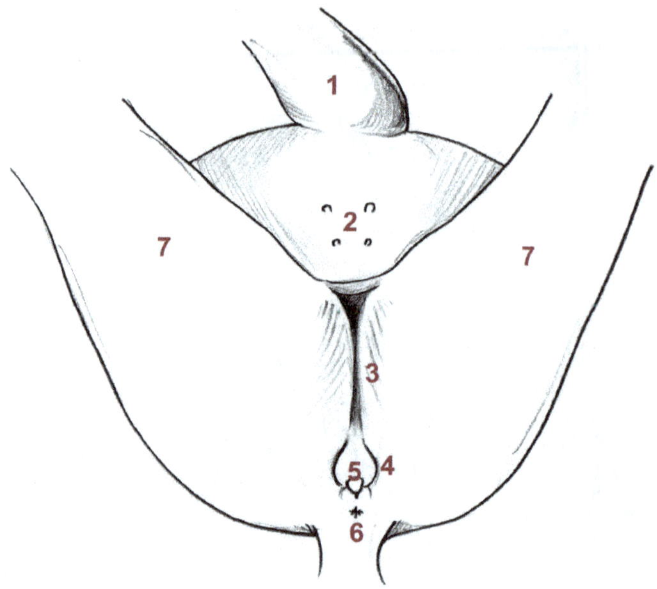

Figure 7.12. Development of the external genital organs in a bovine female fetus at 80 days of gestation (adapted from Barone 1990). 1: Umbilical cord; 2: Rudimentary teats; 3: Perineal raphe; 4: Vulvar labia; 5: Clitoris; 6: Anus; 7: Posterior limbs.

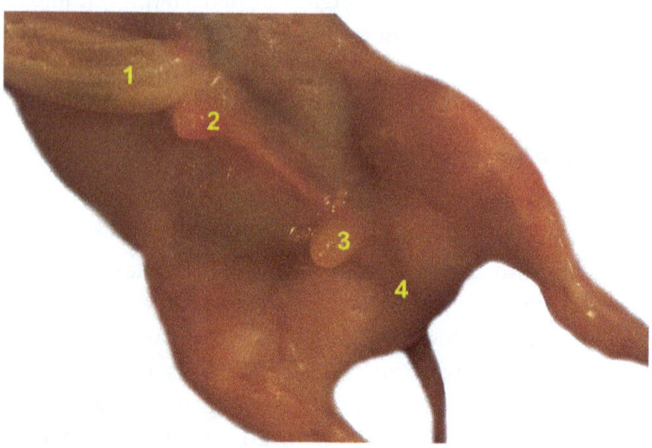

Figure 7.11. Ventral view of a male fetus at 100 days of gestation. The penis and the scrotum are visible. 1: Umbilical cord; 2: Penis and prepuce; 3. Scrotum; 4: Perineal raphe.

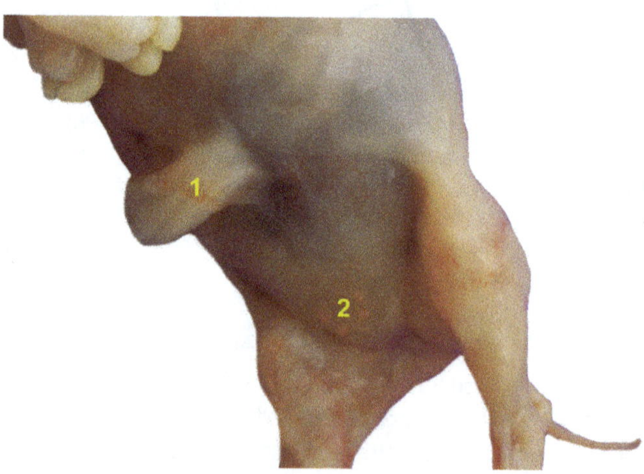

Figure 7.13. Ventral view of a female fetus at 80 days of gestation. The rudimentary teats are visible. 1: Umbilical cord; 2: Four rudimentary teats.

of gestation[11]. Significant fetal movements explain the changes in its location and position within the uterus during gestation. From the 2nd to the 5th months of gestation, the presentation of the fetus can be either anterior or posterior at equal rates[18]. However, anterior presentation predominates starting at the 5th month of gestation (Table 7.3). A definitive anterior presentation occurs on average at 192 days of gestation[11,24].

The position of the fetus in the abdomen and its significant increase in size limit the accessibility of certain body parts to transrectal ultrasound examination during the second half of gestation.

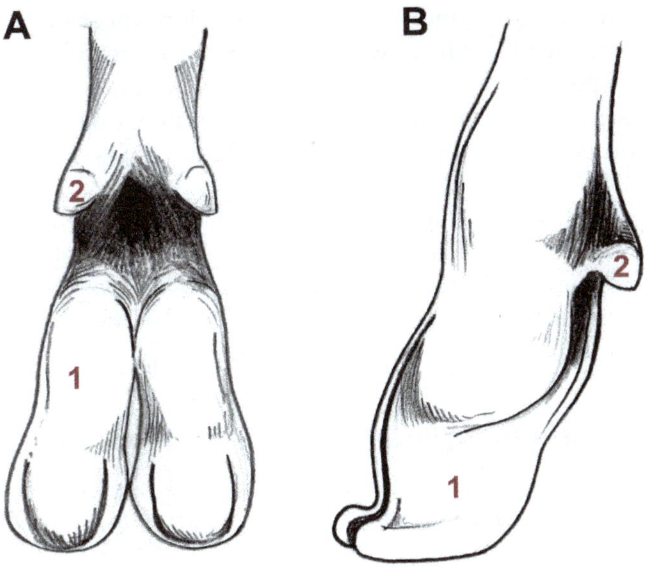

Figure 7.14. Limb extremities of a fetus at 80 days of gestation (adapted from Barone 1990). Posterior view (left) and left lateral view (right). 1: Cornified claw; 2: Dew-claw.

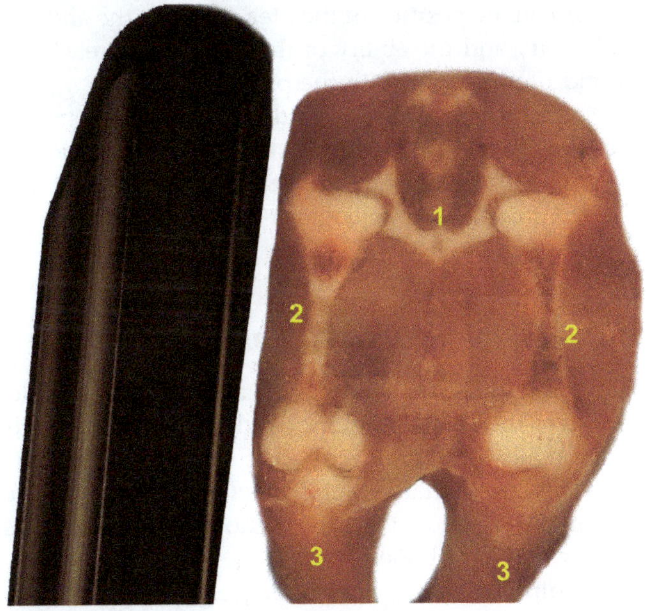

Figure 7.15. Transverse section of the posterior limbs of a male fetus at 100 days of gestation. The linear probe is located on the right side of the fetus. 1: Pelvis; 2: Femur; 3: Posterior limbs.

Ultrasound Fetal Sexing

Ultrasound fetal sexing is helpful to beef and dairy breeders in many ways. Purebred breeders can use this tool to know as early as 60 days of gestation the sex of the upcoming calf resulting from an embryo transfer or the insemination of a cow of high genetic value. It can also be used as a verification to evaluate the accuracy of embryo-sexing or semen-sexing technologies without having to wait for the confirmation of the sex of the calf at birth. Commercial breeders may include this approach in their culling and herd management decisions.

Ultrasound diagnosis of fetal sex: Three steps[8]

The first step is to locate the fetus in the uterus by scanning the uterine body as well as both uterine horns from their proximal to distal parts or vice versa. Since twin (or even triplet) pregnancies can have a major impact on the next lactation, a careful examination of the uterus is needed to confirm the number of fetuses present inside the uterine lumen (see Chapter 6).

The second step is to make sure that the fetus is alive and normal. The different signs showing the presence of a dead fetus were already presented in Chapter 6. Keep in mind that in certain situations the only sign of the death of the fetus might be the absence of a heart beat, especially if the fetal death occurred very recently. Although many clinical malformations are difficult to identify at an early stage, such as 60 days of pregnancy, it is also part of the diagnostic procedure to make sure that the fetus looks normal (see the section on fetal anomalies in this chapter).

Finally, the operator will be ready to complete the procedure with the determination of the sex of the fetus.

Examination of the cow can be done between days 54 and 100 of pregnancy, but the ideal window of opportunity is between days 60 and 70.[6,7,25] Even though the genital tubercle is visible as early as day 45, it does not reach its definitive position until day 58 in most animals. Migration may sometimes occur more rapidly, enabling definitive diagnosis at day 54 or 55. The possibility of establishing an accurate diagnosis at a later stage of the pregnancy (90 to 100 days) will depend on the position of the uterus within the abdominal cavity and the ability of the operator to reach the gravid uterine horn with the probe.

Diagnostic accuracy depends on the experience of the practitioner, the quality of the equipment, and the working conditions. Under ideal conditions, an experienced practitioner will get a definite and accurate diagnosis in almost 100% of the cows.

Appearance of the genital tubercle

The genital tubercle in both the male and the female, as well as the genital swellings and the urogenital folds in the male, are highly echogenic structures. Both the male and the female genital tubercles appear on the screen as bilobed structures whose echogenicity is similar to that of bone tissue.[6]

The ultrasound appearance of the genital tubercle is the same in both the male and the female, at least from 58 to 65 days of gestation. However, its position determines the diagnosis.[7,8,25] In Chapter 2, a description of the scanning technique showed how the position of the probe on the uterus has an impact on what will be seen on the monitor.

Male in different scanning views

At around day 58 of gestation, the genital tubercle reaches its final position, slightly caudal to the umbilicus (Figures 7.16, 7.17).

Between 65 and 70 days of gestation, most of the male fetuses will show a change in the appearance of the genital tubercle. The two-lobed structure observed earlier gives way to a four-lobed structure representing the genital tubercle and the urogenital folds (Figure 7.18).[6]

At this stage, the genital swellings are fused near the midline. These structures are at the origin of the scrotum and appear in the form of two small white lines on each side of the median line between the hindlimbs (Figure 7.19).[6]

Female in different scanning views

At around day 58 of gestation, the genital tubercle reaches its final position, under the tail (Figures 7.20, 7.21).

Identifying external genitalia after day 70

Differentiation of the female tract is completed by about day 70 and mammary glands are 0.6 to 3 mm in diameter on days 80 to 130. Descent of the testis in the bovine fetus is complete at about days 90 to 130. Because of these observations, the term *external genitalia* should be used after day 70, and the term *genital tubercle* should be discontinued.[11]

In the male, the genital tubercle, the urogenital folds and the genital swellings are at the origin of the penis,

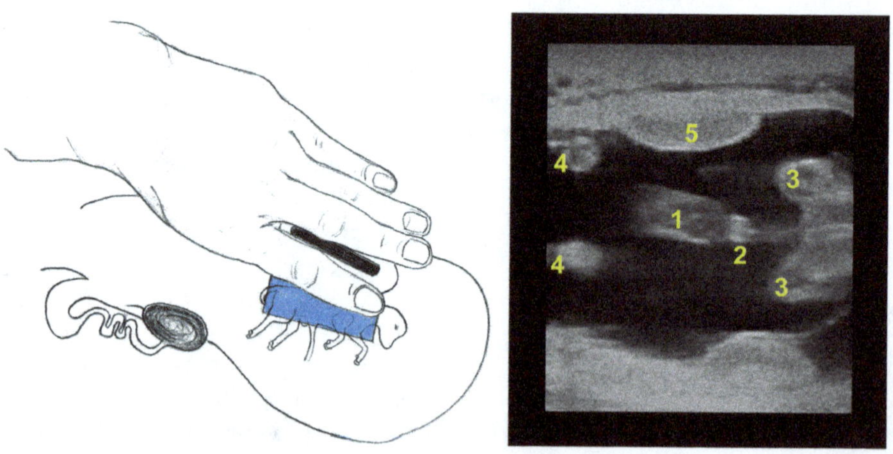

Figure 7.16. Male fetus at 65 days of gestation in longitudinal plane. The left side of the figure shows the position of the probe in relation to the fetus inside the uterus. The right side of the figure shows what will be seen on the screen at the same moment. Please note that the free part of the probe appears on the left side of the ultrasound image. 1: Umbilicus; 2: Genital tubercle; 3: Hindlimbs; 4: Forelimbs; 5: Placentome.

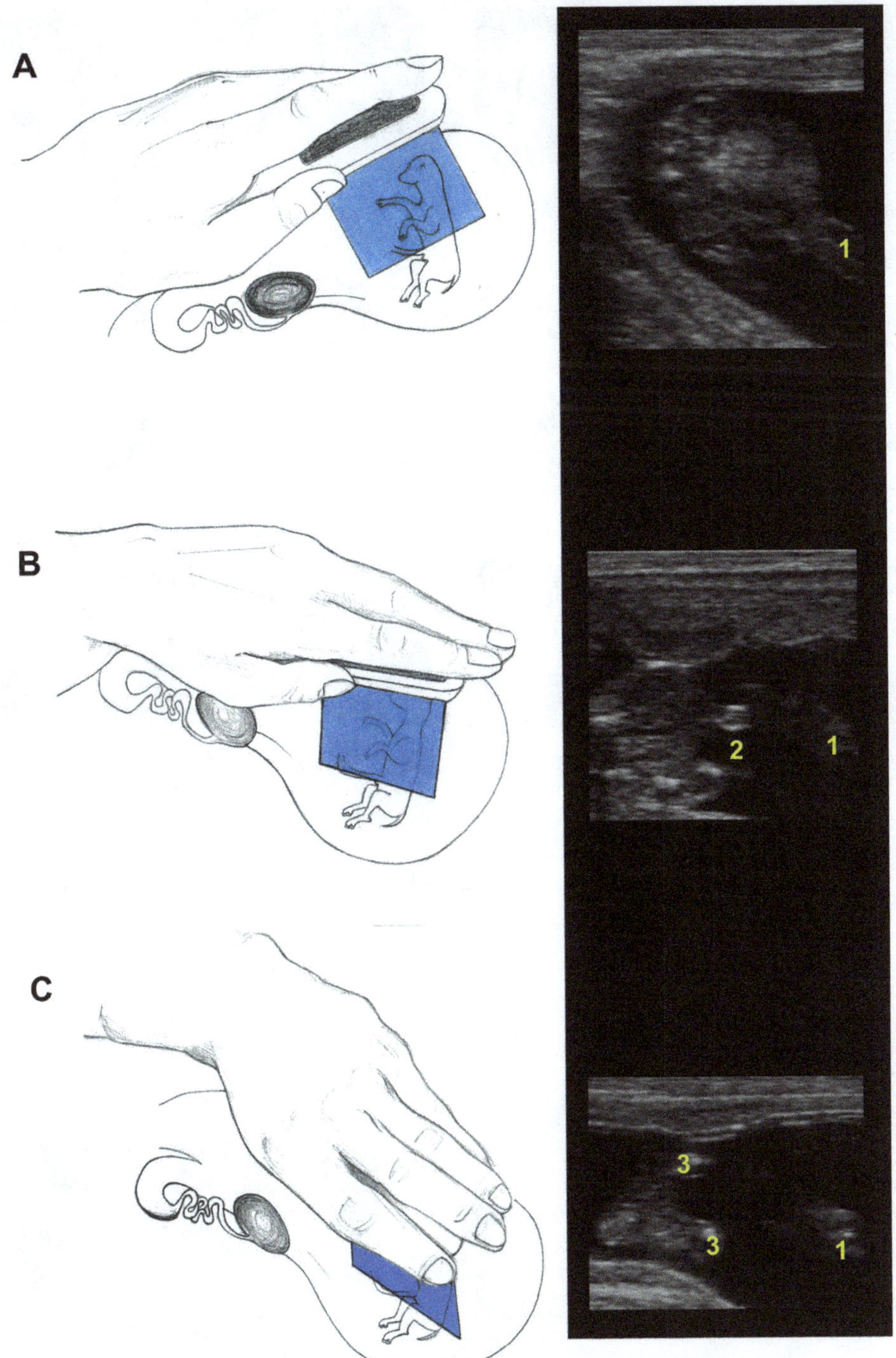

Figure 7.17. Male fetus at 60 days of gestation in three consecutive transversal planes. The left side of the figure shows the position of the probe in relation to the fetus inside the uterus. The right side of the figure shows what will be seen on the screen at the same moment. The probe is moved from the umbilicus (A) to the genital tubercle (B) and the hindlimbs (C). 1: Umbilicus; 2: Genital tubercle; 3: Hindlimbs.

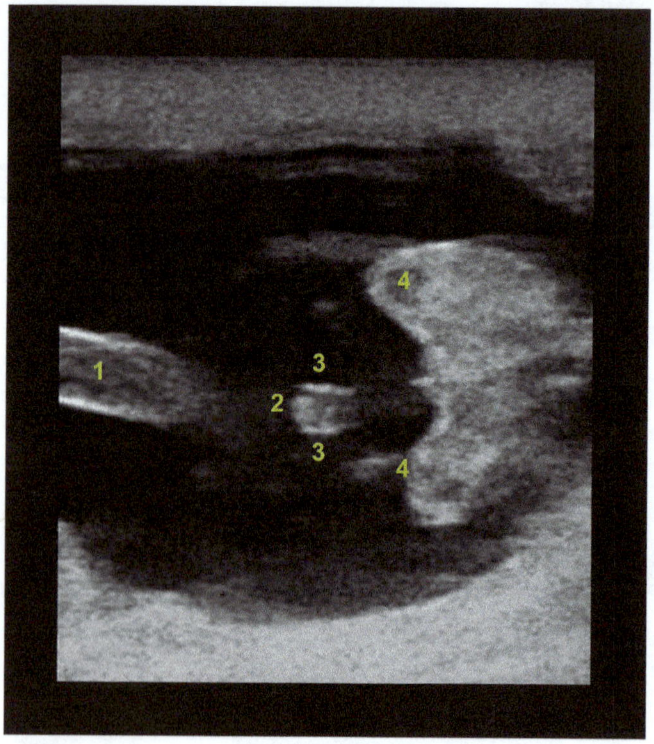

Figure 7.18. Ultrasound appearance of the genital tubercle and the urogenital folds from a male fetus at 68 days of gestation (longitudinal plane). 1: Umbilicus; 2: Genital tubercle; 3: Urogenital folds; 4: Hindlimbs.

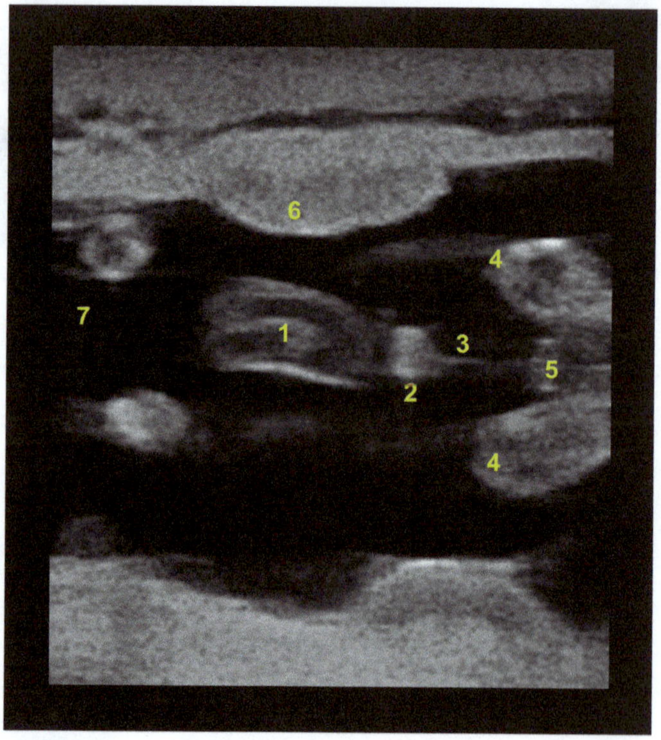

Figure 7.19. Ultrasound appearance of the genital tubercle and the genital swellings from a male fetus at 68 days of gestation (longitudinal plane). 1: Umbilicus; 2: Genital tubercle; 3: Median line; 4: Hindlimbs; 5: Genital (scrotal) swellings; 6: placentome; 7: Forelimbs.

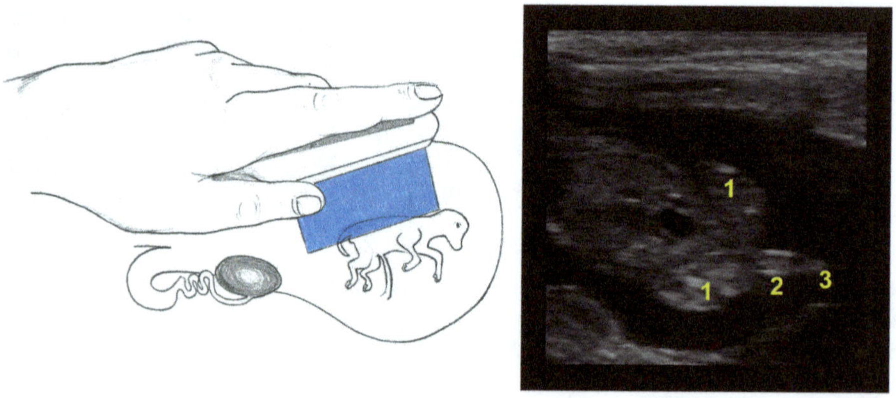

Figure 7.20. Female fetus at 60 days of gestation in longitudinal plane. The left side of the figure shows the position of the probe in relation to the fetus inside the uterus. The right side of the figure shows what will be seen on the screen at the same moment. 1: Hindlimbs; 2: Genital tubercle; 3: Tail.

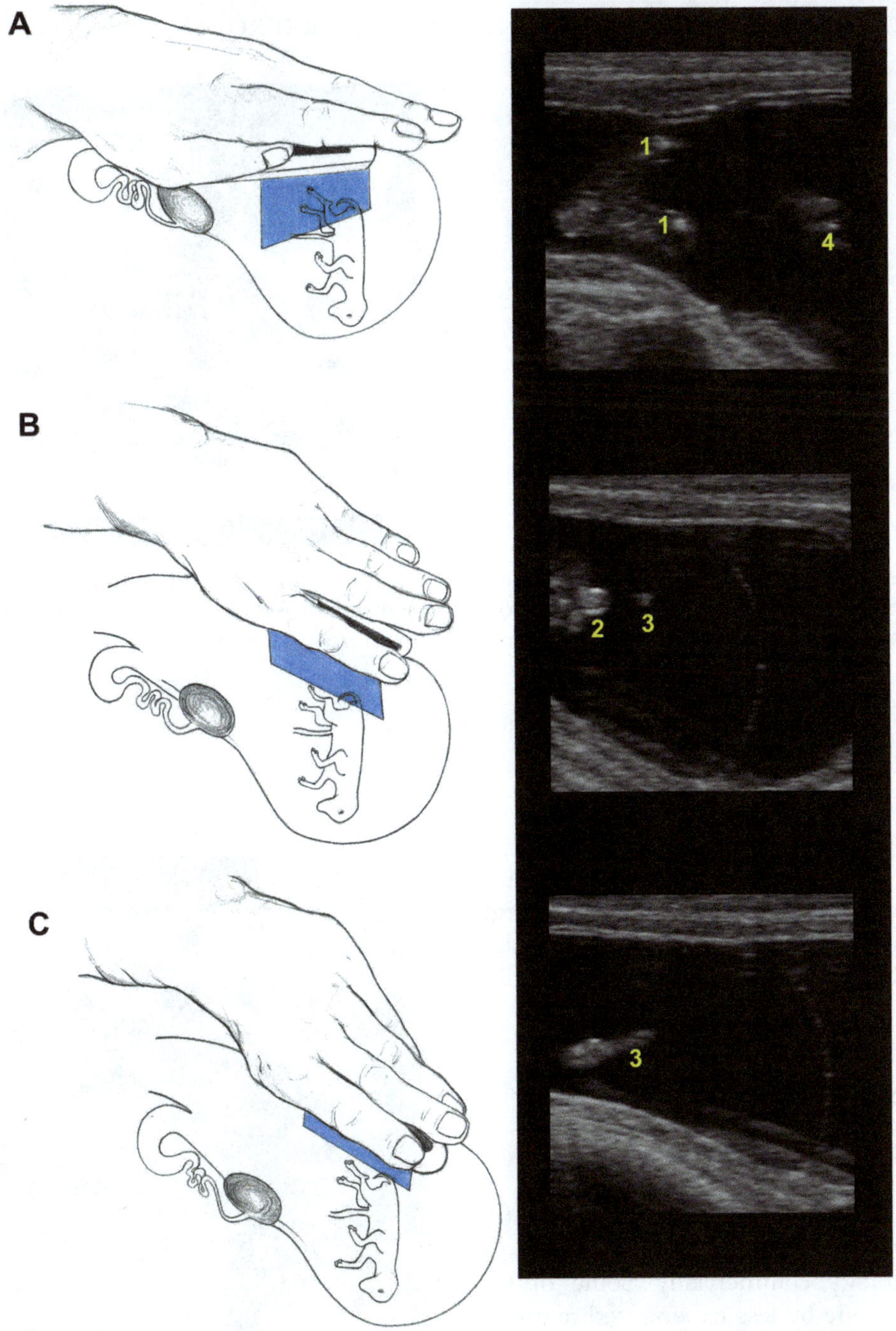

Figure 7.21. Female fetus at 60 days of gestation in three consecutive transverse planes. The left side of the figure shows the position of the probe in relation to the fetus inside the uterus. The right side of the figure shows what will be seen on the screen at the same moment. The probe is moved from the hindlimbs (A) to the genital tubercle (B) and the tail (C). 1: Hindlimbs; 2: Genital tubercle; 3: Tail; 4: Umbilicus.

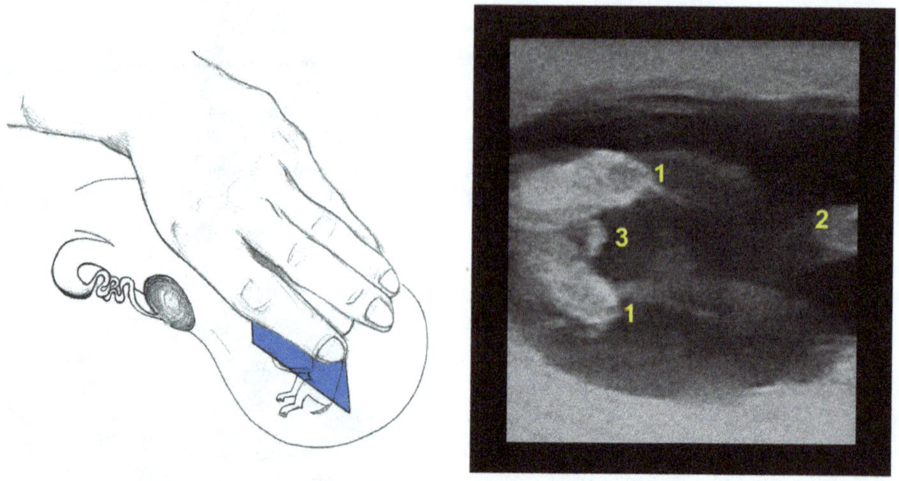

Figure 7.22. Ultrasound appearance of the scrotum of a male fetus at 75 days of gestation (transversal plane). The left side of the figure shows the position of the probe in relation to the fetus inside the uterus. The right side of the figure shows what will be seen on the screen at the same moment. 1: Hindlimbs; 2: Umbilicus; 3: Scrotum.

the prepuce, and the scrotum, respectively (Figure 7.22). In the female, the genital swellings undergo gradual atrophy and eventually disappear around day 50. The genital tubercle becomes the clitoris, and the urogenital folds form the vulvar labia.[6]

Advice for less experienced practitioners

Although highly variable between individuals, it usually takes considerable training and a few months of practice to reach a level of confidence high enough to use this technology commercially. Some of the common mistakes made by less experienced manipulators include confusing the umbilicus with the male genital tubercle or confusing a section of the tail (caudal vertebra) with the female genital tubercle (Figure 7.23). It is also not recommended to confirm a female based on the impression that "nothing was seen in the umbilical region" or a male based on the impression that "nothing was seen under the tail." Make sure that a complete examination of the fetus is done. Accurate knowledge of the fetal anatomy and the ultrasonographic appearance of the different fetal structures will help avoid confusion during the diagnostic procedure. The manipulator should never forget to confirm the number of fetuses as well as the viability of the fetus(es).

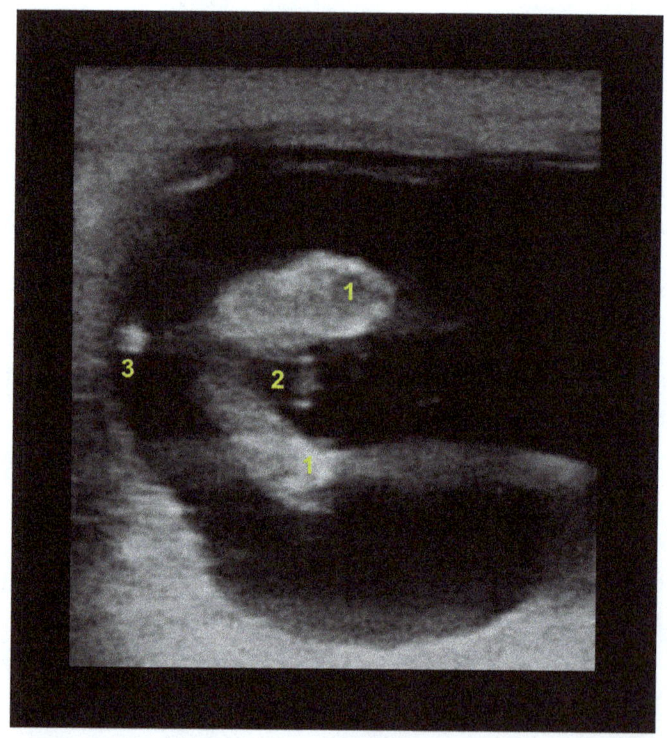

Figure 7.23. Ultrasonogram of a male fetus of 72 days. This image presents a situation where a less experienced manipulator can be misled by an incorrect identification of a fetal structure. For some practitioners, the appearance of the tail (caudal vertebra) on this day 72 male fetus can be misidentified as the external genitalia from a female fetus. 1: Hindlimbs; 2: Scrotum; 3: Tail.

Fetal Anomalies

The incidence of bovine fetal anomalies is very low. It has been estimated at 0.07% or 15 detected anomalies from 21,000 pregnancy examinations over a 5-year period[11]. Most of the reported anomalies were diagnosed at the time of fetal sexing. Often the pregnancy is noted as abnormal during the embryonic stage, but the exact nature of the abnormality cannot be described until the fetal stage. The following are some of the reasons justifying a second ultrasonographic examination after an early pregnancy evaluation:

- Early detection of embryonic and fetal losses
- Confirmation of multiple fetuses
- Evaluation of normal development of the conceptus and fetal viability
- Detection of fetal anomalies

The early detection of fetal anomalies makes it possible to terminate the abnormal pregnancy and allow rebreeding of the cows without too much consequence. Most fetal anomalies have a very poor prognosis for the birth of a live calf, which justifies the termination of the pregnancy.

The most easily detectable fetal anomalies during ultrasonographic exams in cattle are schistosomus reflexus, amorphus globosus (or fetal mole), conjoined fetuses (Siamese twins), a two-headed fetus, and an extrathoracic heart. Some other congenital or acquired anomalies worthy of mention are hydrocephalus, fetal ascites, and pericardial effusion. Figures 7.24–7.28 present some of these anomalies.

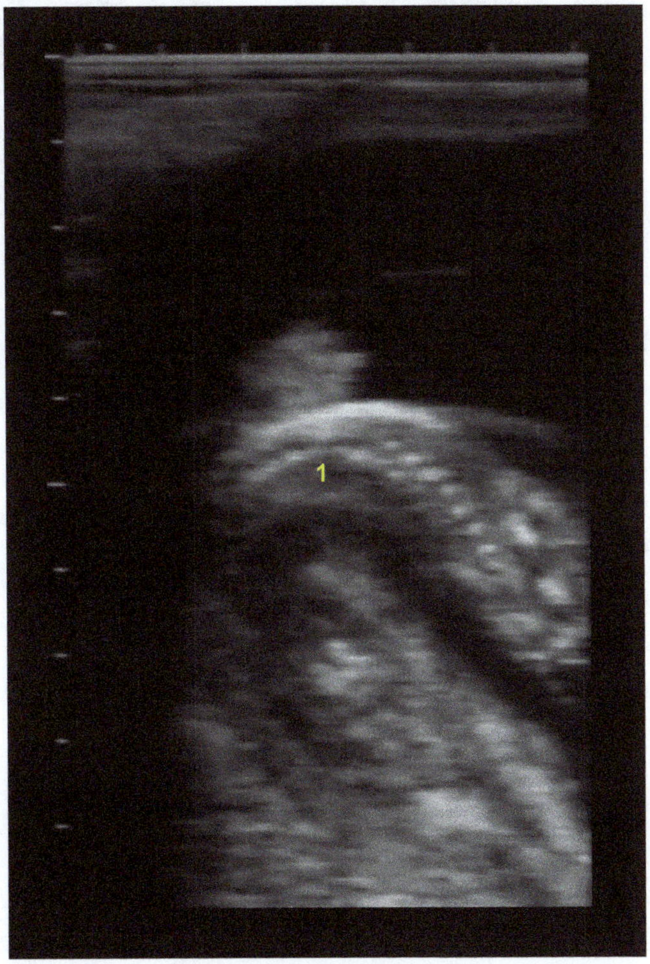

Figure 7.24. Ultrasonographic image of a schistosomus reflexus fetus at 80 days (probe 5 MHz; depth 10 cm). Courtesy of Dr. Sandra Curran. This condition is characterized by acute angulation of the spine so that the tail lies close to the head of the fetus. Schistosomus reflexus (SR) is a rare and fatal congenital disorder. SR fetuses often survive to parturition but cannot be delivered live without a C-section and always result in a dystocia; SR is incompatible with life following birth of the calf. Primarily observed in ruminants, its defining features include a reverse ventro-dorsal curvature of the vertebral column, exposure of the abdominal viscera because the ventral abdominal wall cannot close, limb ankylosis, and positioning of the limbs adjacent to the skull. 1: Acute reverse curvature of the vertebral column.

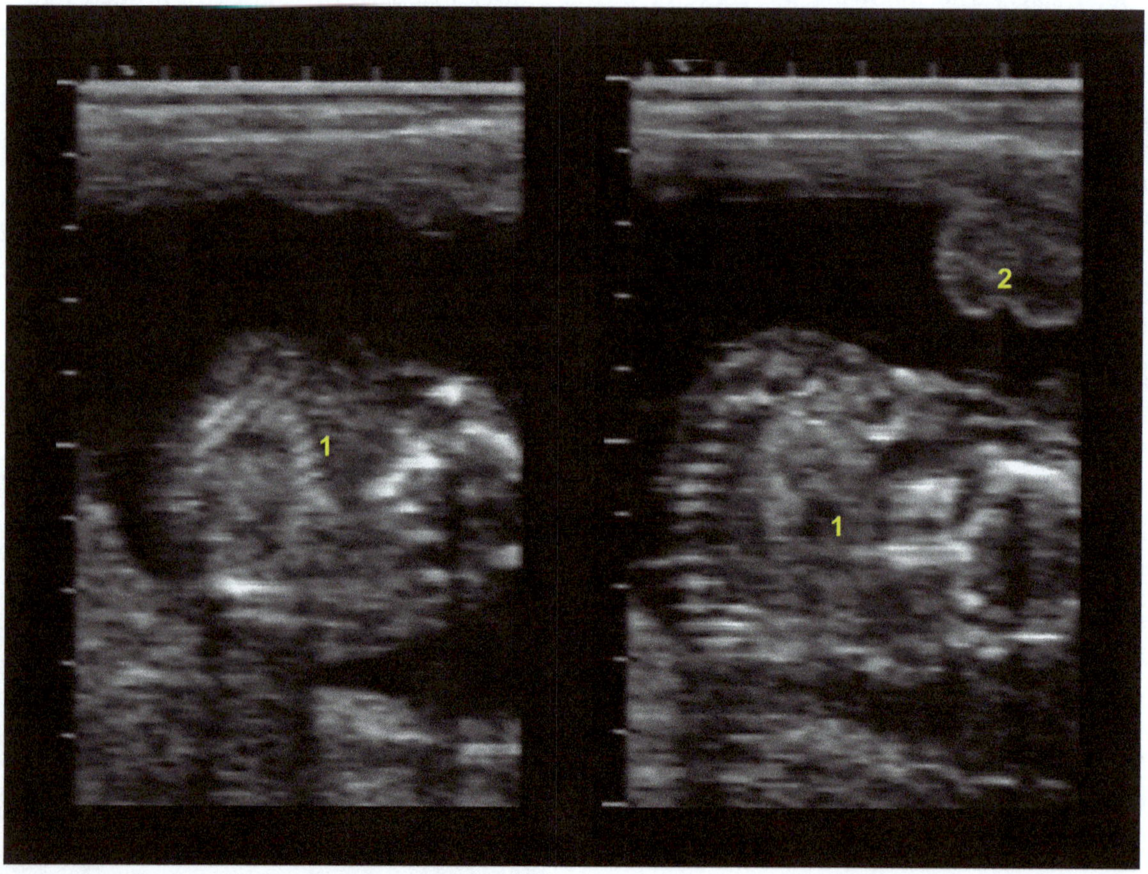

Figure 7.25. Sonograms of an amorphus globosus or fetal mole (probe 5 MHz; depth 10 cm). Courtesy of Dr. Sandra Curran. The amorphus globosus (AM) is a spherical structure of all three basic germ layers covered with normal, pigmented skin typical of the breed. AM may cause dystocia. 1: Heterogenous rounded structure with hyperechogenic bone tissue; 2: Placentome.

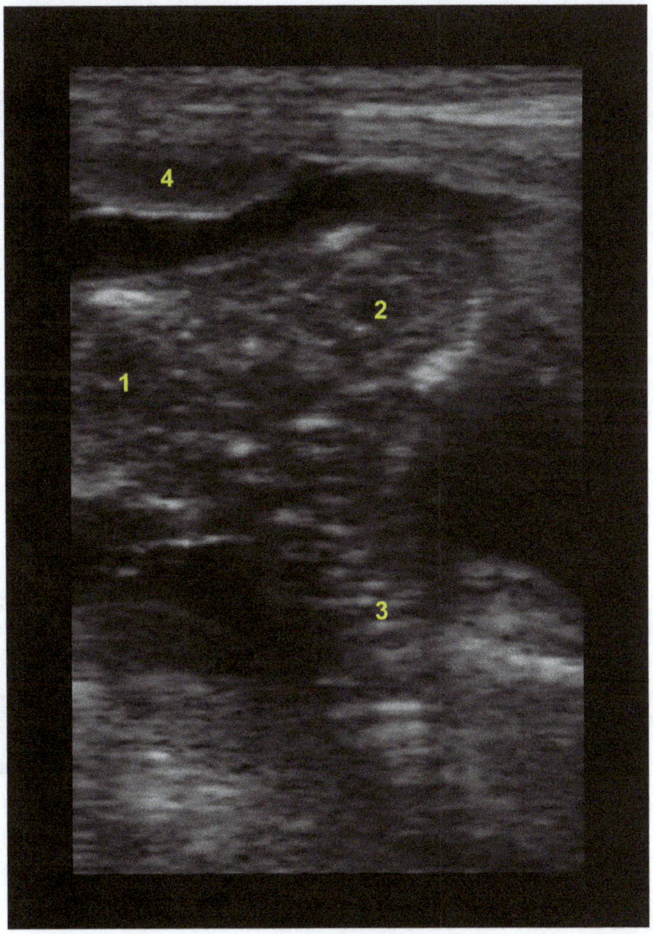

Figure 7.26. Ultrasonographic image of a two-headed fetus of 64 days (probe 6 MH; depth 6 cm). Courtesy of Dr. Sébastien Buczinski. Note that the cervical column splits in two parts from the first thoracic vertebrae. 1: Head #1; 2: Head #2; 3: Base of the neck; 4: Placentome.

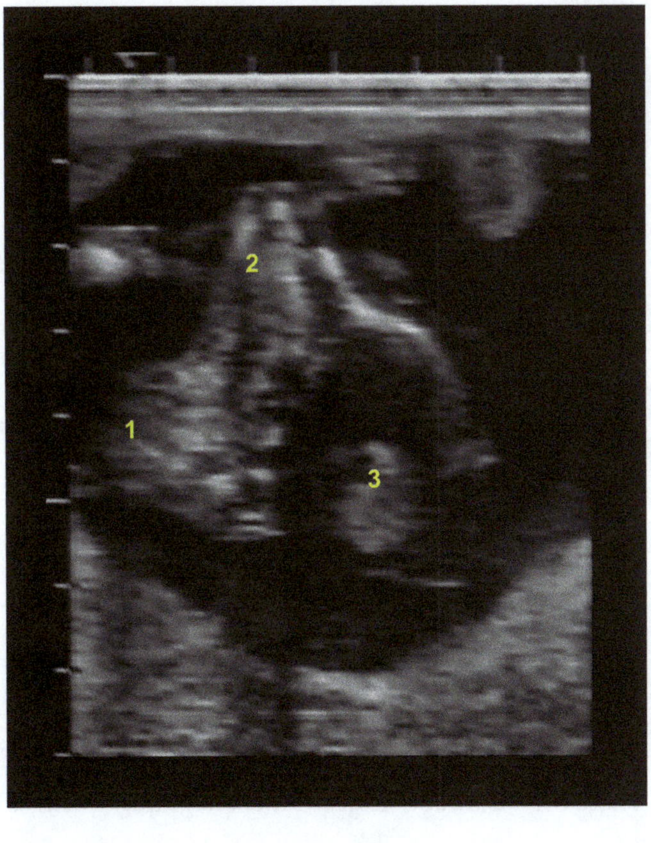

Figure 7.27. Ultrasound image of a bovine hydrocephalic fetus (probe 5 MHz; depth 8 cm). Courtesy of Dr. Sandra Curran. Note the abnormal accumulation of cerebrospinal fluid within the cerebral ventricular system of this 90-day fetus. 1: Neck; 2: Mandible; 3: Brain.

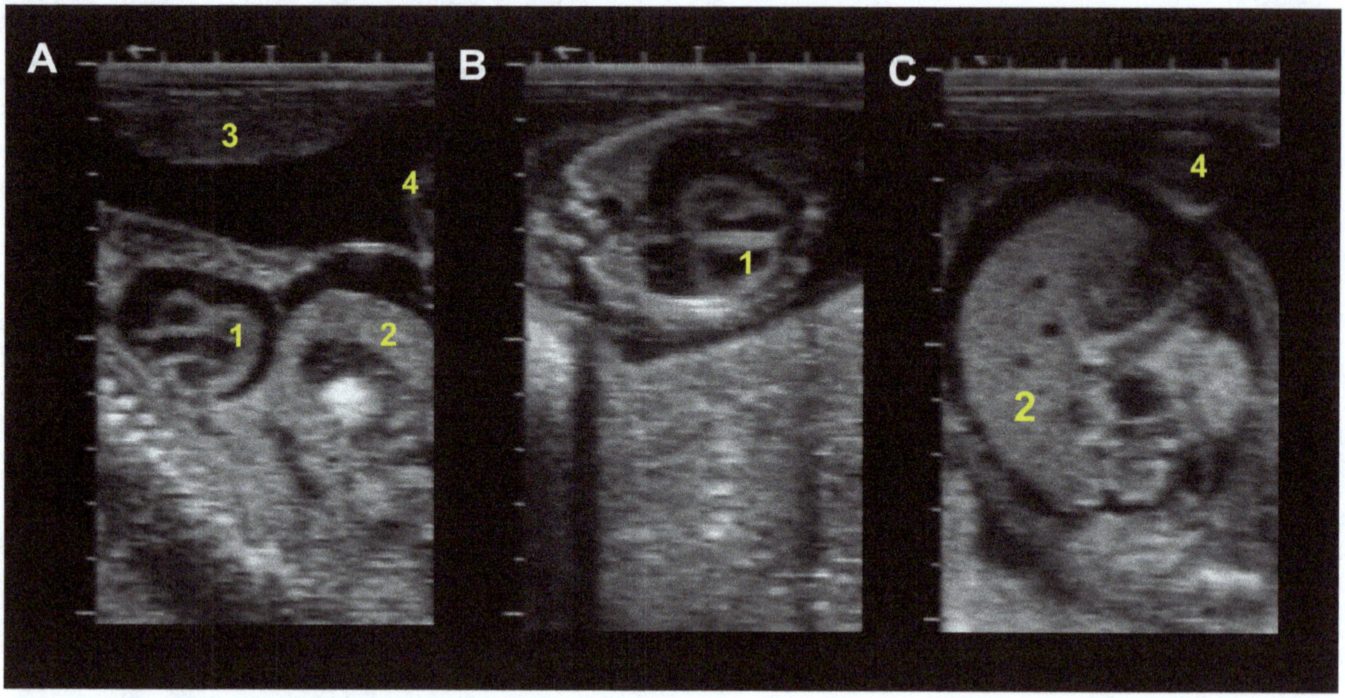

Figure 7.28. Ultrasonograms of fetal ascites and pericardial effusion in a 100-day fetus (probe 5 MHz; depth 10 cm). Courtesy of Dr. Sandra Curran. Note the abnormal accumulation of fluid around the heart (pericardial effusion) (A and B) and in the abdominal cavity (ascitis) (A and C), which permits easy identification of the contour of the organs. The cause of this condition is often undiagnosed but is often fatal to the fetus. 1: Heart; 2: Liver; 3: Placentome; 4: Umbilicus.

Fetal Well-Being During Late Pregnancy (Normal Gestation, Compromised Pregnancy, and Clone)

The ultrasonographic assessment of the feto-placental unit can add highly valuable information concerning fetal well-being.[29] In human pregnancies this examination consists of the evaluation of fetal growth, health status, and early detection of congenital anomalies.[5] There are few studies describing the ultrasonographic appearance of the conceptus in the bovine and equine late pregnancy.[3,13,23]

Practical assessment of fetal well-being during late bovine pregnancy

Two of the difficulties of examination during late gestation are the size of the fetus and the depth of the maternal abdomen. After 5 months of pregnancy the conceptus rests on the ventral abdominal wall. Therefore, transabdominal ultrasonography with a low-frequency probe (2 to 3.5 MHz) must be used to obtain deep images up to 20–25 cm and visualize the fetus and its adnexa (Figures 7.29, 7.30). To improve the quality of the ultrasound images the abdomen is prepared by shaving the area from the lower half of the right flank ventrally to the linea alba and cranially to the xiphoid process. Clipping is followed by rinsing with warm water and application of transducer coupling gel. After the 7th month of pregnancy, pressing the abdomen may help in locating the fetus.

Ultrasonographic parameters that can be assessed with fetal ultrasound

Various parameters are used in different species to assess the fetus and its adnexa (amniotic and allantoic fluids and uterus) (Table 7.4). Of those, the most pertinent are presented in this section.

Depth of placental fluids

The placental fluids (amniotic and allantoic) are highly dependent on the fetus and the annexes for their production. The amniotic fluid contains small echogenic particles in contrast to the allantoic fluid, which is anechoic (Figure 7.31). Their quantity can be affected by various fetal or adnexial disorders. Their quantity is indirectly assessed by the deepest pocket of fluid that can be observed when the ultrasonography is performed (Figure 7.32). The deepest pocket of placental fluid generally exceeds 20 cm after the 7th month of pregnancy.

Placental assessment

The placental assessment is performed by assessing the shape, size, and echogenic aspect of the placentomes. The normal size of the placentomes is 6 by 8 to 10 cm. They are ovoid with a homogeneous echogenicity (Figure 7.33). The allanto-amniotic membrane between the allantoic and the amniotic fluid can be seen when imaging the placental fluids. The thickness of this membrane is usually less than 0.5 cm in healthy cows. The thickness of the allanto-amniotic membrane can occasionally be increased in case of hydrallantois.

Fetal heart rate

The fetal heart rate (FHR) is an interesting indicator of fetal health. The FHR can be measured when imaging

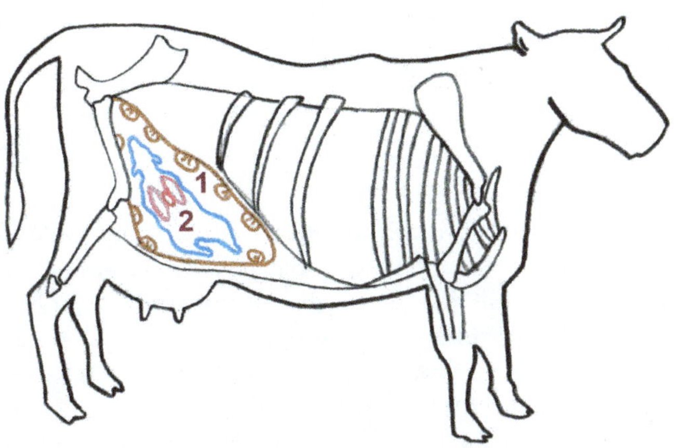

Figure 7.29. Topographic representation of the fetus and uterus in late pregnancy. The right lateral view of the abdominal cavity can be scanned in order to evaluate the fetal viability in late pregnancy. Please note that it is often necessary to prepare the scanning area up to the xiphoid process. 1: Gravid uterus (brown); 2: Fetus (blue).

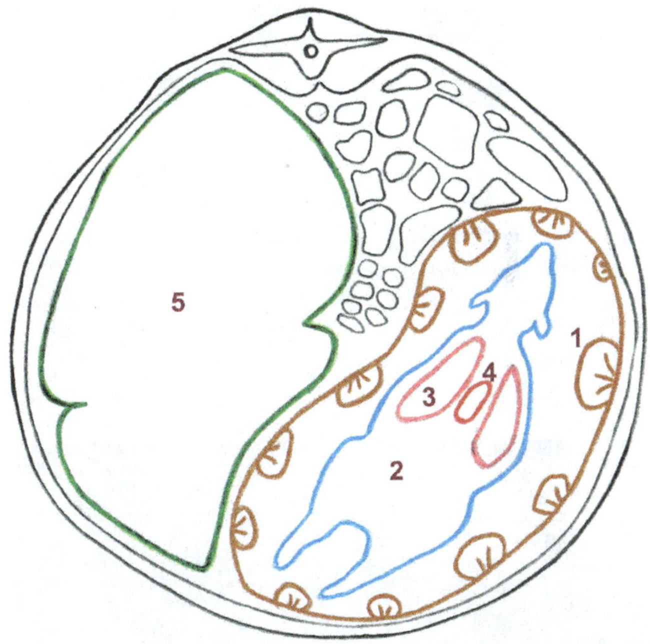

Figure 7.30. Transverse section of the bovine maternal abdomen during late pregnancy. This drawing presents the position of a 7-month fetus in the uterus of a cow and the possible area of interest for transabdominal ultrasonographic fetal viability assessment. Please note that it is often necessary to scan over the midline of the abdomen to achieve a complete evaluation of the fetal well-being. 1: Gravid uterus (brown); 2: Fetus (blue); 3: Lungs (pink); 4: Heart (red); 5: Rumen (green).

Table 7.4.
The different ultrasonographic parameters used in human, equine, and bovine fetal well-being assessment (Buczinski et al. 2006, 2007; Jonker 2004; Reef et al. 1996; Woodward et al. 2005)

Human	Equine	Cattle
Fetal movements	Global fetal activity	Global fetal activity
Heart rate variability	Fetal heart rate variability	Fetal heart rate (3 to 5 measurements)
Deepest pocket of amniotic fluid	Maximal depth of fetal fluids	Maximal depth of fetal fluids, fluid echogenicity
Fetal tone	Fetal aortic diameter	Mean size and aspects of 4 placentomes
Fetal breathing movements	Uteroplacental thickness and aspect	Allanto-amniotic membrane thickness

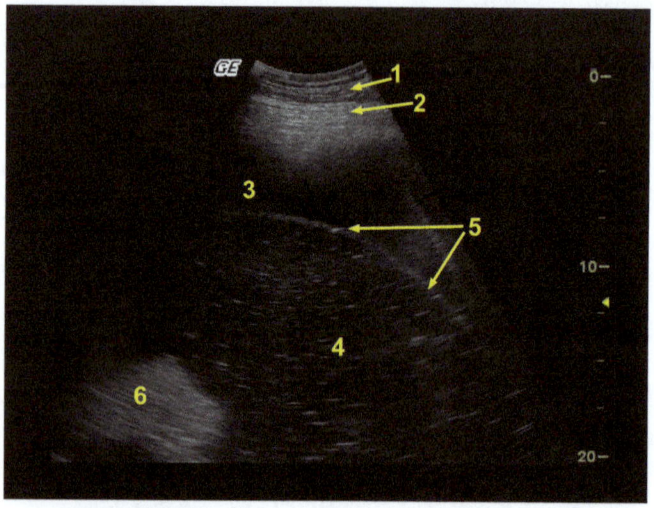

Figure 7.31. Ultrasonographic image for the assessment of the amniotic and allantoic fluid in a pregnant cow of 7 months. Note that the amniotic fluid has numerous echogenic particles compared to the allantoic fluid, which is anechogenous. 1: Abdominal wall; 2: Uterine wall; 3: Allantoic fluid (anechogenous); 4: Amniotic fluid (hyperechogenous particles); 5: Allanto-amniotic membrane; 6: Fetal part of the fetus (moving).

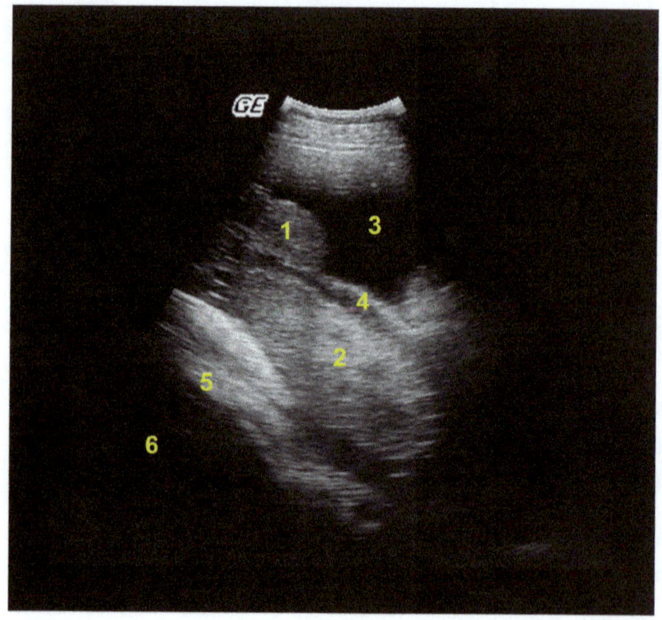

Figure 7.33. Ultrasonographic appearance of normal placentomes in a pregnant cow of 8 months. 1: Normal placentome in transversal view; 2: Normal placentome in longitudinal view; 3: Allantoic fluid; 4: Uterine wall; 5: Fetal bone; 6: Acoustic shadow.

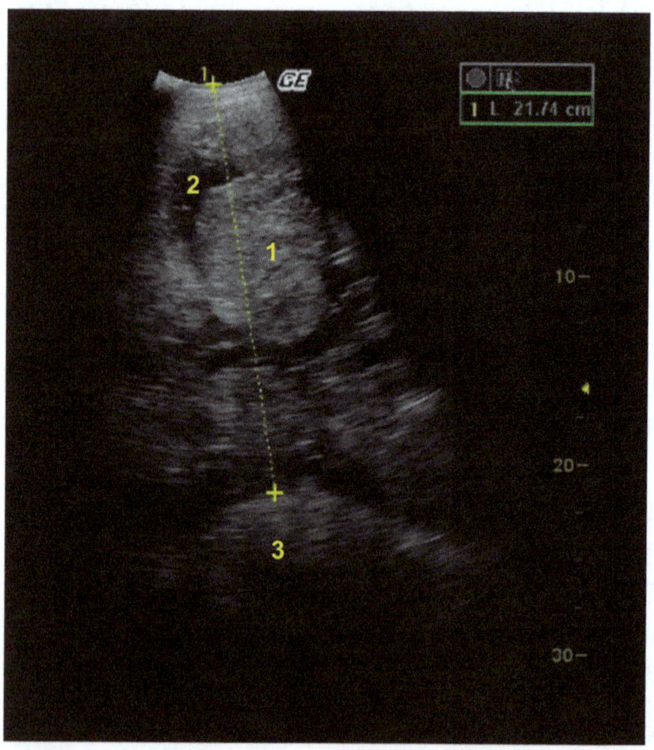

Figure 7.32. Ultrasound evaluation and measurements of the deepest pocket of uterine fluid in a pregnant cow of 8 months. The deepest pocket of placental fluid has been measured at 21.74 cm (yellow calipers). 1: Placentome; 2: Allantoic fluid (anechogenous); 3: Fetus.

the fetal thorax (Figure 7.34) by counting heartbeats for 15 seconds and multiplying the number by 4 to obtain FHR or with M-mode if available. Highly variable FHR (see the normal ranges in the section on ultrasonographic fetal well-being assessment in normal pregnancies during late gestation; see also Chapter 6 concerning early pregnancy) indicates a healthy fetus, which adapts its FHR to its activity with a mature neurologic development. However, ultrasonographic measurements of FHR in late pregnancy have a limited value because the variation of FHR is not easily assessed and can be affected by various stimuli. Continuous recording of the FHR by Doppler ultrasonography could potentially help to assess fetal heart rate variability, but it is not available in most private practices.

Fetal movements

Fetal activity is an important part of the assessment of fetal well-being.[3,5,23,29] As the nervous system develops, the movements of the fetus are accompanied by an increase of the FHR to increase cardiac output.[5] Due to the size of the fetus and the deep abdomen of the dam no gradation of the complexity of the movements can be made. A fetal joint can sometimes be recognized

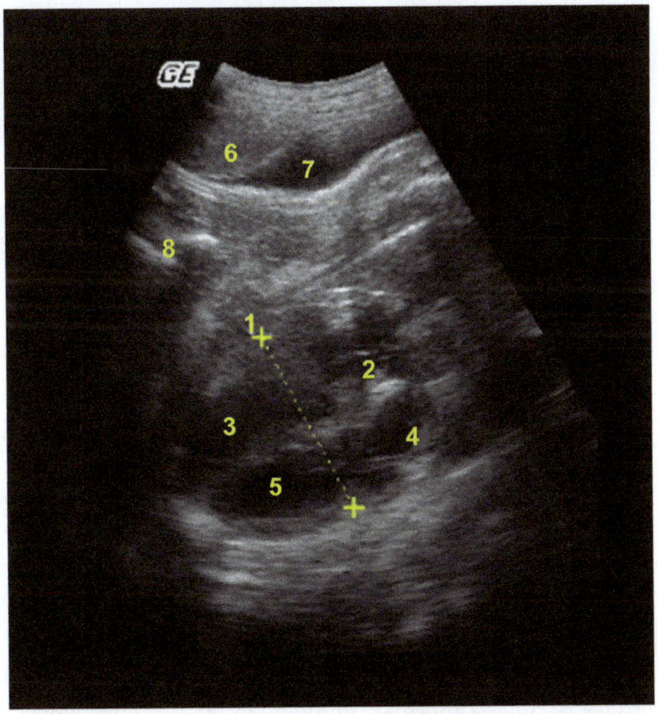

Figure 7.34. Ultrasonographic examination of the heart and thorax of an 8-month bovine fetus. 1: Atrioventricular limits of the heart in long axis view; 2: Left atrium; 3: Left ventricle; 4: Right atrium; 5: Right ventricle; 6: Placentome; 7: Allantoic fluid; 8: Thoracic limb.

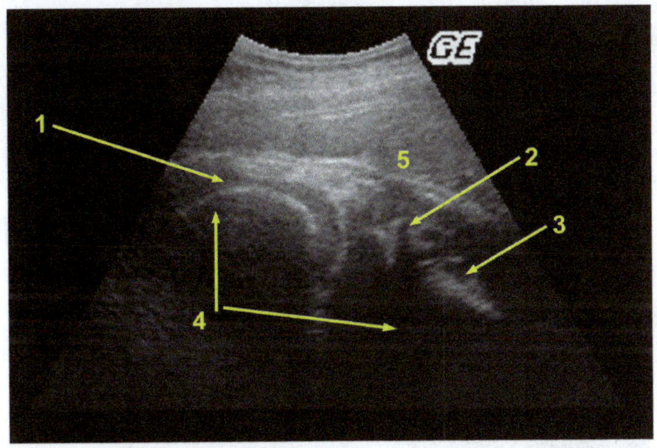

Figure 7.35. Ultrasonographic observation of the fetal limb (fetal stifle) to assess fetal movements in a pregnant cow of 8 months. 1: Femoral condyle; 2: Tibial crest; 3: Tibia; 4: Shadow artifact; 5: Placentome.

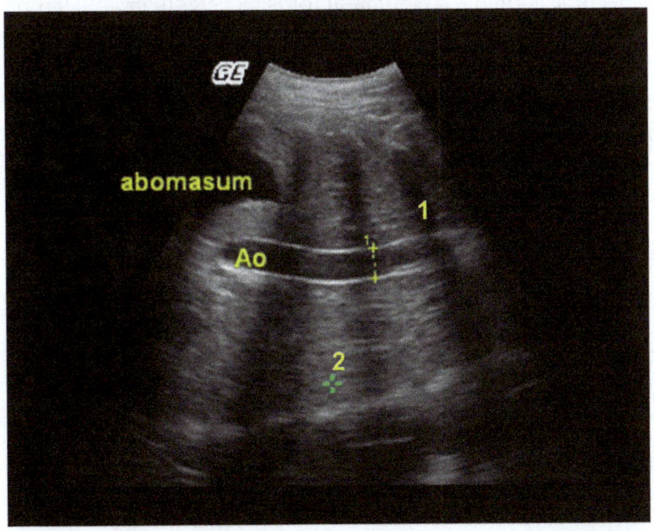

Figure 7.36. Ultrasonographic fetal thorax examination and aortic (Ao) measurement during a fetal well-being evaluation of a pregnant cow of 7 months. Ao: Longitudinal section of the aorta, which has a diameter of 1.28cm. The transversal plane is between the calipers. 1: Acoustic shadow due to costal blockage of the ultrasound beam; 2: Fetal lung parenchyma.

easily (Figure 7.35). However, it is quite easy to record the proportion of time the fetus is moving when performing the ultrasonographic examination. This gross examination of fetal movement is used in equine fetal biophysical profiles.[23] According to the proportion of time that the fetus is moving, a four-grade scale can be used.[23] A score of 0 is given to fetuses that did not move during the 30min period, 1 to fetuses moving less than one-third of the examination time, 2 for fetuses moving more than one-third but less than two-thirds of the time, and 3 for fetuses moving more than two-thirds of the examination time.

Indicators of fetal growth

The ultrasonographic indicators of fetal growth are well known in early pregnancy to midpregnancy when the fetus can be easily imaged (Table 7.2). However, late indicators have not been studied because they are difficult to observe or to measure consistently. The thoracic aortic diameter has been mentioned as a reliable parameter in horses. The aorta is easily observed as an anechoic tubular structure with a hyperechoic wall in the thorax (Figure 7.36). Although mentioned as a possible fetal growth parameter in cattle, it has not been fully validated.[5,13] The only valid indicator of fetal weight in late pregnancy in cattle is the width of the metacarpal or metatarsal bone as measured by transrectal ultrasonography. Those parameters are linearly correlated with birth weight, but can be assessed only

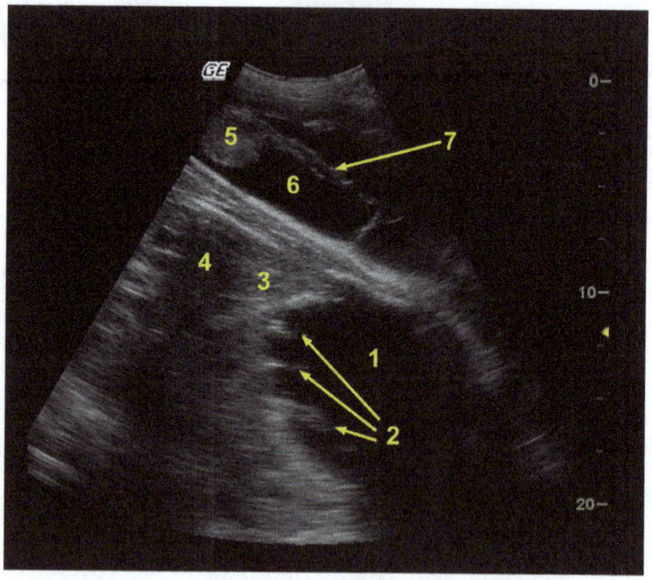

Figure 7.37. Ultrasonographic aspect of the abomasum and liver of an 8-month-old bovine fetus. 1: Abomasum with anechoic content; 2: Abomasal folds; 3: Fetal liver; 4: Fetal rib with acoustic shadow; 5: Placentome; 6: Allantoic fluid; 7: Uterine wall.

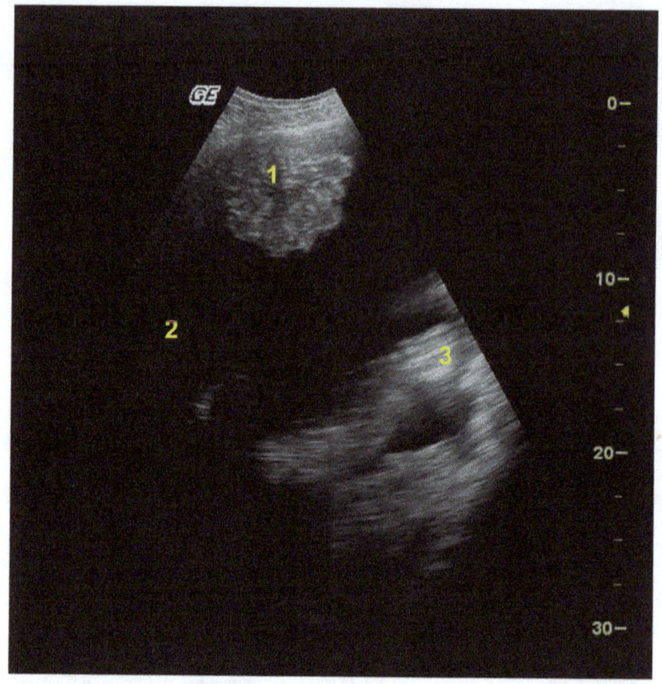

Figure 7.38. Abnormal findings in a 7-month cloned pregnancy with irregular placentomes. Note the irregular shape of the placentome above the fetus. 1: Irregular placentome with a lumpy shape and heterogenic echogenicity; 2: Allantoic fluid (anechoic); 3: Fetus moving during the procedure.

when the fetus is palpable per rectum the last month of pregnancy.[26] Various organs can also be assessed by fetal ultrasonography (Figure 7.37).

Ultrasonographic fetal well-being assessment in normal pregnancies

Preliminary data have shown that ultrasonographic fetal viability assessment can be done in cattle. The mean duration of the examination is 30 min. The FHR is variable in fetuses. The mean FHR is 105 beats per minute (bpm) in the last month of pregnancy and generally varies from 90 to 125 bpm.[5] However, large variations have been recorded, especially when contraction of the uterus occurs during parturition (from 60 to 220 bpm). The fetuses are generally active less than one-third of the total examination time or between one-third to two-thirds of the examination time.

Ultrasonographic fetal well-being assessment in compromised pregnancies

Because any disease of the dam can have an impact on the perfusion of the conceptus and blood supply of the fetus[5] ultrasonographic fetal well-being can potentially be helpful in determining the impact of any disease on the fetus.[4,5] Preliminary data in small numbers of pregnancies have shown that serial measurements of FHR in abnormal pregnancies were not different from normal pregnancies. The absence of a heartbeat when imaging the thorax was indicative of fetal death.[3,17] Inactive fetuses during the examination period or fetuses active throughout the entire examination time were fetuses that had a poor outcome. However, sleeping periods with no detrimental impact on the fetus have been mentioned in mares[23] and women. For this reason, fetal inactivity should be confirmed by repeating the ultrasonographic assessment. If the outcome is the same it should be interpreted as an indicator of fetal distress or death.[5,17] Although hyperechoic particles are frequently observed in amniotic and more rarely in allantoic fluid, permanent visualization of a large amount of those particles in fetal fluids during repeated examinations is indicative of fetal death.[17]

Ultrasonographic fetal well-being assessment in cloned pregnancies

Various anomalies of the dam, the fetus, or its annexes have been reported in cloned pregnancies.[3]

Hydrallantois can develop in those cases and is characterized by progressive enlargement of the abdomen of the dam and great difficulty in imaging the fetus due to the increased quantity of allantoic fluid.[3,13] A thickening of the allanto-amniotic membrane (more than 1 cm) is also often evident. Abnormal placentomes can also be seen with heterogenic echogenicity and lumpy shape (Figure 7.38).

Other potential interest of ultrasonography in late pregnancy

Multiple anomalies have been identified with the help of an ultrasonographic screening during late pregnancy in humans.[29] A decrease of the placental fluid is mainly observed in cases of oligohydramnios when there is a decrease of fluid production or increase of fluid removal (fetal deglutition of amniotic fluid). Various fetal congenital anomalies can also be detected by routine ultrasonographic examination of the conceptus.[29] However, the data are scant concerning this use of ultrasonography in cattle with the exception of the detection of fetal anasarca in one case of cloned pregnancy.[3]

REFERENCES

1. Barone R (1990). Anatomie comparée des mammifères domestiques. Tome 4; Splanchnologie II, Appareil urogénital, foetus et ses annexes, péritoine et topographie abdominale, Vigot Ed., pp. 506–674.
2. Blin PC, Bossavy A, Fournier CL (1963). Dynamique pondérale et linéaire des estomacs, du foie et de l'intestin des foetus bovin et ovin. Econ Méd Animales 4: 141–160.
3. Buczinski S, Fecteau G, Lefebvre RC, Smith LC (2006). Ultrasonographic assessment of bovine fetal wellbeing during late pregnancy in normal, compromised and cloned pregnancies. J Vet Int Med 20: 722–723.
4. Buczinski S, Bélanger AM, Fecteau G, Roy JP (2007). Prolonged gestation in two Holstein cows: transabdominal ultrasonographic findings in late pregnancy and pathologic studies of the fetuses. J Vet Med A 54: 624–626.
5. Buczinski S, Fecteau G, Lefebvre RC, Smith LC (2007). Fetal well-being assessment in bovine near-term gestations: Current knowledge and future perspectives arising from comparative medicine. Can Vet J 48: 178–183.
6. Carrière P, DesCôteaux L, Durocher J (2005). Ultrasonography of the reproductive system of the cow. [CD-ROM]. Faculté de médecine vétérinaire, Université de Montréal, St-Hyacinthe, Québec.
7. Curran S (1992). Fetal sex determination in cattle and horses by ultrasonography. Theriogenology 37: 17–20.
8. Durocher J, DesCôteaux L, Carrière PD (2002). Évaluation échographique du tractus reproducteur bovin: Détermination du sexe du foetus. Le Médecin Vétérinaire du Québec 32: 132–134.
9. Eley RM, Thatcher WW, Bazer FW, Wilcox CJ, Becker RB, Head HH, Adkinson RW (1978). Development of the conceptus in the bovine. J Dairy Sci 61: 467–473.
10. Evans HE, Sacks WO (1973). Prenatal development of domestic and laboratory mammals: growth curves, external features and selected references. Anat Histol Embryol 2: 11–45.
11. Ginther OJ (1998). Ultrasonic Imaging and Animal Reproduction: Cattle. Equiservices Publishing. Wisconsin, 304 pages.
12. Gjesdal F (1969). Age determination of bovine foetuses. Acta Vet Scand 10: 197–218.
13. Heyman Y, Chavatte-Palmer P, LeBourhis D, Camous S, Vignon X, Renard JP (2002). Frequency and occurrence of late-gestation losses from cattle cloned embryos. Biol Reprod 66: 6–13.
14. Hughes EA, Davies DAR (1989). Practical uses of ultrasound in early pregnancy in cattle. Vet Rec 124: 456–458.
15. Inomata T, Eguchi Y, Yamamoto M, Asari M, Kano Y, Mochizuki K (1982). Development of the external genitalia in bovine fetuses. Jpn J Vet Sci 44: 489–496.
16. Jonker FH, van Oord HA, van Geijn HP, van der Weijden GC, Taverne MAM (1994). Feasibility of continuous recording of fetal heart rate in the near term bovine fetus by means of transabdominal Doppler. Vet Q 16: 165–168.
17. Jonker FH (2004). Fetal death: comparative aspects in large domestic animals. Anim Reprod Sci 82: 415–430.
18. Kähn W (1989). Sonographic fetometry in the bovine. Theriogenology 31: 1105–1121.
19. Maneely RB (1952). Note on the ageing of bovine embryos. Vet Rec 64: 509–511.
20. Noden DM, De Lahunta A (1985). Digestive system. In: Noden DM, De Lahunta A (Eds.), The Embryology of Domestic Animals. Verlag Williams et Wilkins, Baltimore, London, Los Angeles, Sidney, pp. 292–311.
21. Noden DM, De Lahunta A (1985). Derivatives of the intermediate mesoderm: Urinary system, adrenal gland. In: Noden DM, De Lahunta A (Eds.), The Embryology of Domestic Animals. Verlag Williams et Wilkins, Baltimore, London, Los Angeles, Sidney, pp. 312–321.
22. Noden DM, De Lahunta A (1985). Derivatives of the intermediate mesoderm: Reproductive organs. In: Noden DM, De Lahunta A (Eds.), The Embryology of Domestic Animals. Verlag Williams et Wilkins, Baltimore, London, Los Angeles, Sidney, pp. 322–342.

23. Reef VB, Vaala WE, Worth LT, Sertich PL, Spencer PA (1996). Ultrasonographic assessment of fetal well-being during late gestation: development of an equine biophysical profile. Equine Vet J 28: 200–208.
24. Scanlon PF (1974). Orientation of cattle fetuses in utero in relation to stage of pregnancy. J Dairy Sci 58: 571–573.
25. Stroud B (1994). Clinical application of bovine reproductive ultrasonography. Compend Contin Educ 16(8): 1085–1097.
26. Takahashi M, Ueki A, Kawahata K, Goto T (2001). Relationships between the width of the metacarpus or metatarsus and the birth weight in Holstein calves. J Reprod Dev 47: 105–108.
27. White IR, Russel AJF, Wright IA, Whyte TK (1985). Real-time ultrasonic scanning in the diagnosis of pregnancy and the estimation of gestational age in cattle. Vet Rec 117: 5–8.
28. Winters LM, Green WW, Comsock RE (1942). Prenatal development of the bovine. Minn Tech Bull 151: 1–50.
29. Woodward PJ, Kennedy A, Sohaey R, Byrne JLB, Oh KY, Puchalski MD (2005). Diagnostic imaging—Obstetrics. Elsevier-Saunders, Amirsys Inc, Salt Lake City, UT.

Points to Remember

- A very good knowledge of fetal anatomy and ultrasonographic appearances of the fetal structures enables the practitioners to recognize the main landmarks of the gravid uterus greater than 55 days.
- The embryonic abdominal cavity is occupied almost entirely by the liver and the mesonephros. On day 65 of gestation, the liver extends past the umbilicus caudally.
- At 2 months of gestation, the stomach is divided into its four compartments. The rumen and the reticulum are similar in size to the abomasum, whereas the omasum is clearly larger.
- The abomasum and the omasum appear as hyperechogenic spots, whereas the rumen is the largest hypoechogenic region in the abdomen.
- Cervical, thoracic, lumbar, and sacral vertebrae begin to ossify starting on days 61 to 65 of gestation, with the coccygeal vertebrae starting on day 86 of gestation.
- The first centers of ossification in the skull, which appears very echogenic on the ultrasound image, appear toward the end of the 2nd month of gestation.
- Ultrasound fetal sexing diagnosis involves three steps. The first step is to locate the fetus (or fetuses) in the uterus, the second is to make sure that the fetus is alive and normal, and the third step is to complete the procedure with the determination of the sex of the fetus(es).
- Examination of the cow for ultrasound fetal sexing can be done between days 54 and 100 of pregnancy, but the ideal window of opportunity is between days 60 and 70.
- In the male, the genital tubercle, the urogenital folds, and the genital swellings are at the origin of the penis, the prepuce, and the scrotum, respectively.
- In the female, the genital swellings undergo gradual atrophy and eventually disappear around day 50. The genital tubercle becomes the clitoris and the urogenital folds form the vulvar labia.
- Most of the reported fetal anomalies were diagnosed at the time of fetal sexing and were probably not detectable at the embryonic stage.
- Although rare, the most easily detectable fetal anomalies that can be seen during ultrasonographic exams in cattle are schistosomus reflexus, amorphus globosus, conjoined twins, two-headed fetuses, and extrathoracic heart.
- Transabdominal ultrasonography examination with a low-frequency probe (2 to 3.5 MHz probe) is necessary to obtain good images when evaluating fetal well-being in late pregnancies.
- The ultrasonographic evaluation of fetal movements, heart rate, placental fluids, and placentomes are good indicators for the assessment of fetal well-being and are helpful to identify compromised pregnancies.
- Inactive fetuses during the entire ultrasonographic examination period or fetuses active throughout the entire examination time are fetuses that have a poor outcome.
- Fetal inactivity should be confirmed by repeating the ultrasonographic assessment. If the outcome is the same it should be interpreted as an indicator of fetal distress or death.
- Although hyperechoic particles are frequently observed in amniotic and more rarely in allantoic fluid, permanent visualization of a large amount of those particles in fetal fluids during repeated examinations is indicative of fetal death.

Summary Questions

1. Starting at what month of gestation do the testicles descend into the scrotal sac of the fetus?
   a. 2 months
   b. 3 months
   c. 5 months
   d. 8 months

2. Which compartmentalized cavity 2–3cm wide is located in the left section of the abdomen in this transverse section of the lower abdomen, taken at the level of the penis of a bovine male fetus at 100 days of gestation? The 10cm linear probe is located on the left side of the fetus.
   a. Reticulum
   b. Abomasum
   c. Urachus
   d. Dorsal and ventral sacs of the rumen

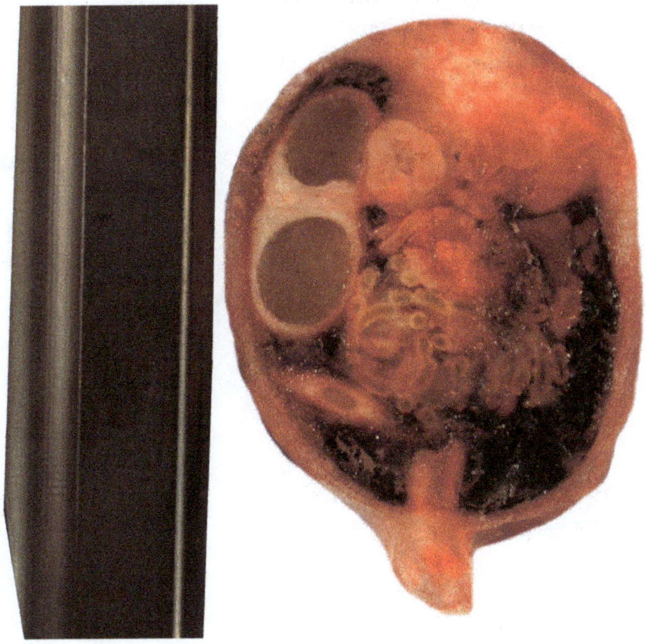

3. Identify the statement that is false regarding the scanning techniques when performing fetal sexing in cows.
   a. The ideal window of opportunity for fetal sexing is between 60 and 70 days of pregnancy.
   b. The possibility of establishing an accurate diagnosis at a later stage of the pregnancy (90 to 100 days) will depend on the position of the uterus within the abdominal cavity and the ability of the operator to reach the gravid uterine horn with the probe.
   c. Since the genital tubercle reaches its definite position only after day 58, it is never advisable to diagnose gender before that period of the gestation.
   d. It is an important step of the procedure to make sure how many fetuses are present in the uterus.

4. Looking at the ultrasonographic appearance of the genital tubercle from this male fetus in transversal plane, identify its approximate age (probe 7.5MHz; depth 6cm).
   a. 54 days
   b. 61 days
   c. 72 days
   d. None of the above

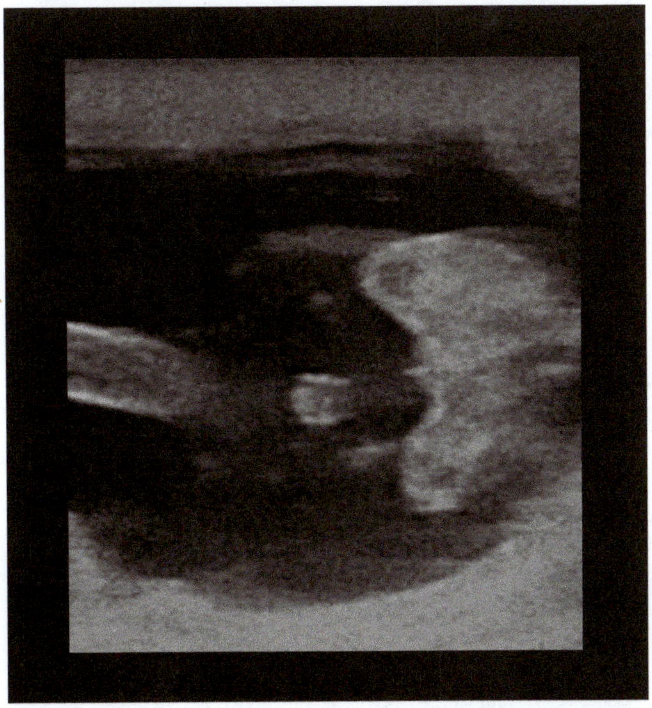

5. Identify the following structures from this day 60 female fetus in longitudinal plane: genital tubercle (GT), placentome (PL), tail (TL).
   a. 1 = GT / 2 = PL / 3 = TL
   b. 1 = PL / 2 = GT / 3 = TL
   c. 1 = TL / 2 = GT / 3 = PL
   d. 1 = PL / 2 = TL / 3 = GT

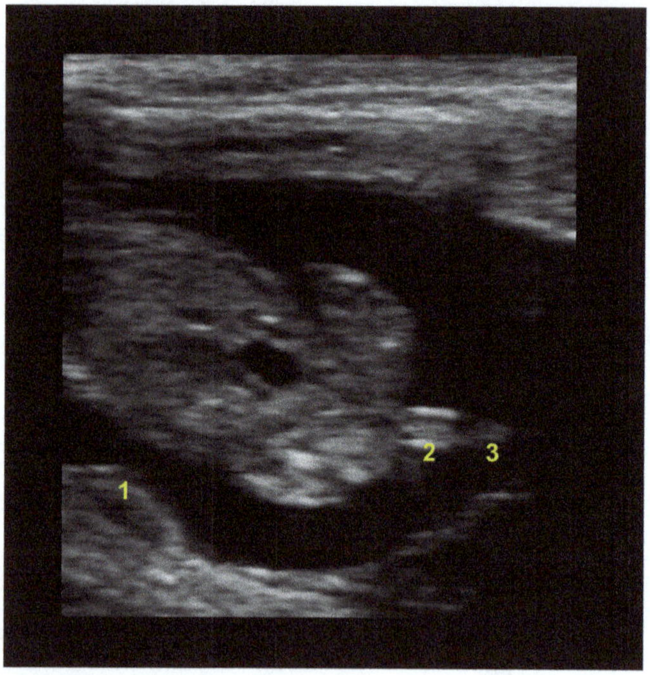

6. Observing a high variation of fetal heart rate measurements (90–125 bpm) during the ultrasonographic fetal viability assessment is
   a. Compatible with fetal distress and should be interpreted as a compromised pregnancy
   b. Compatible with normal nervous development and maturation of the fetus and can be an indicator of a healthy fetus
   c. Compatible with a disease of the fetus and is frequently observed in abnormal cloned calves
   d. Not conclusive

7. Which of those parameters is not indicative of fetal death when performing the ultrasonographic fetal well-being (UFWB) assessment in late gestation?
   a. The absence of fetal heart beat when imaging the fetal thorax
   b. Repeated fetal inactivity when performing UFWB
   c. Permanent imaging of echoic particles in allantoic and amniotic fluid
   d. Absence of visualization of the fetus when performing the UFWB

Answers

1. c
2. d
3. c
4. c
5. b
6. b
7. d

CHAPTER EIGHT

Bovine Embryo Transfer, in vitro Fertilization, Special Procedures, and Cloning

Brad Stroud and Jean Durocher

Introduction

An embryo transfer (ET) practitioner uses transrectal palpation for most diagnostic procedures related to the technology, i.e., corpus luteum (CL) counts and early pregnancy diagnosis. However, there are several clinical situations where real-time transrectal ultrasonography provides additional information to the veterinarian, which affects the technical and financial outcome of the ET process.[6,7] Whether it be a donor female on her first day of a superovulation protocol, a superovulated donor female in estrus, a donor female on embryo collection day, a recipient on transfer day, early pregnancy diagnosis for rapid recipient turnaround, or fetal sexing of the conceptus, ultrasound has become an essential tool for critical decision making that palpation alone cannot achieve in progressive embryo transfer operations. The images from this chapter are typical examples in which reproductive ultrasound has been proven over the past 20 years to aid in reproductive diagnostics in progressive ET programs.

It takes years of experience to become an accomplished bovine reproductive ultrasonographer. The authors realize that some proposed applications may vary between bovine practitioners. Although ultrasonography gives the practitioner an elegant view of both the anatomical and the physiological state of the reproductive tract at a given moment in time, one should always combine the information visible on a sonogram in conjunction with past and recent reproductive history before making critical diagnostic decisions or predicting outcomes. There are exceptions to several of the predicted outcomes illustrated in this chapter and many recommendations on ET come from the clinical experiences of the first author.

Notes About the Images

Most of these images were collected with an Aloka 3500 unit equipped with a small 3.75 cm (1.5 inch) curvilinear transducer (probe) of 10 MHz. This transducer is designed for use in human liver surgery to scan the surface of the liver for abscesses or tumors. The first author prefers this transducer over a straight linear transducer because the total contact of the probe with rectal tissue is 3.75 cm (1.5 inch) as compared with 10 cm (4 inches) for the linear probe, which creates a nicer image without black air space or reverberation artifacts (see Chapters 1 and 2 for more details) due to noncontact areas often seen when using a linear probe. However, a standard linear probe is used with success for these examinations by most practitioners.

Most of the images were taken in BB-mode, but a few were taken in B-mode. When in BB-mode, the left half of the image is always the left ovary and the right half of the image is always the right ovary. When in B-mode it could be either ovary, but only one ovary will be shown.

The reader should bear in mind that each image represents only a 1 mm slice of the ovary in a given plane (see Figures 2.3 through 2.5 in Chapter 2). More follicles or even an entire CL may be present on the ovary but may not be visible in a single still image.

Along both the left edge and bottom side of each image there are several green dashes that can be used to estimate sizes and/or distances on the image produced by the Aloka 3500. The distance between two large dashes is 10 mm. There is also a small green dash between every two large dashes, and the distance between a small dash and a large dash is 5 mm.

The follicles were categorized based on their sizes. Large follicles are ≥8 mm in diameter, medium ones are 4 to 7 mm in diameter, and small follicles are less than 4 mm in diameter. This categorization is also used in all other bovine chapters.

Embryo Donors

Day 1 of a superovulation protocol

Beginning with ET donor females on day 1 of a superovulation protocol, transrectal ultrasound gives the technician some insight into the number of small, medium, and large follicles that are present on both ovaries. Additionally, the presence of a CL indicates that the donor is in a physiological state of diestrus. The evaluation of the amount of small and medium sized follicles on the ovaries on day 1 of a superovulation protocol is a useful tool to predict the number of embryos at the time of embryo collection. Cows with a low number of small and medium-sized follicles at the onset of the hormonal stimulation protocol will usually give fewer embryos than the ones with an average or a high count.[3] Nevertheless, the ultrasonographer should be cautious in predicting the outcome of an embryo collection because there is variability in the fertilization rate from one flush to another. A highly significant correlation between the number of small and medium-sized follicles on the ovaries before the initiation of hormonal stimulation and the number of follicles at oocyte collection, as well as the number of transferable embryos produced from IVF is reported.[2,5] Also, large pathological cysts in the absence of a CL can persuade the veterinarian to strongly consider eliminating her from the donor pool. Cystic ovaries have been covered in Chapter 4 of this atlas.

Figures 8.1 to 8.3 present ultrasonograms of follicles before a superovulation protocol.

Ovarian response to superovulation from day 1 until embryo collection day

The superovulation protocol includes the administration of FSH twice daily during four consecutive days with prostaglandin $F_{2\alpha}$ being given in the AM and PM of day 3 along with the fifth and sixth FSH injections. Very few ET practitioners will enjoy the opportunity to scan donors every day throughout a superovulation protocol. However, there are a few points of noticeable changes of which the ultrasonographer should be aware. First, the antral follicles present on day 1 of the protocol do not show appreciable growth until day 3 (about the time of the first prostaglandin injection). Second, the most rapid follicular growth phase occurs between the first prostaglandin injection and the onset of estrus. Third, when using a high-resolution ultrasound unit, the regressing corpus luteum that was present at the onset of the superovulation protocol can still be visible at the time of estrus. This can be confusing to an ultrasonographer who is asked by an owner to scan the cow for estrus that otherwise may not be

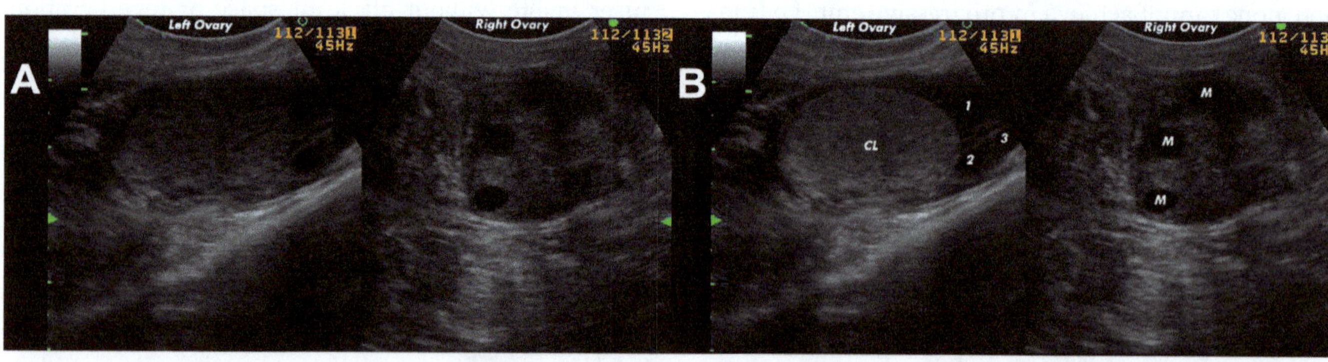

Figure 8.1. Ultrasonographic images in BB-mode with a low number of small follicles on day 1 of the first FSH injection in a donor cow. The left ovary has a 6 mm medium-sized follicle on the upper-right edge of the ovary (1). About 5 mm below that follicle is another 4 mm medium-sized follicle (2). The very far right tip of the edge of the ovary has a small 2–3 mm follicle (3). It sits between, and to the right of, the two medium-sized follicles. The remainder of that ovary consists of a large corpus luteum (CL). The right ovary has three medium-sized follicles (M).

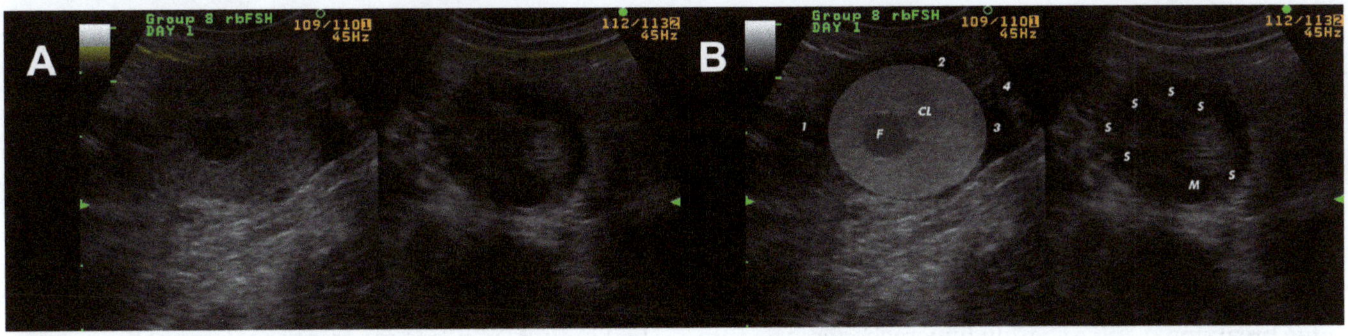

Figure 8.2. Ultrasonographic images in BB-mode with an average number of small and medium-sized follicles on day 1 before the first FSH injection of a superovulation protocol. The left ovary has a medium-sized cavitated CL with a 6mm fluid-filled center (F). It has three medium-sized follicles (1, 2, 3) plus a small follicle (4). Notice that the medium-sized follicles are flattened. That could be due to the ultrasonographer pressing the transducer too firmly against the ovary. The right ovary has one medium-sized follicle (M), and six small follicles (S).

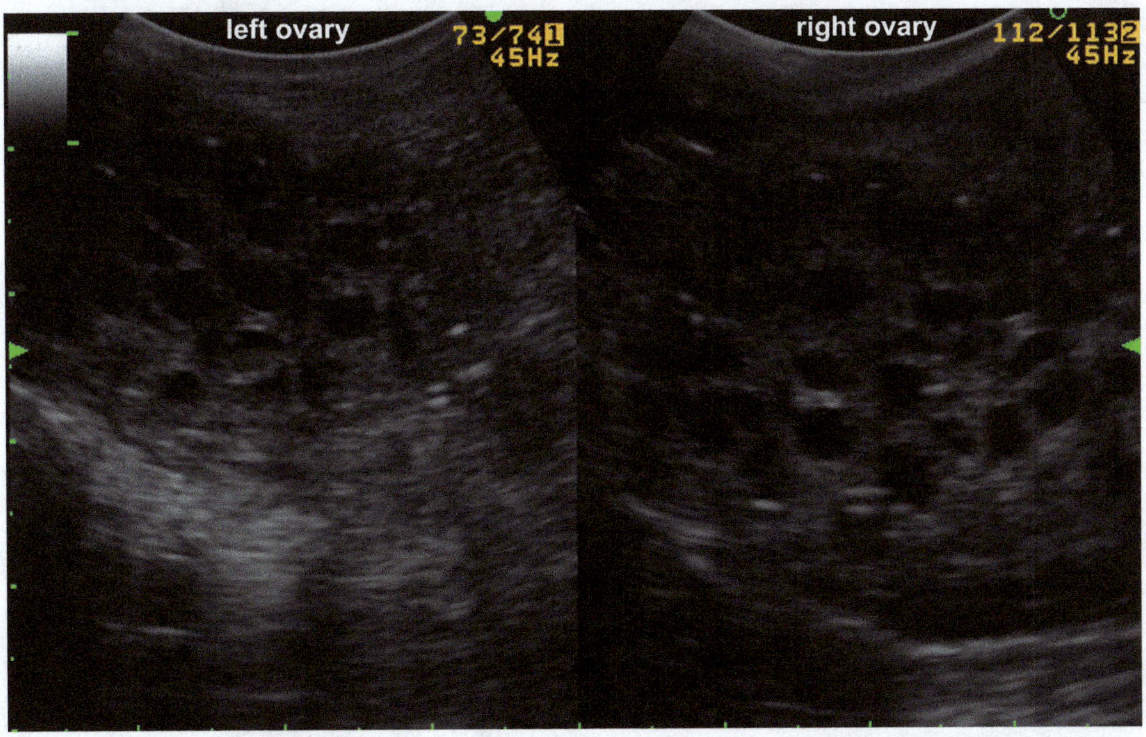

Figure 8.3. Ultrasonographic images in BB-mode with numerous small follicles on day 1 of the first FSH injection in a donor cow. This sonogram is self-explanatory. Both ovaries have numerous medium-sized and small follicles.

exhibiting signs, or that may be in standing heat with the need to predict a stimulatory response. The practitioner should be careful telling an owner of a donor that the cow is not going to come into estrus because the CL is still visible. It is very common for the CL to still be visible 12 to 18 hours after the onset of estrus. Close examination of the CL will reveal peripheral edge breakdown and a slightly hyperechogenic texture to the body or remnant of the regressing CL.

The following series of ultrasound images taken from the same cow demonstrate the evolution of the recruitment and growth of follicles in response to superovulation (Figures 8.4 to 8.8).

Response to superovulation at the time of insemination

By the onset of estrus, or certainly by 12 hours after the first mount, an ultrasonographer can count the number of ovulatory-sized (≥8 mm) follicles by carefully scanning back and forth across the ovaries. This is an important factor in determining whether to use rare or

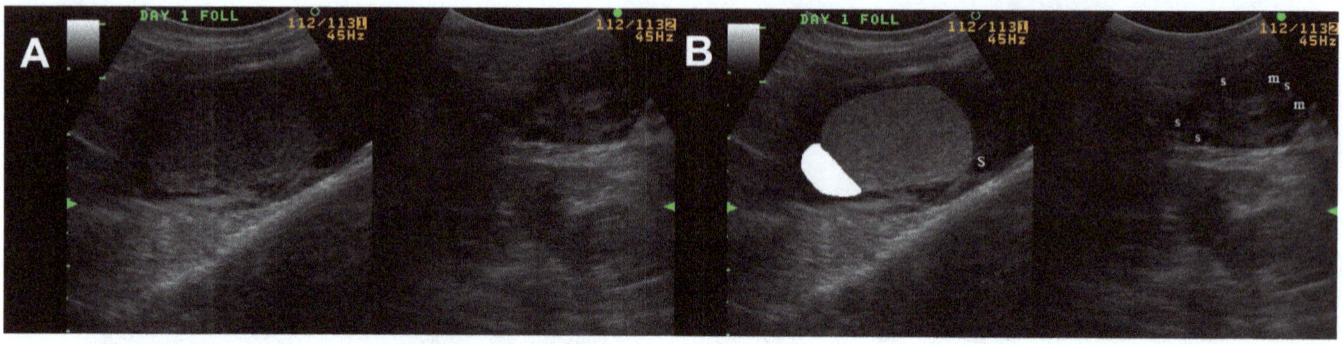

Figure 8.4. Ultrasonographic image taken on day 1 of the superovulation protocol. This image was recorded at the time of the first FSH injection. Left ovary: The left ovary image shows the luteal tissue of a CL that is approximately 3 cm in width (translucent white highlight). The lower-left corner of the CL is the ovulatory papilla (opaque white), which is that portion of the CL that protrudes above the surface of the ovary and is readily discernible by rectal palpation. The lower-right corner of the left ovary has one small (3 mm) follicle (S). Right ovary: The far right side of the right ovary has two medium-sized follicles (m) that are somewhat flattened by pressure exerted on the ovary by the ultrasonographer. The rest of the ovary has four small follicles, one of which is sandwiched between the two medium-sized follicles (s). The other tiny small black figures scattered across the ovary are cross sections of blood vessels. It is often difficult to distinguish between very small follicles and blood vessels.

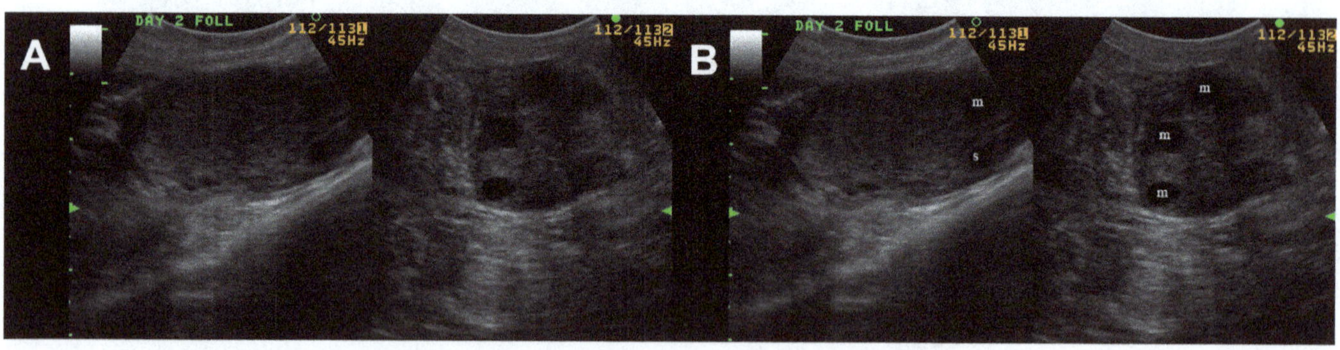

Figure 8.5. Ultrasonographic image taken on day 2 of the superovulation protocol. This image was taken on the second day of a 4-day FSH injection protocol on the same cow as in Figure 8.4. The left ovary is almost in the same position as it was during the scan of the previous day. However, it now shows a medium-sized follicle (m) immediately above the small follicle (s) on the right side of the ovary. This follicle is not a result of growth from the FSH injections of the previous day. It was present the day before, but it was not in the plane of the image captured the day before. The right ovary has three easily recognizable medium-sized follicles (m). When comparing the right ovary of day 2 with the right ovary of day 1 it is easy to see that the ultrasonographer has the probe or transducer in a different plane. Because ovaries are not perfectly round (many are oval and flattened), one plane will make the ovary appear larger than the other. Generally, follicles do not show noticeable growth after only 24 hours of stimulation.

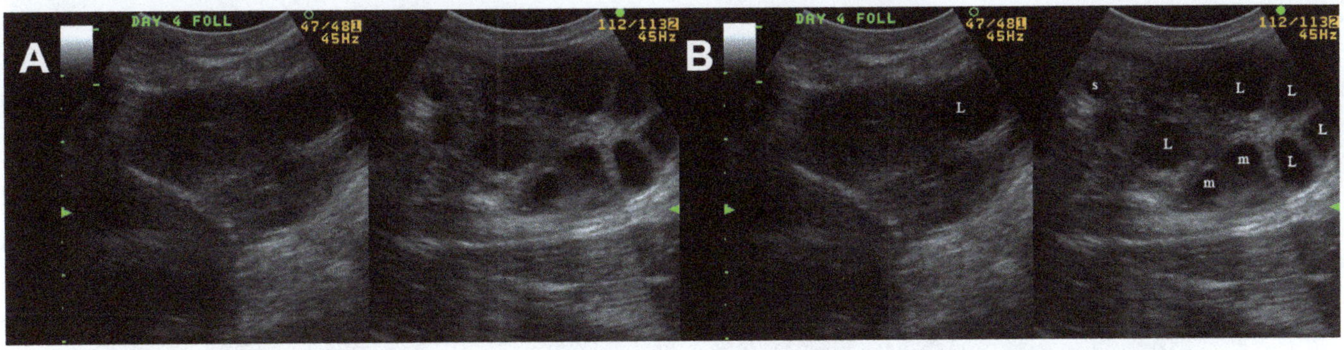

Figure 8.6. Ultrasonographic image taken on day 4 of the superovulation protocol. An image from day 3 was skipped, which was also the day that prostaglandin was given to the donor. Notice that the CL on the left ovary is noticeably smaller due to the effect of the prostaglandin the day before. The left ovary has a large 8 mm follicle (L) that was medium-sized 2 days previously. The right ovary now has five large follicles (L), three medium-sized follicles (m), and one small follicle (s). Recruited follicles from superovulation have their steepest growth curve 24 to 48 hours after prostaglandin has been administered. Notice that the right ovary has grown substantially in diameter. This is due to the growth of follicles globally from within that ovary. One must not forget that this image represents only a 1 mm plane through the ovary. By scanning the entire ovary an ultrasonographer would see about twice the number of large follicles as shown in this image. As a point of reference, this image was captured 21 hours before the onset of estrus of the donor.

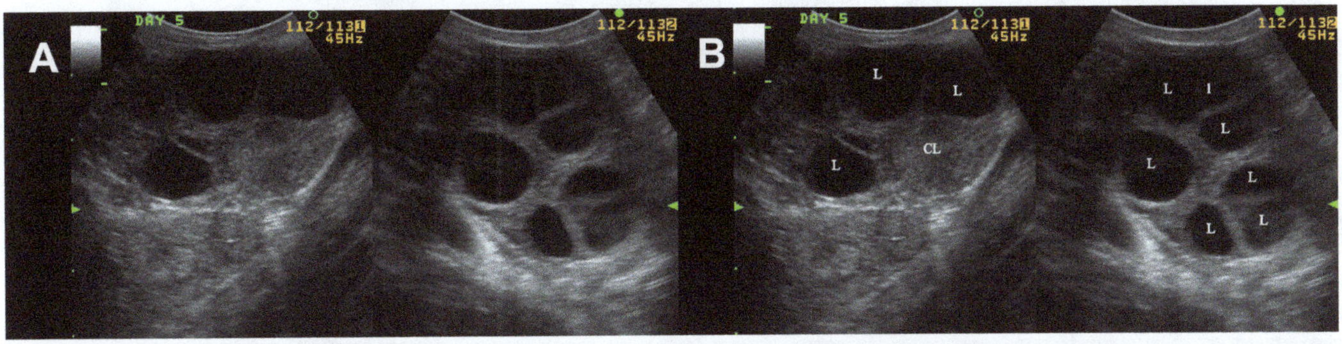

Figure 8.7. Ultrasonographic image taken on day 5 of the superovulation protocol. The donor had been in estrus for 3 hours when the cow was examined by the ultrasonographer. Note that the ovary has been inverted or flipped by the practitioner when compared to the day 1 image. The corpus luteum (CL) on the left ovary is still visible, but it is only half its original size. The left ovary now has three large follicles (L). The right ovary has seven large follicles (L) in the plane of this image. The upper-right follicle (l) appears to be medium-sized, but was labeled large because this view captures only a portion of that follicle. A slight rotation of the transducer in the rectum revealed this follicle to be greater than 12 mm in diameter.

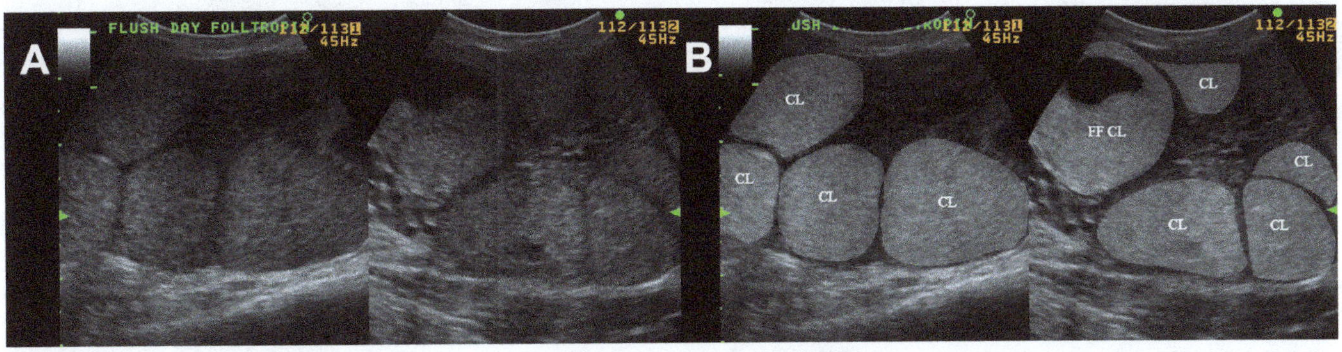

Figure 8.8. Ultrasonographic images captured on collection/flush day of the superovulated donor, which was 7 days after the onset of standing heat. The follicles that were present on day 5 at the onset of estrus have ovulated and formed CLs. The left ovary has four CLs (CL) and the right ovary has five CLs in this particular plane. A more thorough scan to other sections of the ovary will reveal more CLs. The right ovary has a large CL on the upper-left that is labeled FF CL. That CL has a fluid-filled center surrounded by luteal tissue (cavitated CL), and is considered normal. It is very common to see fluid-filled CLs on embryo collection day.

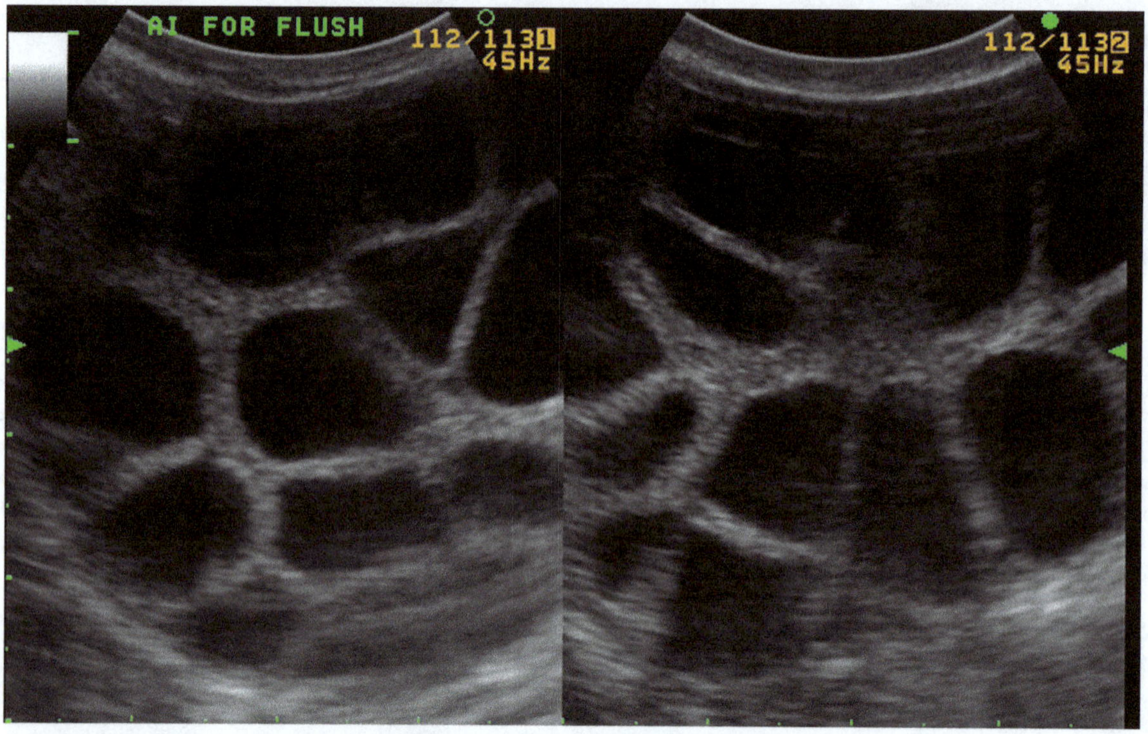

Figure 8.9. Ultrasonographic images of a superovulated donor in estrus after a heavy hormonal stimulation. This image is composed of numerous large follicles on both ovaries. A thorough scan of the ovaries of this cow through all geometrical planes revealed a total of 40 follicles. This could be helpful information when deciding to use rare or expensive frozen semen for a donor.

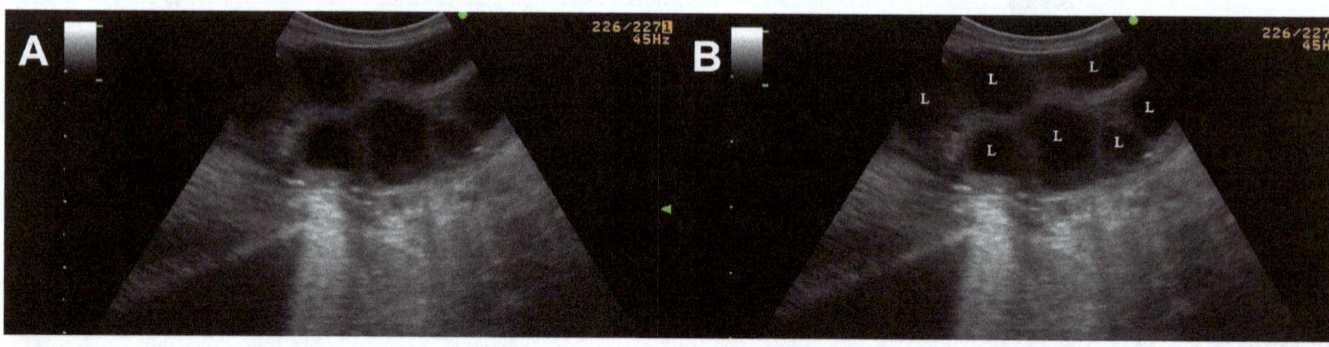

Figure 8.10. Ultrasonographic image of the right ovary of a superovulated donor in estrus after a moderate hormonal stimulation. The other ovary of this donor revealed a similar stimulation. This is a more moderate FSH stimulation than the one on the cow presented in Figure 8.9. This type of stimulation generally produces healthier ova than a heavily stimulated donor.

otherwise expensive semen on a superovulated donor female. A low number of ovulatory-sized follicles, as determined by ultrasound, is a consistently reliable diagnosis. On the other hand, just because there appears to be a high number of large follicles, that does not mean they will all ovulate and/or produce healthy viable embryos (Figures 8.9 to 8.10). It does, however, mean that there is a reasonable chance for a good superovulatory response and that the donor may be a good candidate for expensive semen.

Day after ovulation

This is perhaps the most difficult time to evaluate the status of the reproductive tract of a superovulated female, particularly the ovaries. The day after ovulation is difficult to define because ovulation can occur over a 24-hour period. To confuse matters more, in a strict sense, ovulation does not necessarily mean that the follicular fluid is expelled along with the oocyte and associated cumulus cells. In a classical ovulation most often the follicular fluid is expelled with the ovum. The removal of the follicular fluid occurs over a period of several hours, but endoscopy reveals that the cumulus oocyte complex is picked up off the surface of the ovary before the follicle fluid is completely expelled. One day postsuperovulation will often reveal a few day 1 CLs, plus some apparently unovulated follicles (intrafollicular fluid present). Day 1 CLs are often difficult to delineate since the luteal cells are just beginning to form the CL. The outer edge of the CL has not been fully formed/defined the day after ovulation, which makes it really difficult to identify or count them. The superovulated ovary at this stage of the cycle is mostly a confused mass of very early CLs without a well-defined outer edge, along with some apparently large unovulated follicles (not to be confused with very small follicles of the next follicular wave). In some cases, the follicular fluid remains for 7–10 days or more.

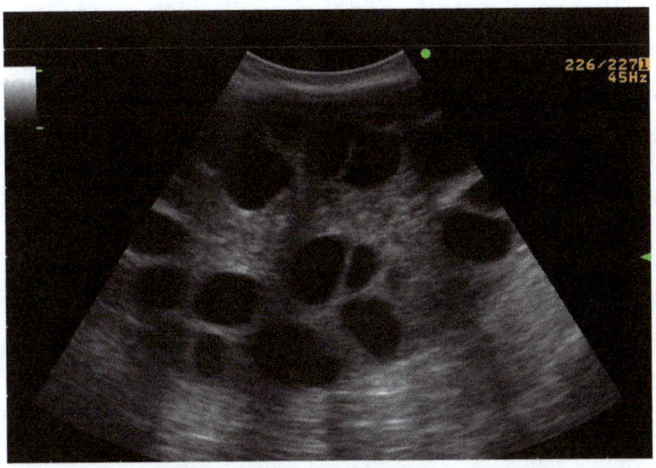

Figure 8.11. Ultrasonographic image from the right ovary of a superovulated donor cow in estrus. At least 14 large follicles are visible on this image of the ovary of a cow 12 hours after the first mount of a superovulated estrus.

This series of three images follows the same superovulated donor female from estrus to 60 and 72 hours postestrus to illustrate the complexity of ovulation from the point of view of an ultrasonographer (Figures 8.11 to 8.13).

Superovulated ovaries on embryo collection day

This is a situation where an ultrasonographer can have a tangible impact on an ET program. Counting CLs by rectal palpation can be unrewarding and sometimes embarrassing. A diagnosis by palpation can be either under- or overestimated. An ultrasound count is much more accurate, especially in the case of classical CLs that appear homogeneously echogenic. Often a palpator will diagnose more CLs, but the collection will reveal fewer total unfertilized ova, degenerate embryos, and viable embryos than CLs. Sometimes the palpator

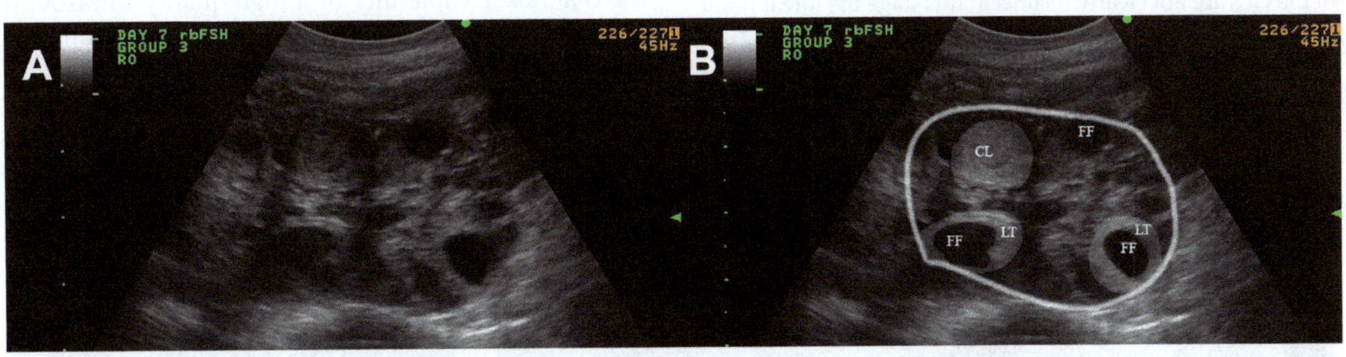

Figure 8.12. Ultrasonographic image from the right ovary of the same superovulated donor cow in Figure 8.11 examined 60 hours after the onset of standing estrus. Ovulation is one of the most difficult situations for a bovine reproductive ultrasonographer to evaluate or diagnose. Not every follicle expels all of its follicular fluid (FF) within 36 hours postestrus, especially after superovulation. Luteal tissue (LT) at this early stage postovulation can be difficult to distinguish from ovarian cortical stroma. In some cases the follicular fluid of an ovulated follicle will take several days to resolve and be replaced by luteal tissue. In other cases almost all of the follicular fluid from individual follicles will still be present on embryo collection day (7 days postestrus). Ultrasound units without high-quality resolution make accurate diagnostics difficult at this stage. CL: Corpus luteum.

will predict only a few CLs, and the embryo harvest will be double or triple the number that was predicted. A careful ultrasound exam will accurately reveal all the classical CLs, even the small nonpalpable ones that reside between the larger ones. The first author, as a matter of routine, relies on ultrasound to count CLs prior to the collection or flush. When the flushing process is complete, at least by feel, the embryo filter is rinsed and the total number of ova and embryos are counted. In the meantime, the Foley catheter remains in place inside the uterus of the donor. If the total number of embryos and/or ova count is less than the predicted CL count, the uterus of the donor is flushed several more times until the CL and total ova count are close. These repeated flushes result in an extra 0.9 viable embryo per collection over the course of a year. In the practice of the leading author in 2007, that resulted in 900 extra embryos being recovered from donors.

A clinical situation where ultrasound is extremely important on embryo collection day is when the palpator diagnoses only one CL. Very often ultrasound reveals more CLs than the palpator diagnosed. Prior to using ultrasound the first author elected to not flush these low CL count donors, and, in some cases, leave them pregnant with "one" embryo as a means of reproductive therapy. After numerous cases of twinning—and in two cases, triplets—ultrasound became an essential diagnostic tool in donors with low CL counts.

Perhaps the most unrewarding situation using ultrasound on embryo collection day is trying to diagnose anovulatory follicles. Unfortunately, an ovum can leave the follicle while the follicular fluid remains within the follicle. Even 7 days postestrus on embryo collection day ultrasound can reveal multiple large follicles on both or either ovary without any apparent classical CLs with luteal tissue. However, embryo collection may reveal a healthy number of viable embryos. As previously mentioned, the follicle fluid is not necessarily completely expelled along with the ovum from the follicle during ovulation, especially in superovulated females. As a result, the authors recommend flushing donors that ultrasonically are presented with large apparently fluid-filled follicles, but no classical homogenous CLs. Obviously, even though not visible via ultrasound, those fluid-filled structures are CLs with little or no visible luteal tissue along their borders.

The group of images that follows clearly illustrates the diagnostic capability of a high-quality ultrasound unit (Figures 8.14 to 8.19). Palpation can sometimes be inadequate when counting CLs. The use of ultrasound

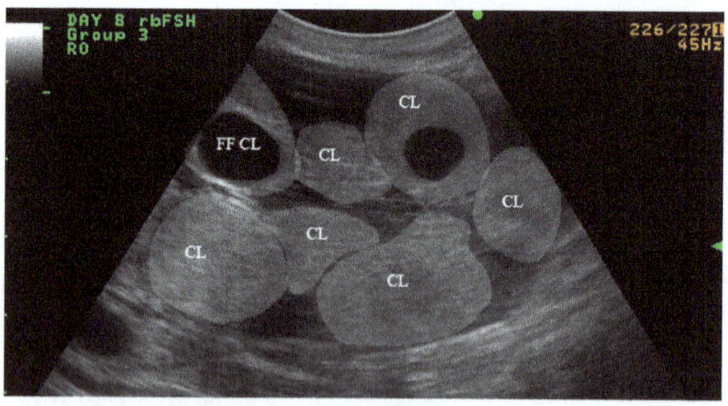

Figure 8.13. Ultrasonographic image from the right ovary of the same superovulated donor cow in Figure 8.11 examined 72 hours after the onset of standing estrus. The CLs at this stage are beginning to take shape. Although the edges of the CLs are not clearly distinct at this stage the luteal tissue is obvious. There are seven CLs in this image of the right ovary, two of which have a fluid-filled center (cavitated CL).

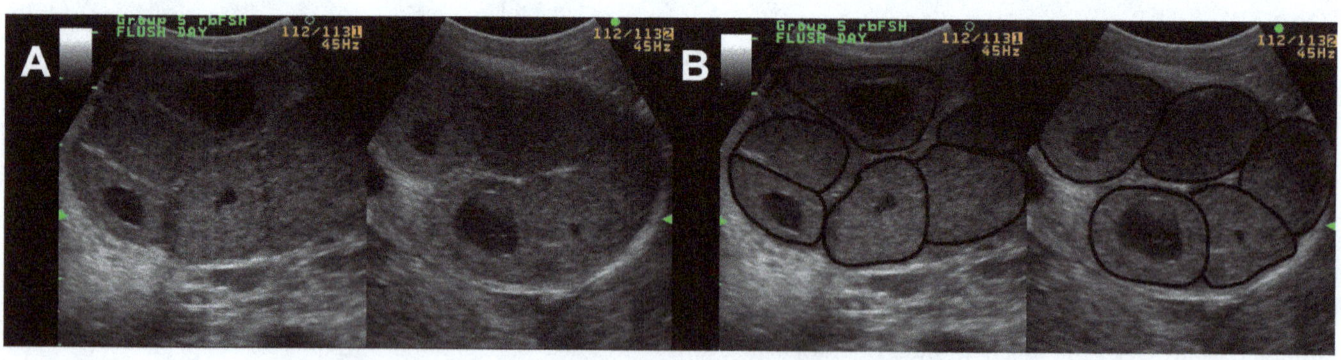

Figure 8.14. Ultrasonographic images of a good ovarian response to superovulation on the day of the embryo collection. There are five distinct CLs on each ovary. A few have fluid centers, which have no negative physiological effect on oocyte quality or eventual embryo development.

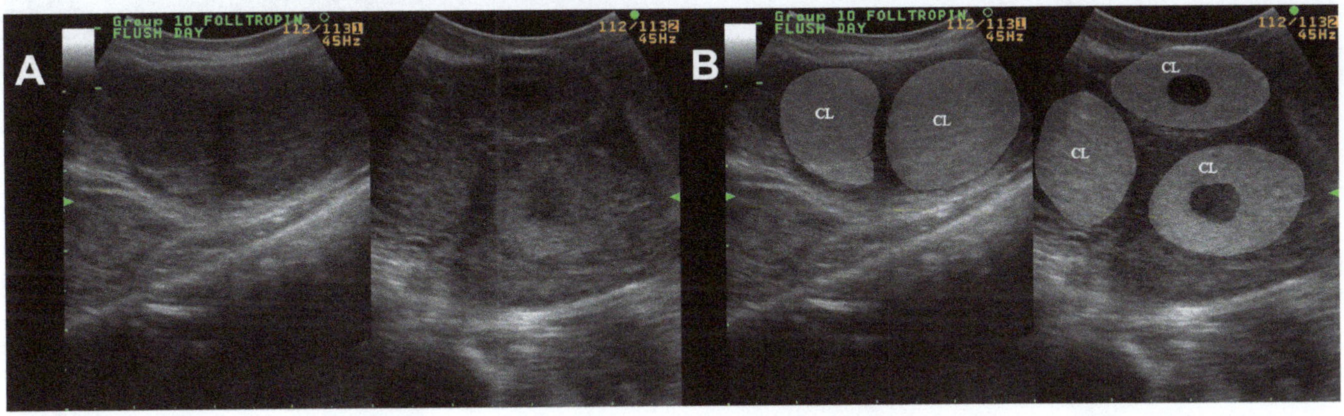

Figure 8.15. Ultrasonographic images of a mediocre ovarian response to superovulation on the day of the embryo collection. The left ovary has two distinct CLs, and the right ovary has three CLs.

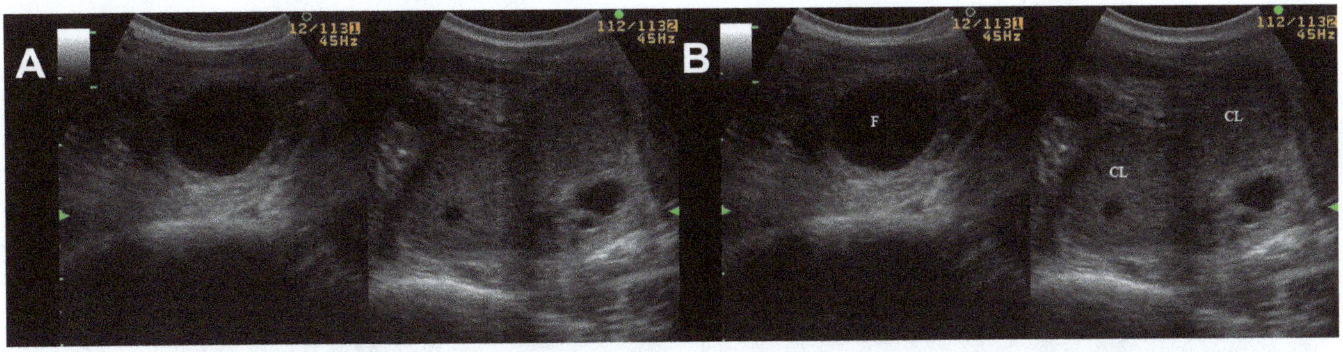

Figure 8.16. Ultrasonographic images of a poor ovarian response to superovulation on the day of the embryo collection. The left ovary has one large follicle (F), and the right ovary has two distinct CLs. A total of two ova could be expected to be recovered.

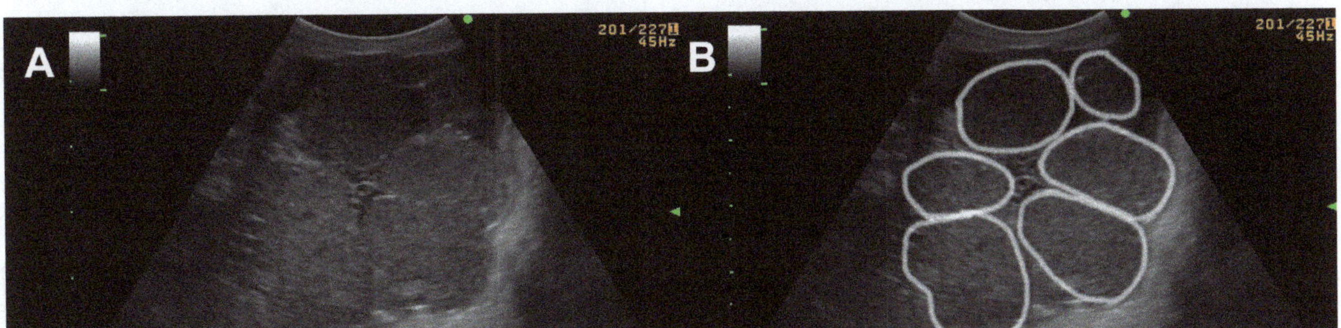

Figure 8.17. Ultrasonographic image in B-mode of one ovary with the presence of six solid or compact corpus luteum (CLs) on the embryo collection day.

gives a more accurate count of the expected embryo recovery rate.

Figures 8.14 to 8.16 present ultrasonograms of a good, mediocre, and poor ovarian hormonal response to superovulation on the day of the embryo collection.

Figures 8.17 and 8.18 illustrate the possible appearance of corpus luteum and follicles (Figure 8.19) on the ovaries on the day of the embryo collection. The presence of anovulatory follicles on embryo collection day is a potentially embarrassing diagnostic scenario for a bovine practitioner. It is sometimes difficult, if not impossible, to determine whether a follicle has ovulated. Sometimes there is a rim of luteal tissue surrounding the follicle that alerts the ultrasonographer that ovulation may have occurred. In other cases, there

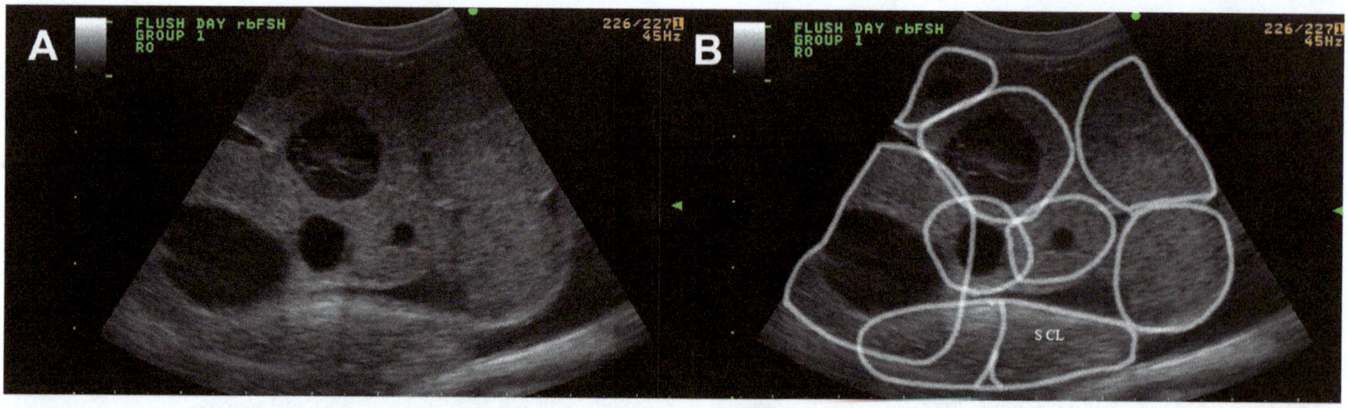

Figure 8.18. Ultrasonographic image in B-mode of one ovary with the presence of solid and fluid-filled corpora lutea (CLs) on the embryo collection day. This image clearly shows a healthy mixture of both solid CLs (S CL) and cavitated or fluid-filled CLs (FF CL).

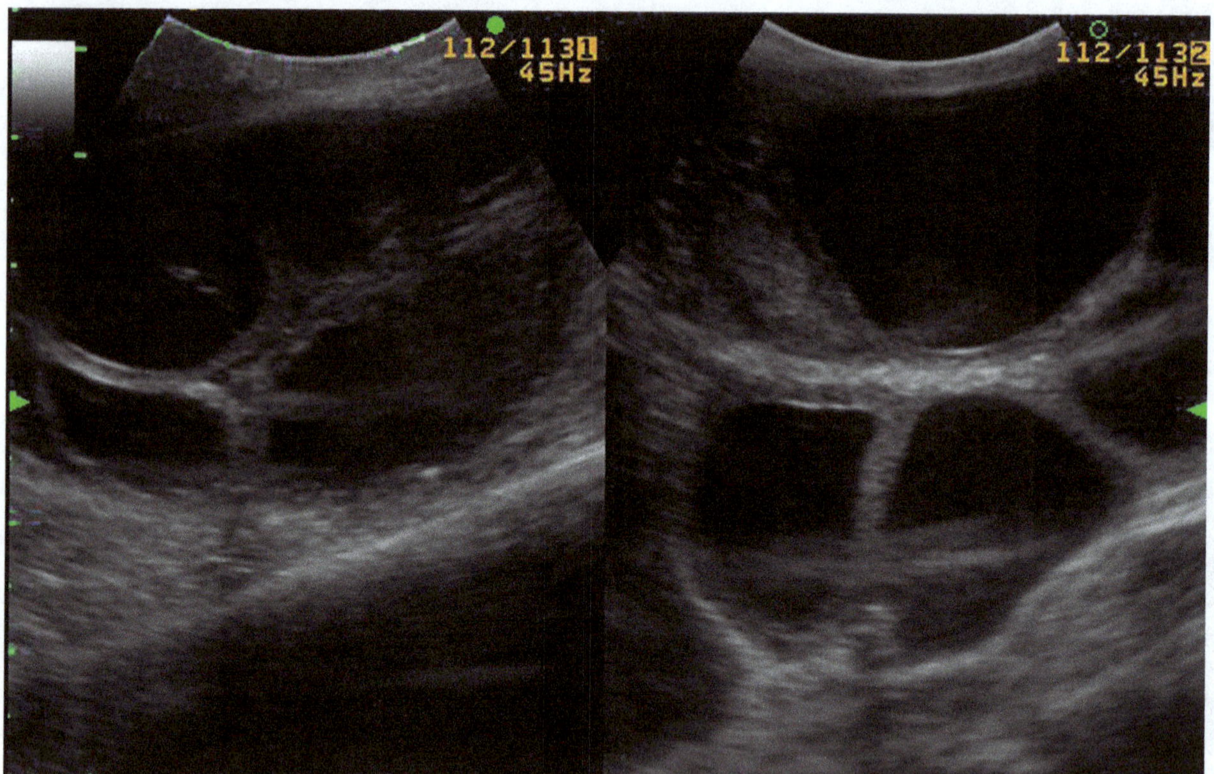

Figure 8.19. Ultrasonographic images in BB-mode of the ovaries of a cow with apparent anovulatory follicles on the embryo collection day. This image represents an actual donor that was flushed. On ultrasound examination there were only a couple of distinct solid CLs. However, the embryo collection revealed 15 total ova with 12 grade one embryos. The practitioner had told the owner to expect nothing from the flush. The reader can compare the luteal tissue on the outer perimeter of these follicles to those of the superovulated donor in estrus with a heavy stimulation in Figure 8.9.

is no apparent luteal tissue, and yet ovulation has occurred, which is proven by embryo recovery. Finally, follicles of a cow in estrus can appear to have a small rim of luteal tissue, which confuses matters even more. The description of Figure 8.19 illustrates this potentially embarrassing situation.

Oocyte Collection for in vitro Fertilization

In vitro fertilization (IVF) became a commercial adjunct to embryo transfer in the early 1990s after the advent of ovum pickup (OPU) with a transvaginal ultrasound probe. Using an elongated needle guide and a curvilinear transducer strategically angled at the anterior end of a plastic holder (collectively called a *vaginal probe:* Figure 8.20), the ultrasonographer guides the probe to the ovary, which is secured via transrectal manipulation with the opposite hand (Figure 8.21), where antral follicles are easily visible. Then by pushing an elongated 17 or 18 gauge needle through the vaginal wall and into the follicle, the ultrasonographer gently aspirates the contents of the follicle, including the cumulus oocyte complex and follicular fluid, into a collection vessel.

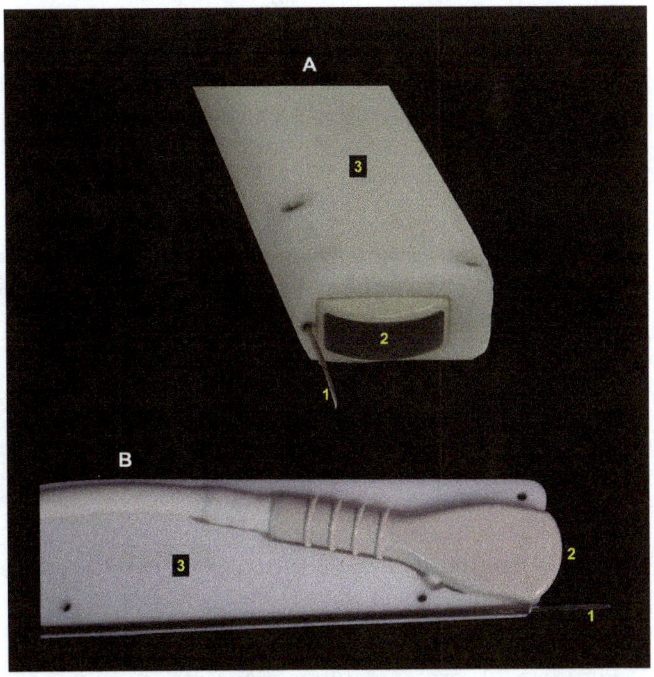

Figure 8.20. Photographs of the vaginal probe necessary for the ovum pickup procedure in cows. A: This picture demonstrates how the needle (1) enters the field of view into the edge of the curvilinear probe (2). B: Vaginal probe, which includes an elongated needle guide and a curvilinear transducer strategically angled in the anterior end of a plastic housing.

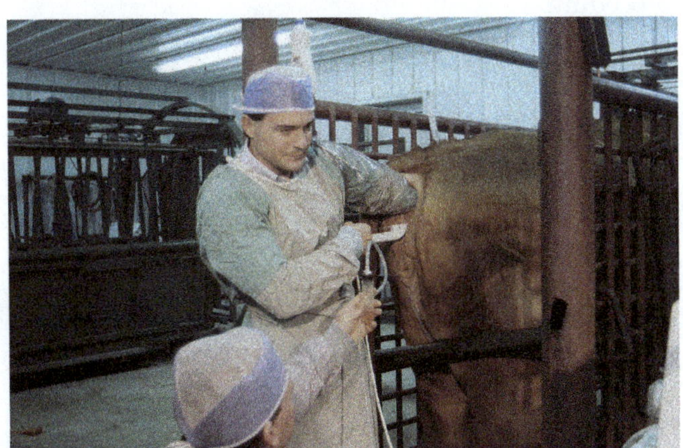

Figure 8.21. Demonstration of the technique to illustrate the ovum pickup procedure in a cow with a special curvilinear vaginal probe equipped with an elongated needle guide. Please note that the ultrasonographer guides the vaginal probe to the ovary, which is secured via transrectal manipulation with the opposite hand.

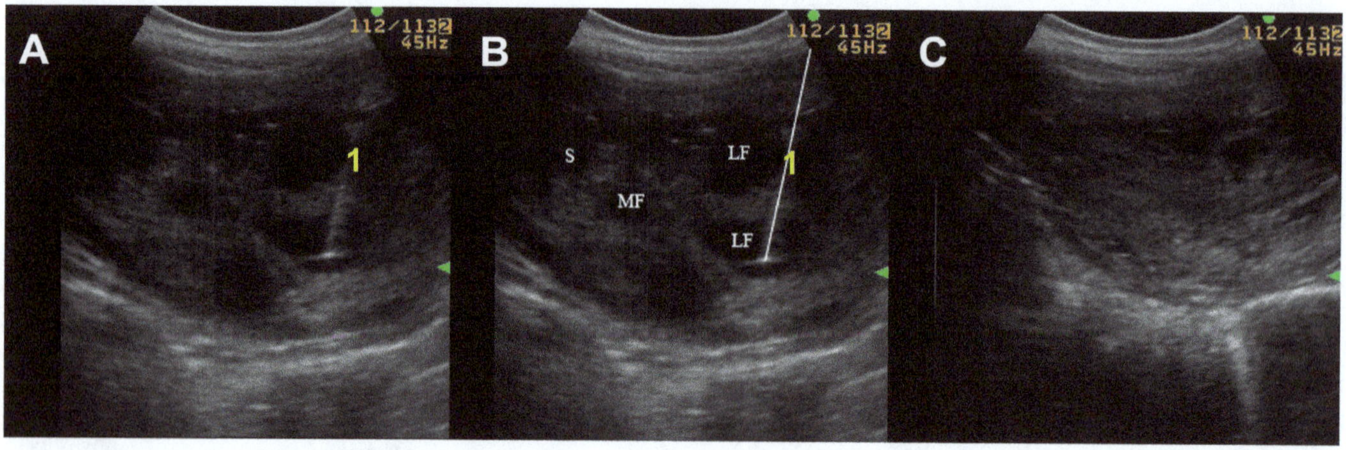

Figure 8.22. Ultrasonograms of the right ovary of a cow during and after an ovum pickup (OPU) procedure with the use of a special vaginal curvilinear probe equipped with an elongated needle guide like the one in Figure 8.20. A and B: The elongated needle (1) passes through the vaginal wall and into the right ovary where the practitioner guides it into a follicle to retrieve a cumulus oocyte complex (COC). The tip of the needle has been slightly scratched at the factory to elicit a hyperechogenic effect to help guide the ultrasonographer. Once the needle enters the follicle, slight aspiration is applied to retrieve the follicular fluid and oocyte complex; C: Ultrasonogram immediately after the OPU procedure. The follicles are no longer present on the right ovary. However, frequently the larger aspirated follicles will fill back up with blood making them appear not to have been evacuated. An inexperienced OPU practitioner may reaspirate these blood-filled follicles creating a very bloody collection. LF: large follicle; MF: medium follicle; S: small follicle.

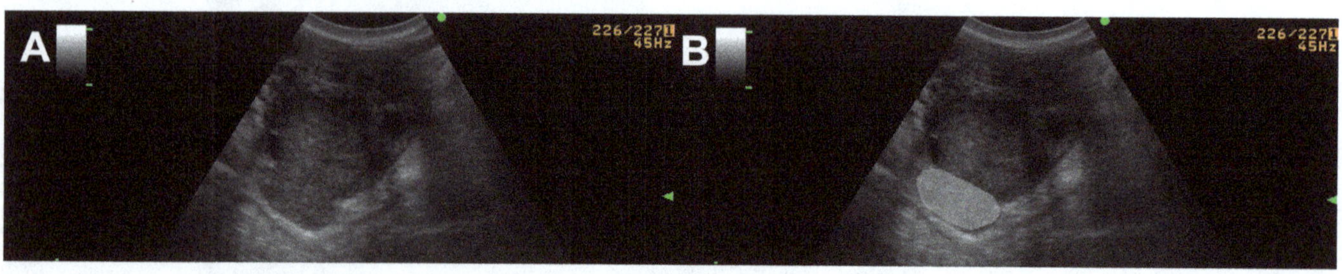

Figure 8.23. Ultrasound image of a corpus luteum (CL) with a papilla that is readily palpated. The papilla is the portion of the CL that protrudes above the surface of the ovary and is easily palpated. This type of CL is considered to be of good quality. The papilla is highlighted white in the right image.

Figure 8.22 presents ultrasonograms of a needle puncturing a follicular during the ovum pickup procedure.

Recipients

Ultrasound is of great benefit in choosing potential recipients. The first examination prior to synchronizing recipients assists in confirming that the recipients are indeed cycling. Many anestrous females will respond (show estrus) to progesterone-containing devices, but conception rates on embryos transferred into induced anestrous females are lower than conception rates in recipients that are cycling when synchronized with such devices. About 80% of CLs are diagnosed by rectal palpation and almost 100% by ultrasound.

At the time of embryo transfer an ultrasound examination to confirm the presence of an appropriate CL is as important as the ET gun itself. The decision to use ultrasound will often make a difference between an acceptable pregnancy rate of 60% and an unacceptable rate of 50% with fresh embryos. The extra effort to confirm the CLs by ultrasound could be the difference between retaining or losing the business of a client. Figures 8.23 to 8.27 present different qualities of CLs and highlight the advantages of ultrasonography over transrectal palpation.

Additionally, a quick scan of the uterus can pick up pathologies that would not have been diagnosed by transrectal palpation. Figures 8.28 and 8.29 illustrate

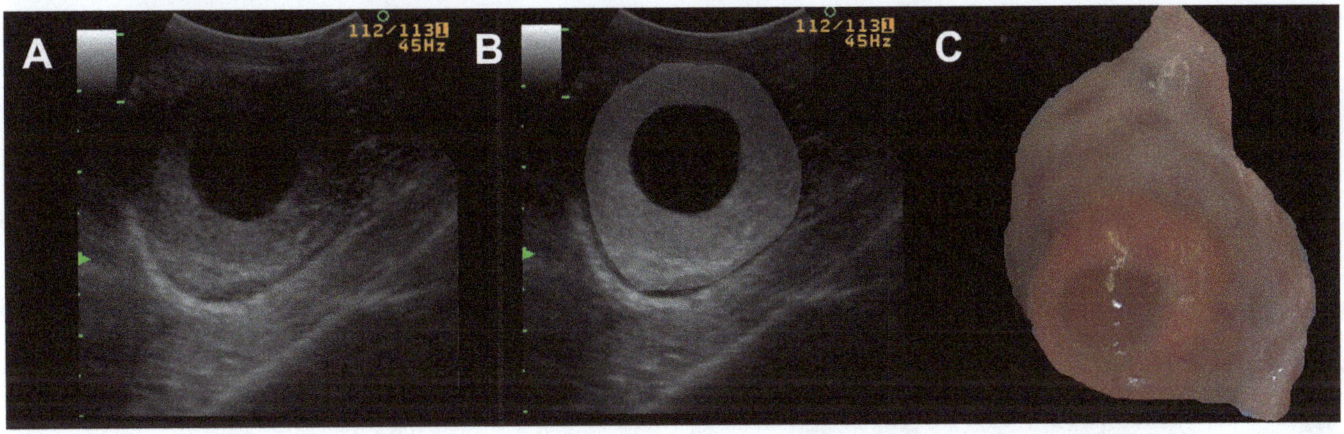

Figure 8.24. Ultrasound image of a cavitary or fluid-filled corpus luteum (CL) and its anatomical appearance. The center of this large CL is fluid-filled. It is considered a good quality CL. Pregnancy rates on recipients with fluid-filled CLs are equal to recipients with compact or solid CLs.

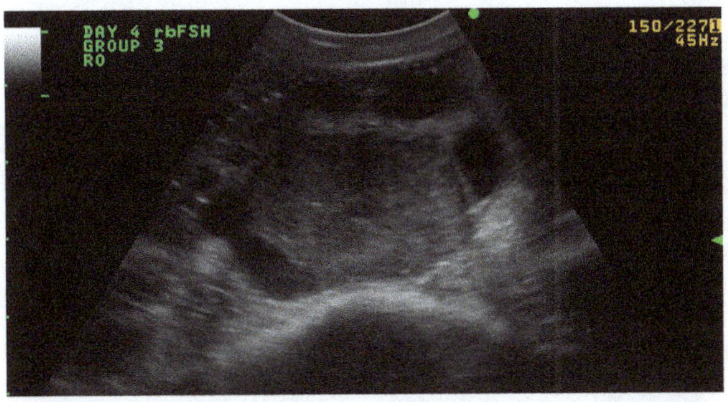

Figure 8.25. Ultrasound image of a nonpalpable corpus luteum (CL) surrounded by follicles. The CL in this image does not have a palpable papilla. It is also surrounded by several medium-sized follicles, which makes the CL very difficult to diagnose by transrectal palpation alone. The ovary will feel enlarged relative to its contralateral mate, but ultrasound is required to make a definitive diagnosis. The homogeneous echogenic luteal tissue is unmistakable.

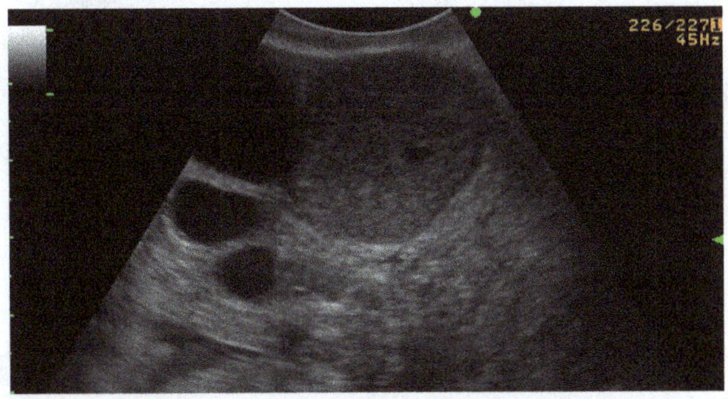

Figure 8.26. Ultrasound image of a large corpus luteum (CL) flanked by three follicles. Although the CL in this picture does not have a papilla and is not completely surrounded by follicles, one side is flanked by two large and one medium-sized follicle. Palpation alone requires a little guesswork under these anatomical circumstances whereas real-time ultrasonography confirms the diagnosis.

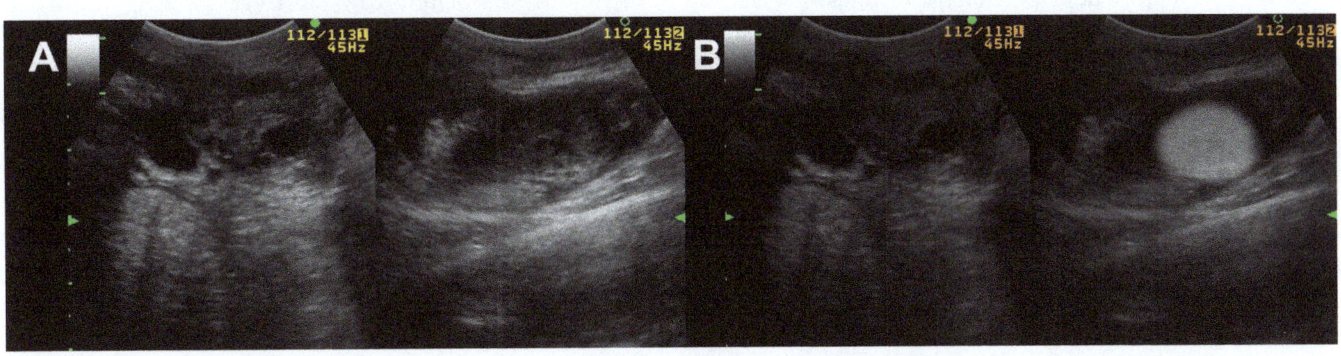

Figure 8.27. Ultrasonographic image in BB-mode of both ovaries of a potential recipient with the presence of a poor-quality corpus luteum (CL). The ovaries on this recipient are small. A CL was not palpable on either ovary although the right ovary was slightly larger. The right ovary has a small CL that is somewhat hypoechogenic compared to larger more homogenous luteal masses. Although there is no evidence to suggest that progesterone levels are lower in females with these types of CLs, it gives assurance to the ET practitioner to see luteal tissue on a relatively small ovary with a nonpalpable CL prior to transferring an embryo into such a recipient.

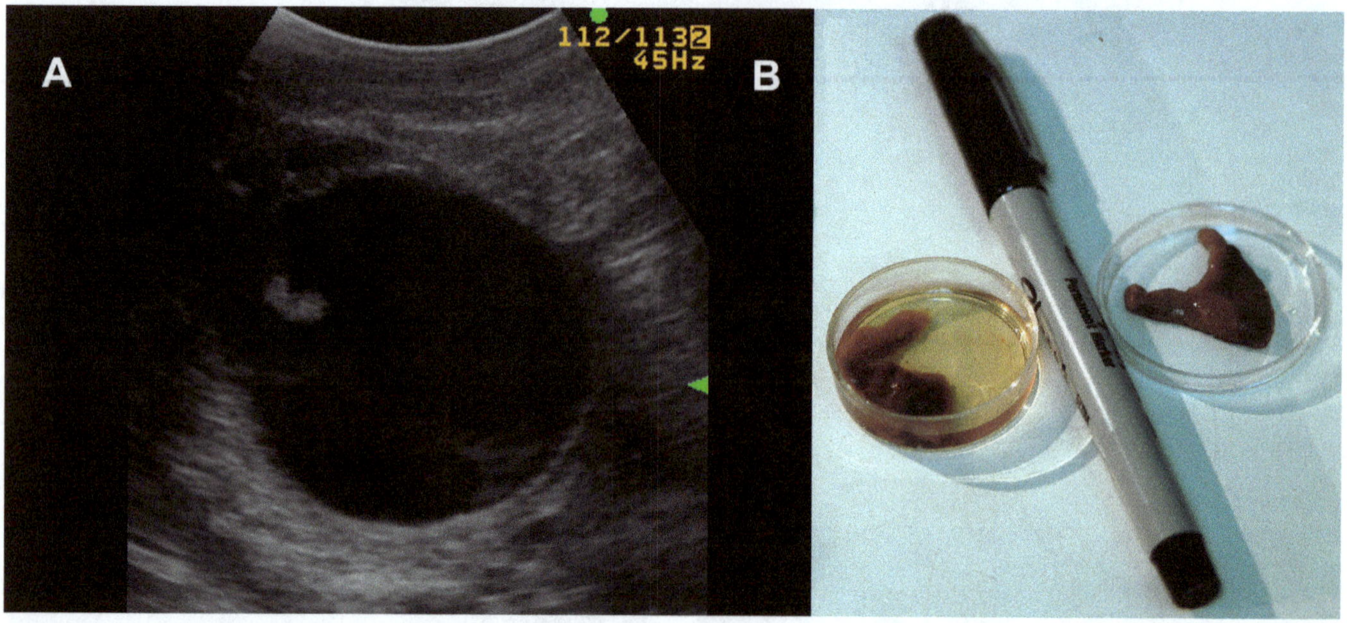

Figure 8.28. Ultrasound image of the uterus of a recipient with the presence of a floating mass within its content. A: Although the volume of fluid exudate in this uterus is palpable, the floating mass of dead myometrial tissue is not. A neophyte ultrasonographer might confuse this pathologic condition with early pregnancy. B: This photograph presents the actual tissue that was recovered via therapeutic flushing of the aforementioned female. Histology revealed myometrium (uterine muscle tissue).

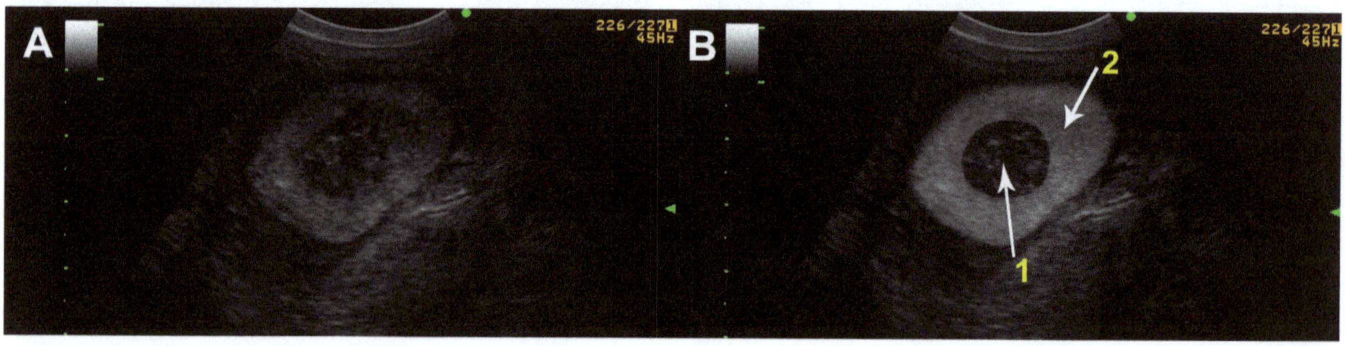

Figure 8.29. Ultrasonographic image in transverse section of the uterus of a mature cow presented as being a problem breeder. The uterine wall is slightly hyperechogenic, but the intraluminal area is abnormal. There are several hyperechogenic specks interspersed in a fairly well-defined and enlarged nonechogenic lumen. Recipients with abnormal uterine scans should be eliminated as candidates for embryos.

some examples of pathological conditions which could not have been diagnosed without the use of ultrasonographic examinations.

Management of Clone Recipients

Cloning is an emerging technology in the bovine industry. On January 15, 2008, after years of detailed study and analysis, the United States Food and Drug Administration has concluded that meat and milk from clones of cattle, swine, and goats, and the offspring of clones from any species traditionally consumed as food, are as safe to eat as food from conventionally bred animals. There was insufficient information for the agency to reach a conclusion on the safety of food from clones of other animal species, such as sheep.[10]

The agency also stated that an animal clone is a genetic copy of a donor animal, similar to an identical

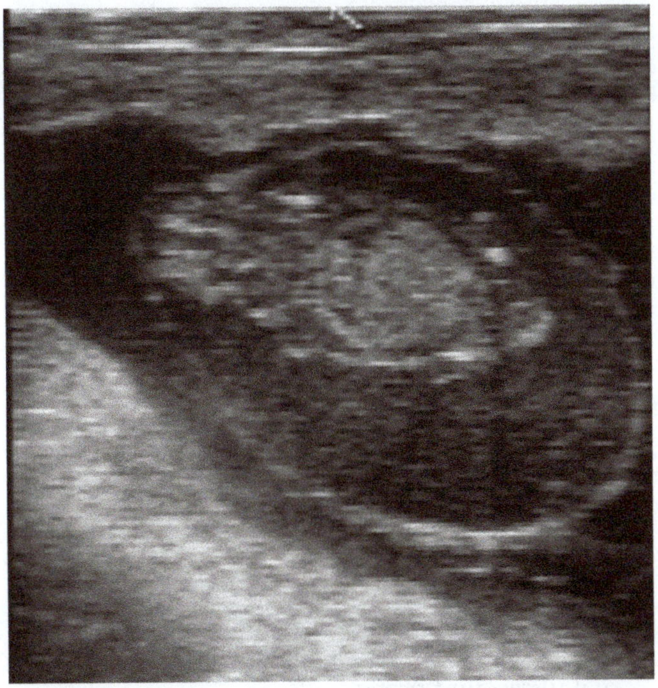

Figure 8.30. Sonogram of a dead clone fetus (probe 7.5 MHz; depth 6 cm). The examination was performed at 70 days of gestation. Although the size of the gravid uterine horn was compatible with a pregnancy of that stage, it is obvious when one looks at the size of the fetus (3 cm) that it died 3 weeks before the examination at around 50 days.

twin, but born at a different time. Cloning is not the same as genetic engineering, which involves altering, adding, or deleting DNA; cloning does not change the gene sequence.[10]

This technology has been in use on a research basis for many years and the management of the clone pregnancies by ultrasonography is a very important component of any cloning program. As observed with other assisted reproductive technologies,[8,9] the embryonic mortality and abortion rate of recipients carrying clone embryos is higher than normal. The conception rate of clone embryos is generally acceptable early in gestation (30 days). The first trimester of the pregnancy is a critical period when a high incidence of fetal death is observed. A follow-up of these pregnancies until 100 days of gestation is very important because many of these fetal deaths will not be followed by immediate expulsion of the fetus. Although the abortion rate will be higher throughout gestation, the prenatal period is another critical time when the evaluation of fetal well-being is crucial.[1] The timing of assisted parturition might be influenced by the evaluation of the near-term fetal well-being (see Chapter 7 for more information). A recent study shows that conception rate following the transfer of a clone embryo drops from 37% (30 days) to 23% (60 days), 18% (90 days), and 10% (270 days).[4] Figure 8.30 is a sonagram of a dead clone fetus.

References

1. Buczinski SM, Fecteau G, Lefebvre RC, Smith LC (2007). Fetal well-being assessment in bovine near-term gestations: current knowledge and future perspectives arising from comparative medicine. Can Vet J 48(2): 178–183.
2. Durocher J, Morin N, Blondin P (2006). Effect of hormonal stimulation on bovine follicular response and oocyte developmental competence in a commercial operation. Theriogenology 65(1): 102–115.
3. Durocher J, Morin N, Blondin P (2006). Using ultrasonography to predict response to superovulation. American Embryo Transfer Association—Canadian Embryo Transfer Association 2006 Joint Convention Proceedings, pp. 45–53.
4. Panarace M, Agüero JI, Garrote M, Jauregui G, Sagovia A, Cané L, Gutiérrez J, Marfil M, Rigali F, Pugliese M, Young S, Lagioia J, Garnil C, Forte Pontes JE, Ereno Junio JC, Mower S, Medina M (2007). How healthy are clones and their progeny: 5 years of field experience. Theriogenology 67(1): 142–151.
5. Sing J, Dominguez M, Jaiswal R, Adam GP (2004). A simple ultrasound test to predict the superstimulatory response in cattle. Theriogenology 62(1–2): 227–243.
6. Stroud BK (1994). Clinical applications of bovine reproductive ultrasonography. Comp Cont Educ 16(8): 1085–1097.
7. Stroud, BK (1997). Bovine reproductive ultrasonogaphy [DVD]. Biotech Productions, Texas.
8. van Wagtendonk-de Leeuw AM, Aerts BJ, den Daas JH, Kemp B, de Ruigh L (1998). Abnormal offspring following in vitro production of bovine preimplantation embryos: a field study. Theriogenology 49(5): 883–894.
9. van Wagtendonk-de Leeuw AM, Mullaart E, de Roos AP, Merton JS, den Daas JH, Kemp B, de Ruigh L (2000). Effects of different reproduction techniques: AI MOET or IVP, on health and welfare of bovine offspring. Theriogenology 53(2): 575–597.
10. http://www.fda.gov/cvm/cloning (FDA Press Release, January 15, 2008). FDA Issues Documents on the Safety of Food from Animal Clones.

Points to Remember

- There are several clinical situations where real-time transrectal ultrasonography provides much more information to the veterinarian, which affects the technical and financial outcome of the embryo transfer (ET) process.
- Ultrasound has become an essential tool for critical decision making in embryo transfer technology that palpation alone cannot achieve. Examples are the evaluation of the donor female on her first day of a superovulation protocol, estimating the response of a superovulated donor female in estrus, estimating the number of potential embryos from a donor female on embryo collection day, evaluating a recipient on transfer day, early pregnancy diagnosis for rapid recipient turn around, and fetal sexing of the pregnant recipient's conceptus.
- The follicular fluid is not necessarily always completely expelled along with the ovum during ovulation, especially in superovulated females. Examination 7 days after superovulation will often reveal a few CLs, plus some apparently anovulatory follicles. Some of the apparently anovulatory follicles did indeed ovulate, but retained fluid. As a result, the authors recommend flushing donors that ultrasonically are presented with large, apparently fluid-filled follicles, but no classical homogenous CLs.
- A thorough ultrasound examination of the ovaries enables the practitioner to detect and accurately count all corpora lutea on embryo collection day. If the total ova count is short of the predicted CL count, the donor's uterus is flushed several more times until the CL and total ova count are close. These repeated flushes result in an average extra 0.9 viable embryos per collection.
- Ultrasound is of great benefit in choosing potential recipients. The first examination prior to synchronizing recipients assists in confirming that the recipients are indeed cycling. At the time of embryo transfer an ultrasound examination must confirm the presence of an appropriate CL and a healthy uterus in order to maximize the conception rate.
- In vitro fertilization (IVF) became a commercial adjunct to embryo transfer in the early 1990s after the advent of ovum pickup (OPU) with a transvaginal ultrasound probe.
- The management of the clone pregnancies by ultrasonography is a very important component of any cloning program. As observed with other assisted reproductive technologies, the embryonic mortality and abortion rate of recipients carrying clone embryos is higher than normal.

Summary Questions

1. From the information obtained from the scanning of the ovaries of these two cows done just before the first FSH injection of the superovulation protocol, which donor do you feel has the best chance of giving a higher number of good-quality embryos at the time of the embryo collection?
   a. Cow A
   b. Cow B

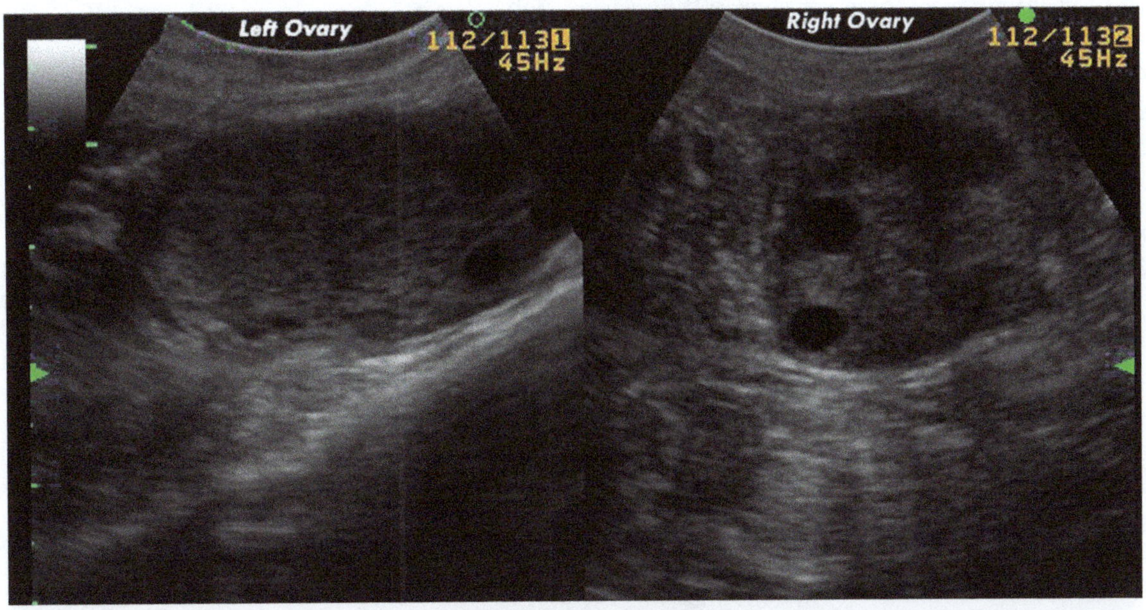

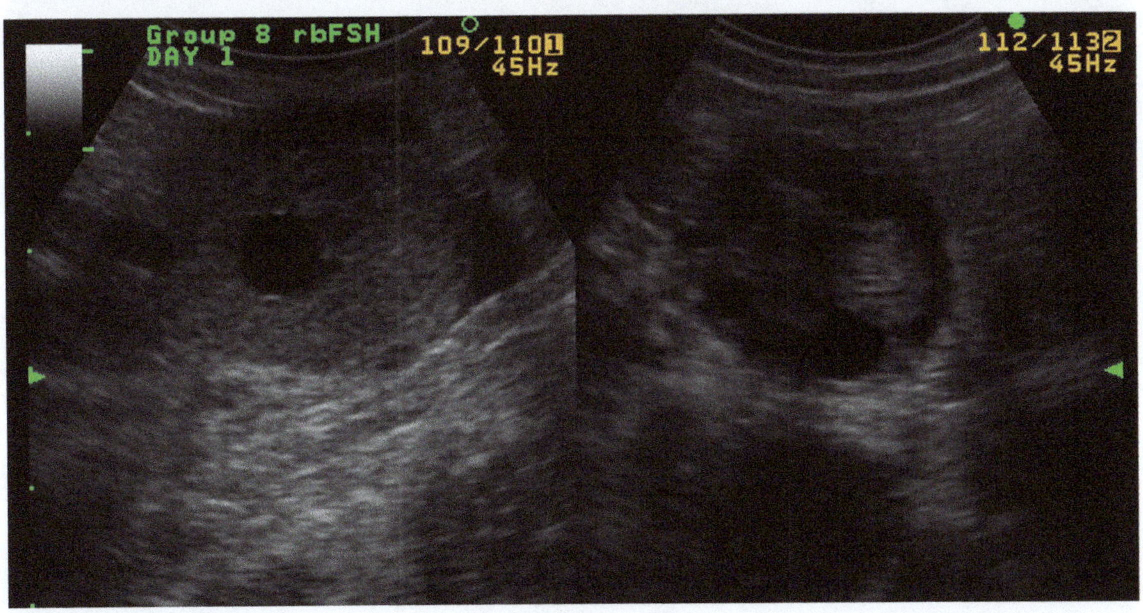

2. Which of the following statements is false? When scanning a donor cow at the onset of heat during the superovulation protocol:
   a. One can predict that a low number of ovulatory-sized follicles will lead to a low number of good-quality embryos at embryo collection.
   b. One can predict that a high number of ovulatory-sized follicles will lead to a high number of good-quality embryos at embryo collection.
   c. A high number of ovulatory-sized follicles might lead to a low number of good-quality embryos at embryo collection if many follicles fail to ovulate.
   d. A high number of ovulatory-sized follicles might lead to a low number of good-quality embryos at embryo collection if the fertilization rate is low.

3. At the time of embryo collection, if the total number of unfertilized eggs, degenerate embryos, and good-quality embryos is low compared to the number of CLs on the ovaries, reflushing the donor cow might be a good idea.
   a. True
   b. False

Answers

1. b
2. b
3. a

CHAPTER NINE

Bull Anatomy and Ultrasonography of the Reproductive Tract

Giovanni Gnemmi and Réjean Lefebvre

Introduction

Fertility is ultimately one of the most important factors for the cattle industry. In the last decade, many studies have reported a decrease in fertility in the commercial model of intensive management and high-producing animals. This reproductive inefficiency in the United States alone causes a loss of from 1 to 5 billion dollars per year[11]. Considering the male/female ratio, fertility of bulls is a key factor in the overall success of the cattle industry and must be maintained at its optimum potential[13]. Breeding soundness evaluation (BSE) is a reliable clinical method to differentiate bulls with high fertility potential from those that are clearly unsatisfactory. However, it does not allow the veterinarian to establish a specific diagnosis and, therefore, estimate a prognosis. Routine BSE is currently based on semen parameters, scrotal circumference, and manual testicular palpation; however, other techniques are often needed to pursue a specific diagnosis. Compared to other more specialized examination procedures (biopsy), ultrasonography is a noninvasive and nontraumatic technique that does not involve risks to the reproductive potential of the bulls[9,10,15]. The most promising application of ultrasonography is to establish precisely the type and the location of the pathological conditions (diagnosis) of the different organs of the male reproductive tract and, consequently, give a prognosis. For valuable individual animals on farms or in bull testing centers, it is worthwhile to pursue a complete diagnostic approach to investigate causes of bull infertility.

Ultrasonographic imaging adds a new dimension to the BSE by effectively allowing clinical assessment of the structures and function of the reproductive tract. Therefore, real-time ultrasonography has significant advantages in the diagnosis of penile, testicular, epididymal, and accessory sex gland abnormalities. The ultrasonographical examination of the male reproductive tract should always be preceded by, at least, a partial BSE and is not mandatory with a satisfactory BSE. It should be performed in specific situations such as the following[7,12]:

- Azoospermia
- Presence of a high number of morphological abnormal sperms
- Pyospermia
- Abnormal size or shape of the reproductive organs
- Unexplained pain

The first part of this chapter presents the ultrasound equipment and techniques that are recommended in order to complete the bull evaluation of the key reproductive organs. The second portion reviews the anatomy, the specific scanning techniques, and the normal appearances of external genitalia and accessory reproductive glands of the bull. Finally, the third section describes and illustrates the most frequent anomalies and ultrasonographic findings of the external and internal reproductive organs of the bull.

Ultrasound Equipment and Techniques

A B-mode (brightness modality), real-time scanner fitted with a 5.0 to 7.5 MHz linear-array transducer

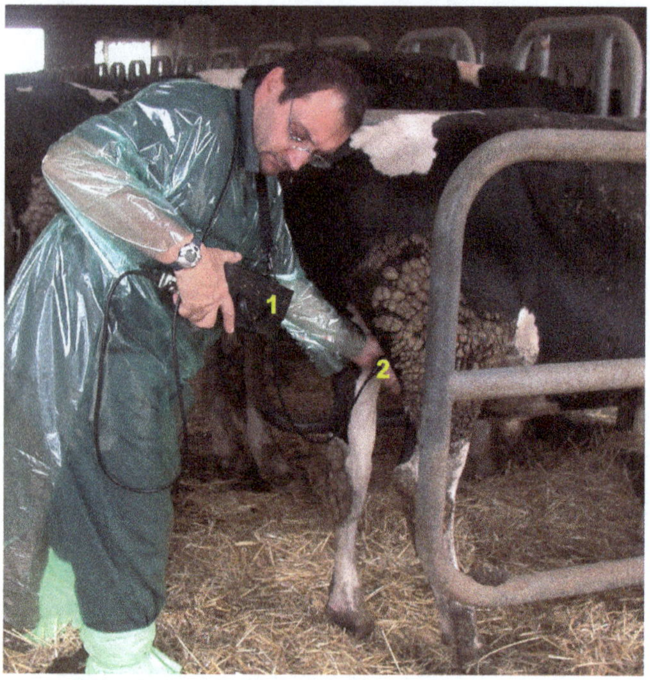

Figure 9.1. Posterior approach to the bull for the ultrasonographic examination of the testicles. 1: Portable ultrasound machine; 2: Linear probe or transducer.

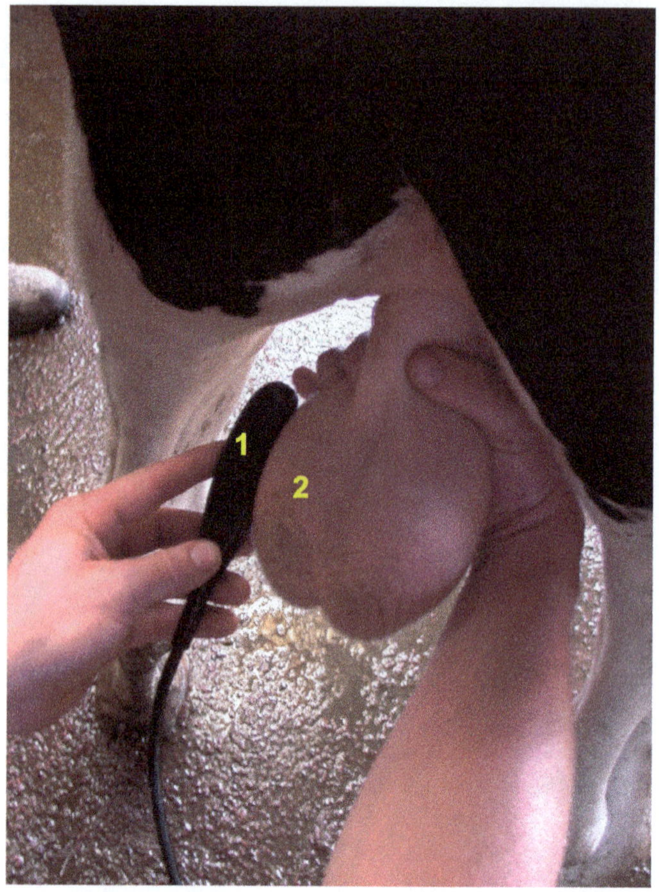

Figure 9.2. Ultrasonographic examination of the testicles of a bull with the use of linear probe. 1: Transducer or ultrasound probe; 2: Left testis.

designed for intrarectal use is necessary for the complete examination of the reproductive tract of the bull. The sector-array transducer (pie-shaped image) is not recommended because of the round shape of the testis. The linear transducer is also more practical in a bovine veterinary practice because of its versatility for both transrectal and surface use. A portable, sturdy, and battery-operated unit is a great advantage because it can be carried anywhere on the farm and can withstand field conditions. The choice of transducer is very important because it determines the tissue penetration of the sound waves and the image resolution. The 7.5 MHz transducer offers additional applications over a 5.0 MHz transducer in more sophisticated ultrasound studies. Studies of degenerative tissues, small masses or evaluation of anomalies of the spermatic cord, are good examples of situations where the 7.5 MHz transducer is valuable.

Scanning technique

External scanning

A visual appraisal of the scrotum is performed while the bull is relaxed. While approaching the bull for ultrasonography, the same precautions as for any examination are required. In the posterior approach (Figure 9.1), the restrained bull is touched to evaluate its attitude. In a continuous and slow movement, the testes, the epididymis, and the spermatic cord are located and examined by palpation. While the animal is in standing position, one testis is manually pushed down into the scrotum while the opposite testis is pushed upward out of the scanning plane, stretching the scrotal wall to allow a good contact between the transducer face and the scrotum[7].

After having examined both testicles individually, they are simultaneously pushed down into the scrotum and retained by grasping the spermatic cord at the neck of the scrotum while the other hand is used to move the transducer across the organ (Figure 9.2). This way the testes are easily compared. The sonographer must apply plenty of water-soluble coupling gel on the transducer face and on the scrotum to maximize the contact by excluding air. Normally, it is not necessary to shave the scrotal hair before the examination;

however, in old bulls or in winter it may be necessary to do so before applying the gel[7].

For a complete ultrasonographic examination, each testis with its respective epididymis must be examined. Two ultrasonographic views must be performed. For the transverse view, the transducer is placed perpendicularly to the longest testicular axis to assess the testicular parenchyma, the tunica vaginalis, the diameter of the testis, the head and tail of the epididymis, and the spermatic cord. Acomparative assessment of both testes is possible when they are scanned simultaneously. For the longitudinal or sagittal view, the transducer is apposed to the longest testicular axis to assess the testicular parenchyma, the tunica vaginalis, the length of the testis (if the transducer is long enough), and the head and tail of the epididymis. In both views, the head and tail of the epididymis are not always easily visible. For the tail, the lateral and caudal planes are usually the easiest approach[7].

Internal scanning

For the examination of internal reproductive organs (bulbourethral glands, pelvic urethra, prostate, ampullae, and vesicular glands), all precautions that apply to transrectal palpation are applicable to transrectal scanning. See Chapter 2 for scanning technique information. In rare cases, aggressive bulls will require stall restraint and sedation (xylazine, 0.01 to 0.02 mg/kg IV). With aggressive bulls, semen collection before the ultrasonography may relax the animal and facilitate the ultrasonographic examination, but it empties the ampullae. All feces should be removed from the rectum prior to the introduction of the transducer. Always carry out a preliminary exploration of the topography, size, and consistency of the organs before performing the actual ultrasonography examination. Transrectal palpation will reveal information impossible to assess by ultrasonography alone.

For biosecurity security reasons (Johne's disease, leukosis, BVD) and to protect the transducer for a prolonged functional life, the transducer can be placed in a plastic sleeve with ultrasound gel both inside and outside the sleeve. A very thin layer of gel is needed between the transducer face and the plastic sleeve; excessive or inadequate gel may reduce the quality of images and cause artifacts (see Chapters 1 and 2 for more details). The transducer face is pressed firmly against the rectal mucosa to allow good transmission. While the index finger directs the transducer the other fingers help to identify and locate the different structures. A two-dimensional image of each accessory sex gland is produced on the monitor, frozen on the screen, and saved on storage device or as hard copy for the description and analysis of the architecture at a later point in time.

Anatomy of the Reproductive System (Figure 9.3)

The following subsections review the anatomy, present the scanning techniques, and illustrate the normal sonograms of key reproductive organs of the bull. The main external reproductive structures (testis, epididymis, testicular cord, and penis) are presented first, followed by the description of the internal reproductive organs (bulbourethral glands, pelvic urethra, prostate, vesicular glands, and ampullae).

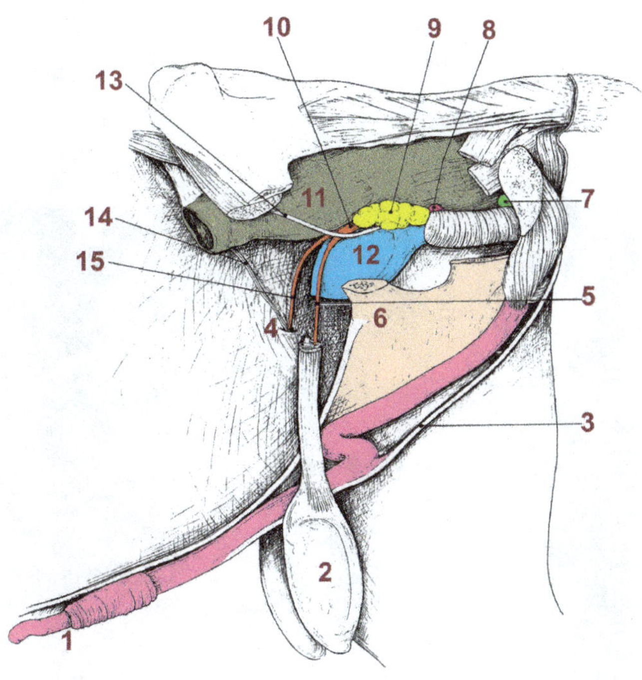

Figure 9.3. Anatomy of the reproductive tract of the bull. Permission to reproduce the image from Le Médecin Vétérinaire du Québec, Volume 35 (4), page 159. 1: Penile gland; 2: Testis; 3: Penile retractor muscle; 4: Right vaginal ring; 5: Left deferent duct; 6: Ischial bone (cut); 7: Bulbourethral gland; 8: Prostate body; 9: Vesicular gland; 10: Left ampulla of deferent duct; 11: Rectum; 12: Urinary bladder; 13: Left urethra; 14: Right testicular vein and artery; 15: Right deferent duct.

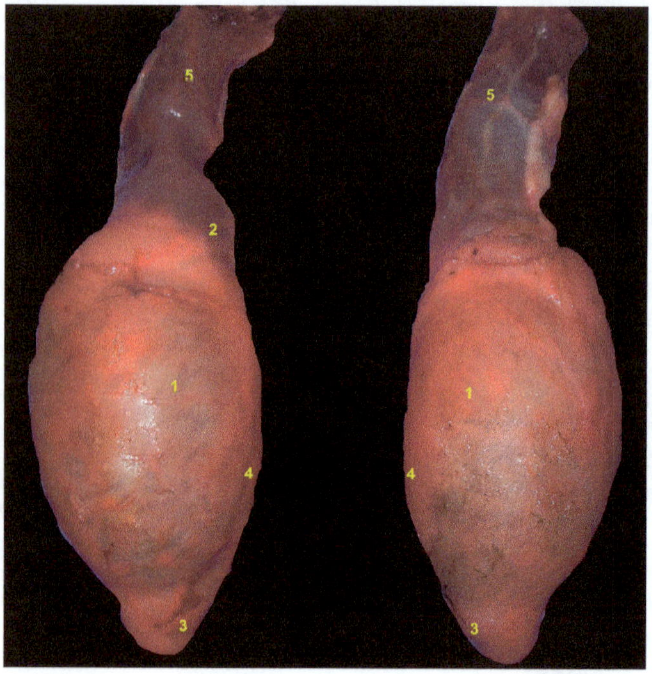

Figure 9.4. Right and left bull testes. 1: Testis; 2: Head of the epididymis; 3: Tail of the epididymis; 4: Body of the epididymis; 5: Testicular cord.

Testis (Figure 9.4)

Anatomy

The testis of a mature bull is an ovoid-shaped organ with a long vertical axis (10 to 12 cm) and a short caudo-cranial (Ca-Cr) axis (6 to 8 cm). The scrotum is modeled upon the testes to form a median groove corresponding to the internal division between the testes and a narrower neck dorsal to the testes. The head of the epididymis is located proximoanterolaterally to the testis with its body running medially and its tail running ventrally.

On visual examination, the tunica should be relaxed enough to see the neck of the scrotum and the convex abaxial contour of the scrotum. The testicular length is roughly two times its diameter. The testes should be firm on palpation.

Ultrasound technique and imaging

Compared to internal organs, ultrasonographic examination of the external genital organs is easier because of better eye-to-hand coordination (Figure 9.5). Prior to

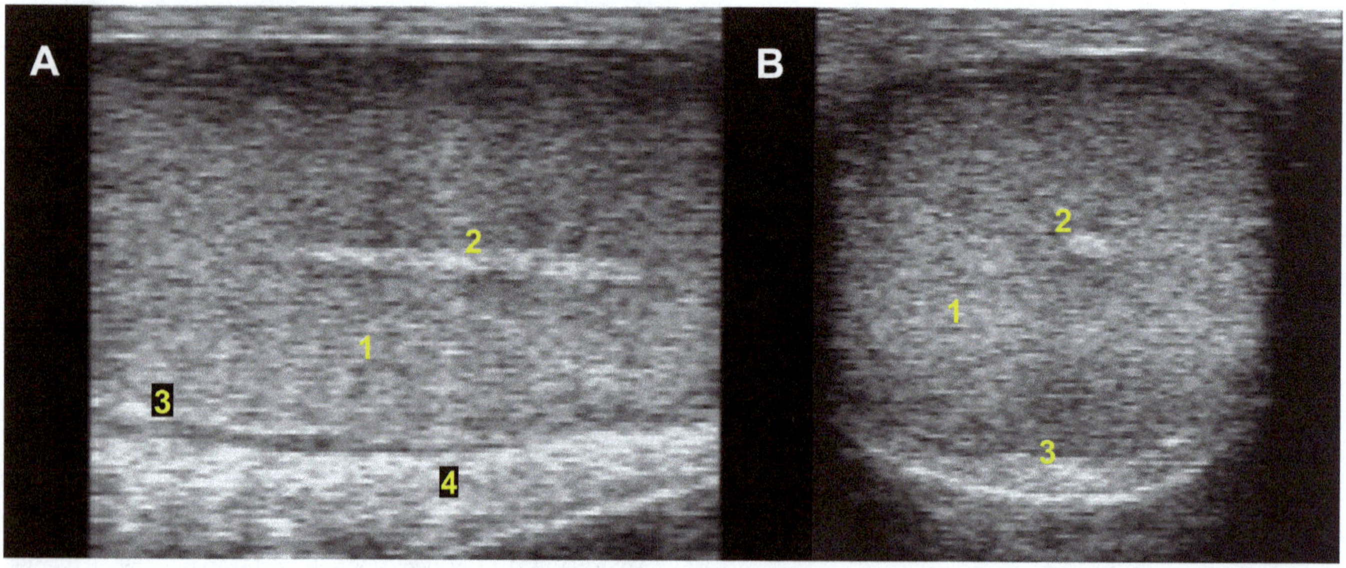

Figure 9.5. Ultrasonographic images of the testes in longitudinal (A) and transverse (B) views (7.5 MHz probe; depth of 6 cm). Normally, the parenchyma is moderately echoic and has a fine, homogeneous echotexture with a hyperechoic mediastinum. The mediastinum appears as a central line on longitudinal view and a dot in transverse view. The border of the testes is characterized by a smooth and hyperechoic tunica albuginea. On the outside an anechoic line, the cavum (<2.0 mm), appears between the parietal and visceral layers of the tunica vaginalis. Blood vessels appear as anechoic circular structures on transverse view. 1: Parenchyma; 2: Mediastinum; 3: Tunica albuginea; 4: Scrotal septum.

examination the testes must be pushed to the bottom of the scrotum to remove skin folds. One hand is used to keep the testes in place and the other one to hold the transducer. The rete testis is central and the most echoic structure of the testicular parenchyma. It is a useful landmark to identify the largest diameter. Longitudinal and transverse images of the testicular parenchyma of both testes must be obtained for comparative purposes.

In a 24-month-old bull, the tunica albugenia, the mediastinum, and the testicular width are about 0.3, 0.5, and 5.75 cm thick, respectively[8]. The echogenicity of the testes increases between 20 and 40 weeks of age of the bull, representing the most active phase of growth of the seminiferous tubules[4]. The testicular parenchyma has a moderate homogeneous echogenicity compared to the hyperechoic mediastinum. The testicular tunics are hyperechoic as well with an apparent anechoic line between the parietal and visceral layers of the tunica vaginalis. Ultrasonography can be used to predict testicular volume and sperm production[5]. In older animals with normal testes, small hyperechoic foci representing testicular septa are occasionally visible. Hyperechoic dots may appear and could represent fibrosis or mineralization secondary to insults.

Epididymis

Anatomy

The head of the epididymis is flattened and close to the dorsal aspect of the testis. The thin and elongate body of the epididymis runs on the medial face of the testis to the tail. The tail is the most obvious of the three segments of the epididymis, located ventrally and forming a firm conspicuous conical swelling (Figure 9.4).

Ultrasound technique and imaging

Examination of the entire epididymis in one plane is impossible. The head and the tail of the epididymis are more difficult to study because images are recorded from an oblique plane near the proximal and distal poles of the testis, which requires repositioning of the transducer. Applying the transducer to the lateral face of the testis generally improves visualization of both parts of the epididymis (Figure 9.6).

Spermatic cord

Anatomy

The spermatic cord is identified within the scrotal neck and appears dorsally to the testis. The testis is suspended in the scrotum by the cremaster muscle. Other important structures are the ductus deferens and convoluted arteries and veins (the pampinifom plexus) that provide a thermoregulation mechanism with a counter-current heat exchanger.

Ultrasound technique and imaging

The examined testis is held with one hand and the transducer is applied to the horizontal plane to locate the rete testis. Keeping the transducer in the horizontal plane (transverse view), it is moved dorsally toward the epididymal head. Further dorsally, the pampiniform plexus, the ductus deferens, and the cremaster muscle can be located if too much pressure is not applied on the structures (Figure 9.7).

Penis

Anatomy

The penis and the distal loop of the sigmoid flexure are readily palpated through the skin of the prepuce and perineum, respectively. The penis of mature bulls is about 120 cm in length and 3 to 4 cm in diameter. It is a fibroelastic organ and therefore rigid even when nonerect. The anatomy of the free extremity of the penis is very distinctive (Figure 9.8).

Ultrasound technique and imaging

Because of long hair, shaving the area of examination is necessary before the gel is applied to the skin. The transducer is moved perpendicularly to the long axis of the penis for a transverse view. Ultrasonography is very useful to diagnose conditions associated with enlargement of the penis (hematoma, abscess, urethritis) (Figure 9.9).

The anatomical positions of the key internal reproductive organs of the bull must be remembered by the ultrasonographer before their evaluations (Figure 9.3). The following text presents the scanning techniques and ultrasound images of the accessory glands and organs from the caudal aspect of the pelvic cavity to its cranial aspect.

The constituents of the spermatic cord disperse within the vaginal ring. The ductus deferens extends dorsally and reaches the dorsal aspect of the bladder where the prostate, vesicular glands, and—further caudally–the pelvic urethra and the bulbourethra can be studied (Figure 9.3). Most of the accessory glands lay close together on the pelvic floor, immediately

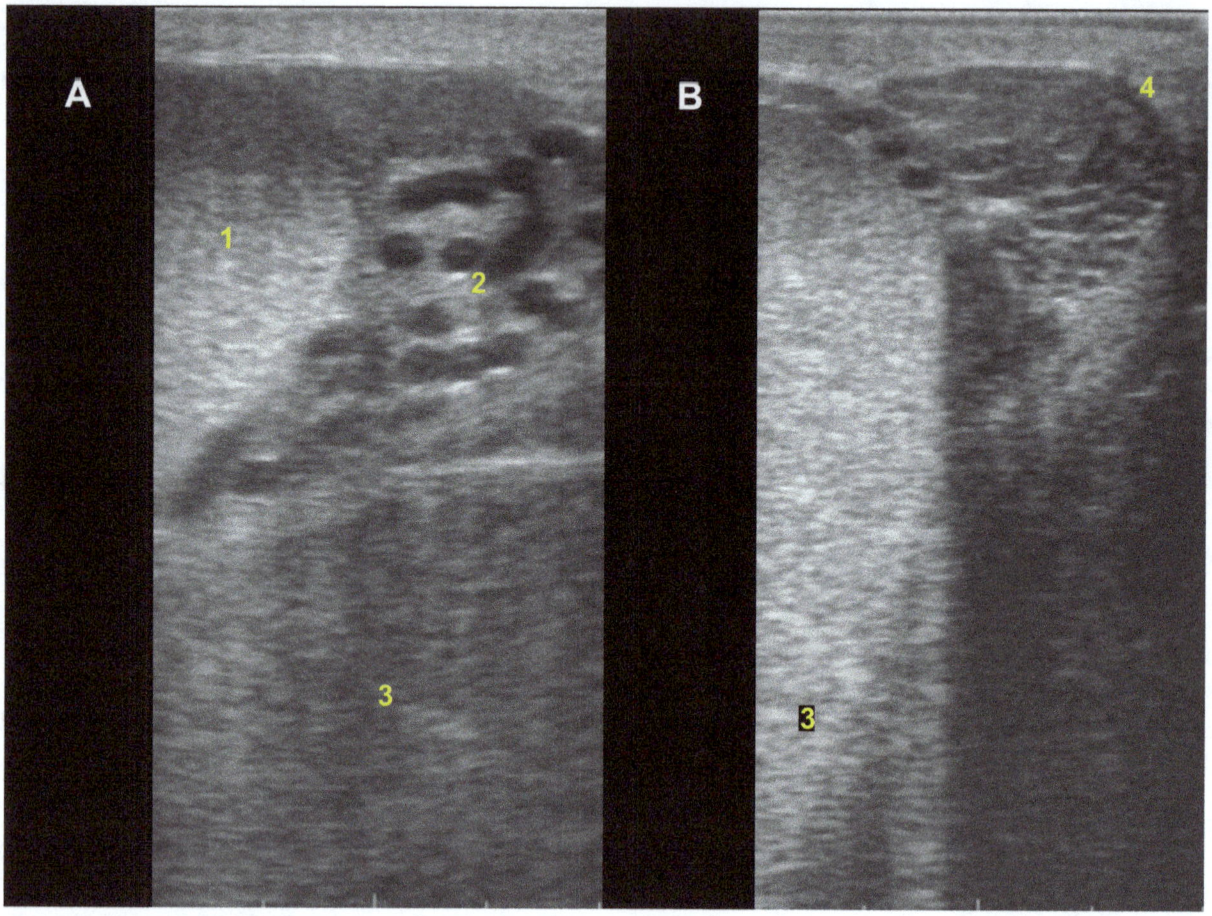

Figure 9.6. Ultrasonograms of the head of the epididymis and the pampiniform plexus (A) and of the tail of the epididymis (B) (7.5 MHz probe; depth of 8 cm). Both head and tail of the epididymis are homogeneous on ultrasonography and present a slightly less echoic and more heterogeneous appearance compared to the testicular parenchyma. They are separated from the testis by an anechoic triangle. 1: Head of the epididymis; 2: Pampiniform plexus; 3: Parenchyma of the testis; 4: Tail of the epididymis.

beneath the rectum. This convenient anatomy allows evaluation of the structure, function, and possible pathology of the internal sex glands.

Bulbourethral glands

Anatomy

The bulbourethral glands are the most caudal accessory glands. Usually, they are not identified by rectal palpation because they are covered by the bulbospongiosus muscle (Figure 9.10). They can also be difficult to visualize with ultrasonography. Bulbourethral glands are ovoid to fusiform with a diameter of about 2.0 cm[6].

Ultrasound technique and imaging

The transducer is pressed ventrally with the caudal pole of the transducer pushed against the inside edge of the sphincter of the anus at a slight lateral angle. This position may cause discomfort to the animal.

Pelvic urethra

Anatomy

The pelvic urethra is cranial to the bulbourethral glands and runs from the ischial arcade to the neck of the bladder. A powerful muscle asymmetrically surrounds the urethra and gives it a cylindrical shape. The ventral portion of the muscle is thicker than the dorsal one.

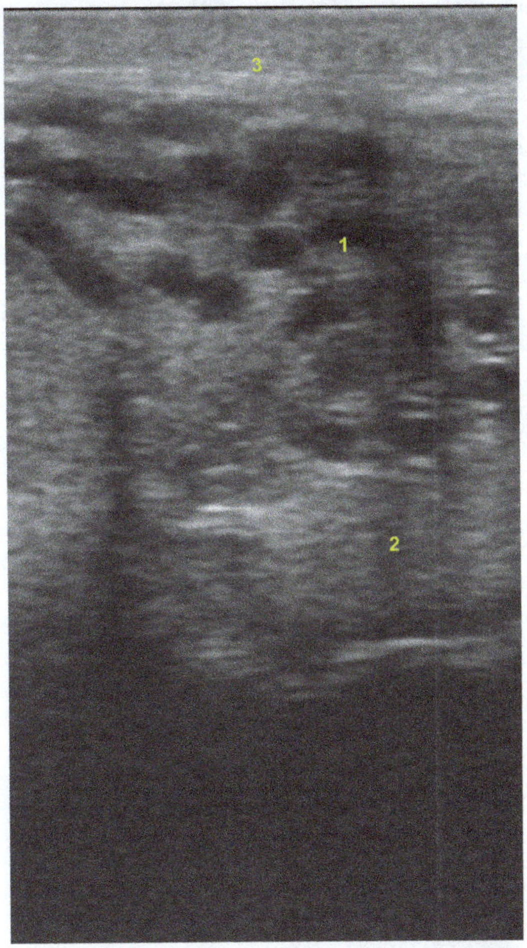

Figure 9.7. Ultrasonogram of the spermatic cord in longitudinal view (7.5 MHz probe; depth of 8 cm). The pampiniform plexus, located on the upper pole of the testis or in the lower part of the testicular cord, appears like a Swiss cheese made of hyperechoic (vessel wall) and anechoic (lumen) dots, representing multiple transverse sections of blood vessels. Sometimes, sections of the vessels appear curved like a banana. The ductus deferens cannot be distinguished from blood vessels. The most external layers of the testis, the vaginal tunic, the spermatic fascia, and the skin are indistinguishable from each other and appear as one hyperechoic layer over the parenchyma. The plexus presents a prominent and complex flow pattern on color Doppler. 1: Pampiniform plexus; 2: Cremaster; 3: Skin.

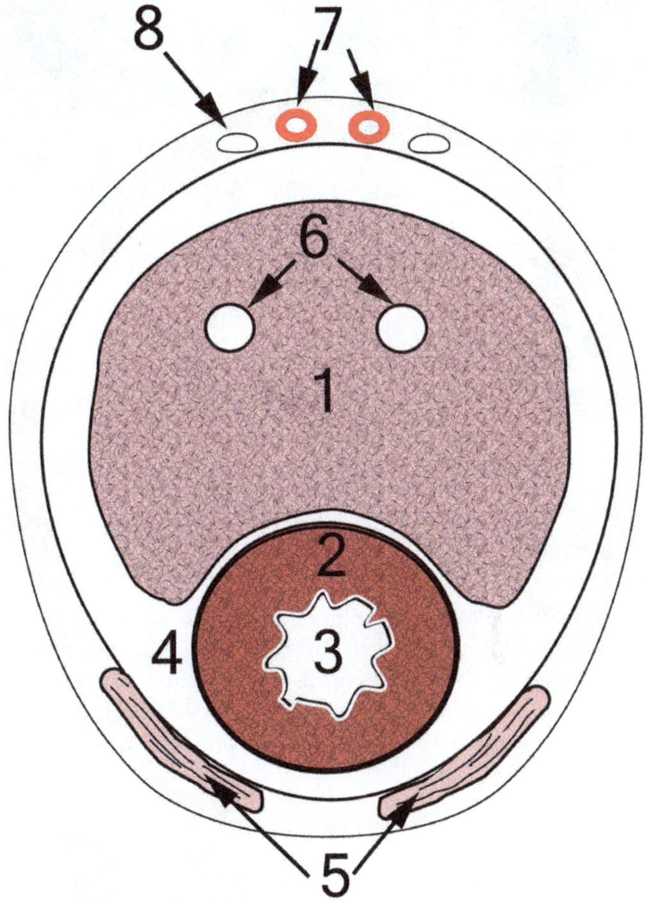

Figure 9.8. Drawing of the transversal section of the penis between the glans and the sigmoid flexure. Courtesy of Dr. André Desrochers (Université de Montréal). Midway between the glans and the sigmoid flexure (Figure 9.3), the urethra is ventral and surrounded by a small amount of corpus spongiosum. Most of the internal space of the penis is occupied dorsally by the corpus cavernosum. The body of the penis is enclosed in a fibrous tunic called the *tunica albuginea*. 1: Corpus cavernosum; 2: Corpus spongiosum; 3: Urethra; 4: Tunica albuginea; 5: Retractor muscle of the penis; 6: Corpus cavernosum veins; 7: Dorsal arteries of the penis; 8: Dorsal vein of the penis.

Contrary to the bulbourethral glands, the pelvic urethra is easy to feel because of its size (3 cm in diameter and 20 cm long) and its rhythmic muscular contractions when stimulated.

Ultrasound technique and imaging

Moving cranially from the bulbourethral glands, the face of the transducer is kept ventrally in the long axis to generate a longitudinal view of the pelvic urethra (Figure 9.11).

Prostate

Anatomy

The prostate is divided in two parts: the body and the pars disseminata. The body of the prostate is divided in two lobes readily palpated transrectally. Dorsal to the neck of the bladder it measures about 3.5 cm by

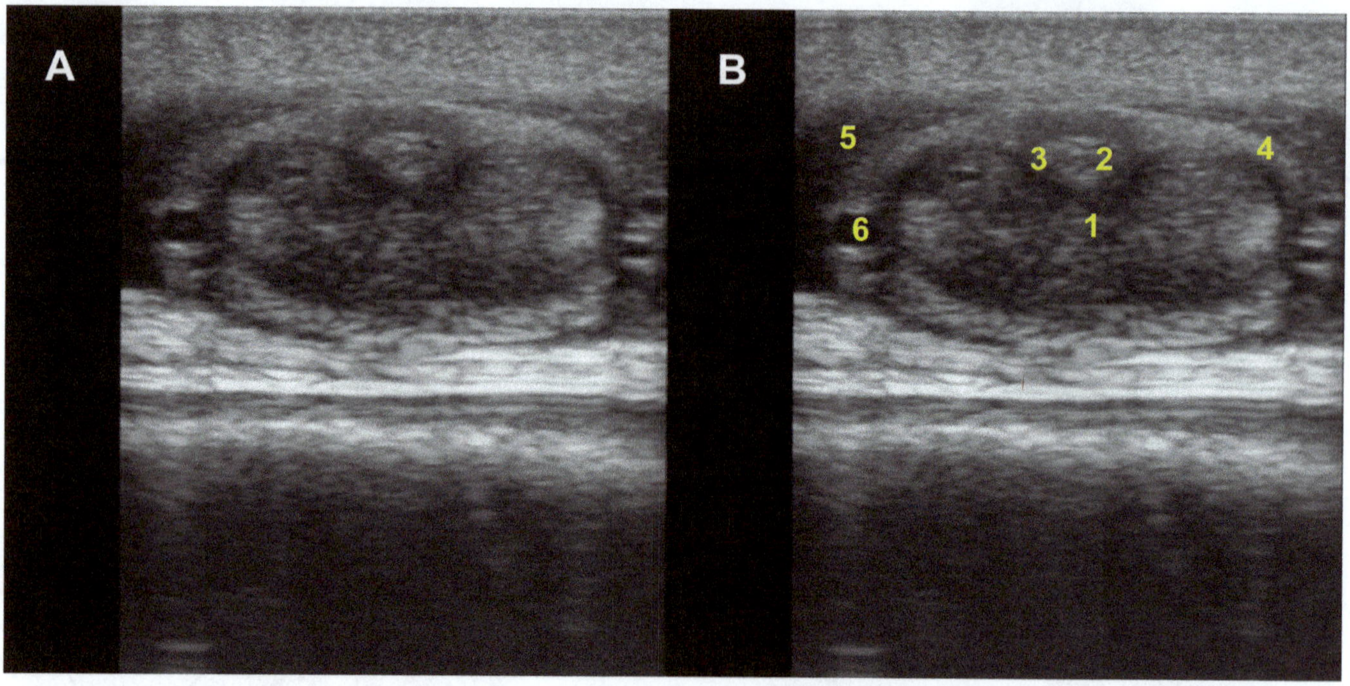

Figure 9.9. Ultrasonography of the penis in transverse view (7.5 MHz probe; depth of 5 cm). The probe is placed on the ventral aspect of the penis in order to obtain this image. In transverse view, the penis consists of a ventral hyperechoic urethra surrounded by the echoic corpus spongiosum and corpus cavernosum. The corpus cavernosum is surrounded by a dense hyperechoic membrane, the tunica albuginea. 1: Corpus cavernosum; 2: Corpus spongiosum; 3: Urethra; 4: Tunica albuginea; 5: Retractor muscle of the penis; 6: Corpus cavernosum veins.

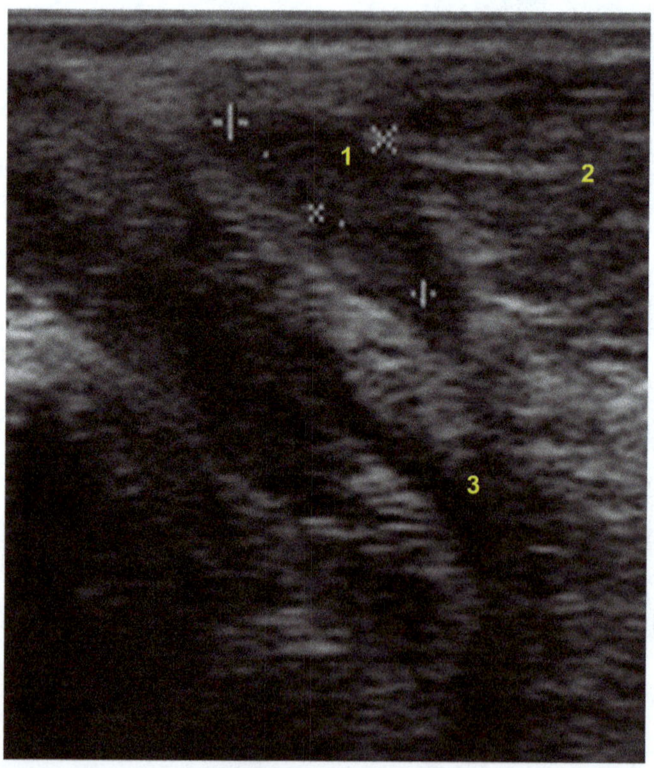

Figure 9.10. Sonogram of a longitudinal view of the bulbourethral gland (5 MHz probe; depth of 7 cm). The bulbourethral glands (2.5 cm by 1 cm) appear homogenously hyperechoic compared to the other accessory glands and less echoic than the surrounding bulbospongiosus muscle, which embeds them and appears heterogeneous with hyperechoic and less echoic bands. 1: Bulbourethral gland; 2: Bulbocavernous muscle; 3: Urethra.

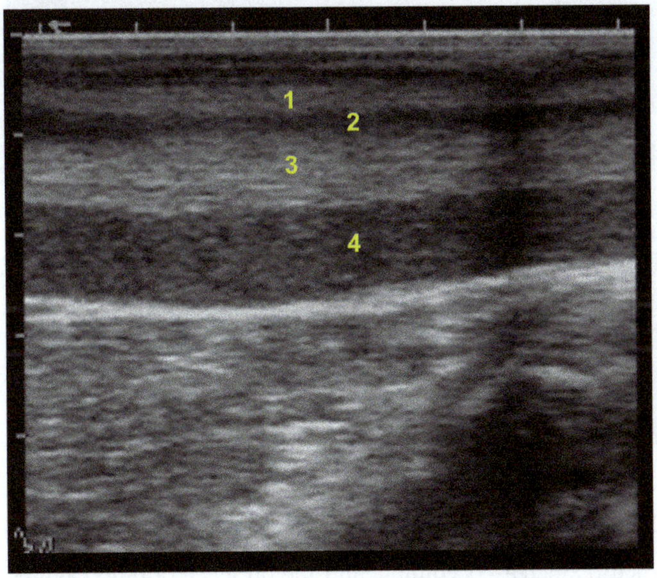

Figure 9.11. Ultrasound image of the nondilated pelvic urethra in longitudinal view (5 MHz probe; depth of 5 cm). The lumen of the pelvic urethra generally appears anechoic when visible or filled with urine compared to the moderately echoic appearance of the surrounding urethra muscle (see Figure 9.12). Forcing urine out of the bladder by pressure or urination allows a better view of the lumen. 1: Rectal wall; 2: Dorsal urethral muscle; 3: Hyperechoic appearance of the prostate pars disseminata (pelvic urethra nonvisible); 4: Ventral urethral muscle.

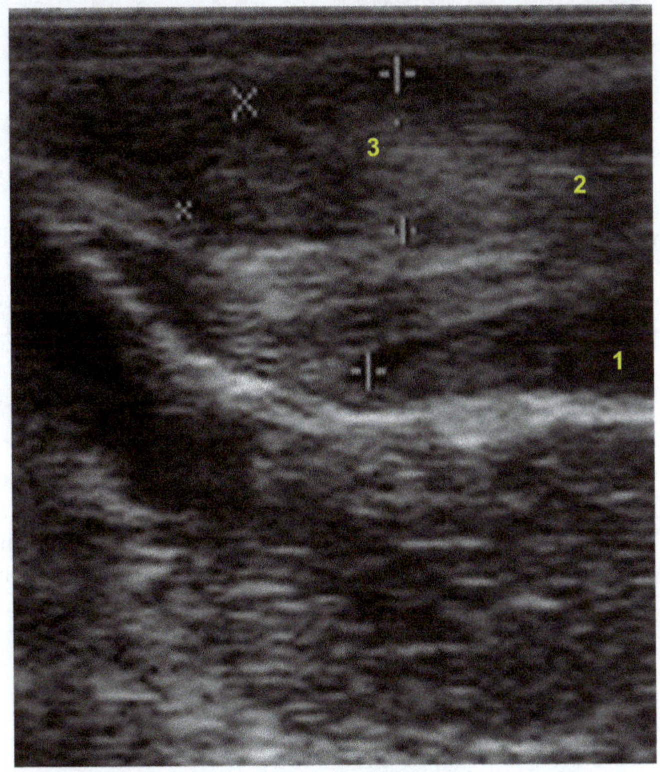

Figure 9.12. Ultrasonographic image of the prostate body in longitudinal view (5 MHz probe; depth of 7 cm). The pars disseminata within the pelvic urethra is continuous with the body of the prostate (see description of the pelvic urethra and Figure 9.11). Ultrasonographically, the prostate body appears as a moderately echoic and homogenous structure located dorsal to the neck of the bladder with smooth margins. On longitudinal view, the shape of the prostate is round to ovoid. 1: Urethra; 2: Pars disseminata of the prostate; 3: Body of the prostate.

1.5 cm. The pars disseminata is about 12 cm long and is not identifiable by transrectal palpation.

Ultrasound technique and imaging

After the examination of the pelvic urethra, the transducer is moved to the cranial pole of the pelvic urethra directly to the body of the prostate where longitudinal and transverse views are performed (Figure 9.12).

Seminal vesicular glands

Anatomy

The paired seminal vesicular glands are free and can be imaged from their proximal attachments close to the neck of the bladder to their dorsolateral segments on each side of the bladder. The irregular and lobed shape of the vesicular glands makes them easy to recognize. Because of their irregular shapes, determining accurately the dimensions of the vesicular glands (VGs) is difficult. However, the mean length of the longest axis of the VGs for a 24-month-old bull is about 12 cm long and 1.7 cm wide[8]. The size of the VGs increases with age more than the other accessory glands[3].

Ultrasound technique and imaging

Once the body of the prostate is imaged, the transducer is advanced cranially and rotated laterally (Figure 9.13).

Ampullae

Anatomy

From the tail of the epididymis, the ductus deferens runs along the medial face of the testis and passes through the inguinal ring dorsally to the bladder to

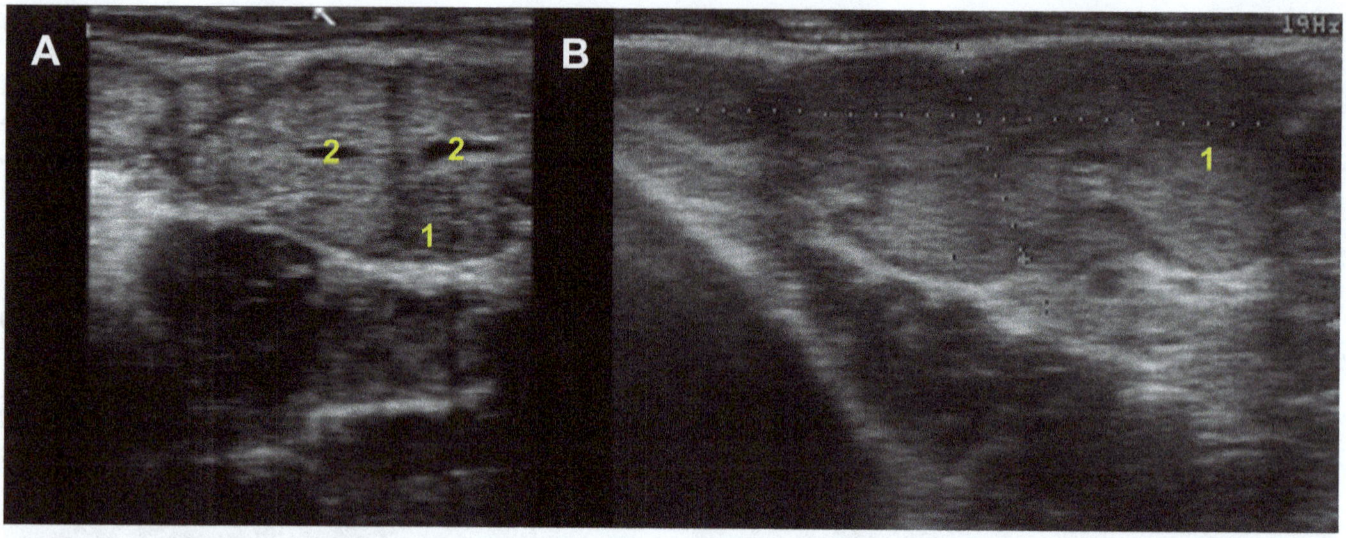

Figure 9.13. Sonograms of the seminal vesicular glands (VGs) in transverse (A) and longitudinal views (B) (7.5 MHz probe; depth of 7 cm). On ultrasonography, VGs are characterized by isoechoic lobes of glandular tissue, separated by hypoechoic regions and hyperechoic borders. The lobular structure of the glands can be identified. The anechoic collection ducts of the VGs can be viewed running from each gland. Loss of lobular structure, increased volume, and the presence of fluid cavities within the gland are the primary signs of vesiculitis. 1: Parenchyma; 2: Lumen of the vesicular gland.

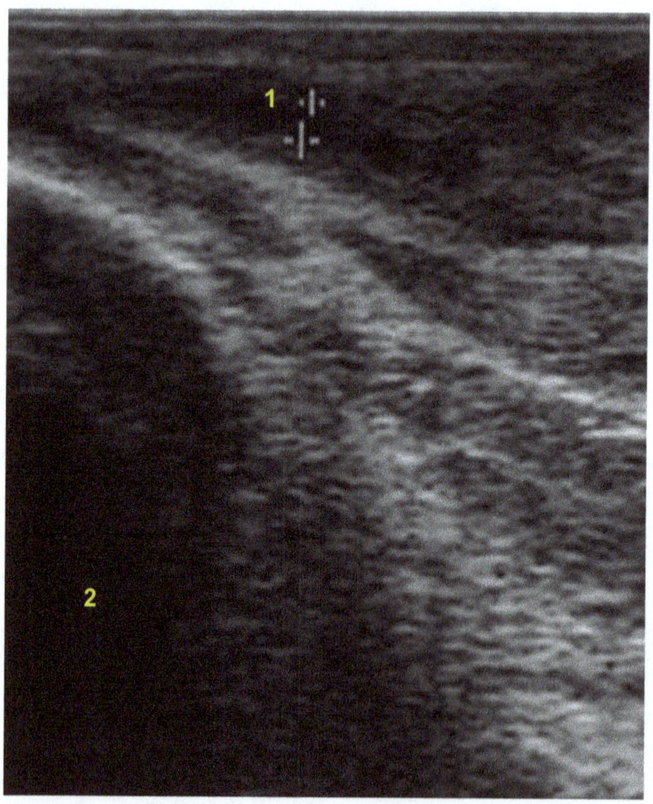

Figure 9.14. Ultrasonogram of the ampulla in longitudinal view (5 MHz probe; depth of 7 cm). The lumen of the ampulla represents 10 to 60% of the whole ampulla diameter[14]. The lumen appears irregular and homogeneously anechoic if filled with semen. Sometimes, valves are seen within the lumen. Closer to the insertion site in the urethra the ampulla gets smaller and terminates in a small and more echoic excretory duct[14]. A transverse view allows an overview of the whole region, including VGs, bladder, and prostate. 1: Lumen of the ampulla; 2: Urinary bladder.

form the ampullae (12 cm long and 1.5 cm wide). Ampullae are the most cranial accessory glands and have a tubular shape with thick walls.

Ultrasound technique and imaging

From the prostate, the transducer is pushed cranially and the depth is increased. For an overview of the ampullae a longitudinal view is recommended (Figure 9.14).

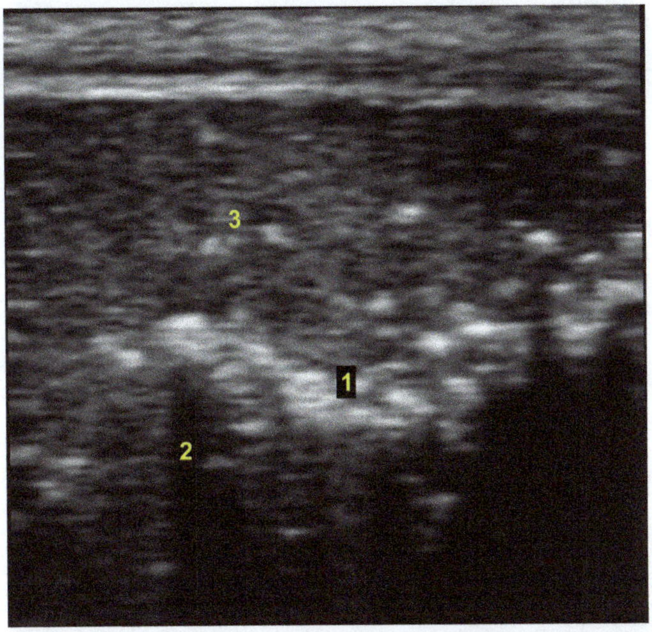

Figure 9.15. Sonogram of chronic orchitis in transverse view (7.5 MHz probe; depth of 6 cm). Depending on the progression of the condition, the ultrasonographic appearance of orchitis may change. The transverse view shows enlargement of the affected testis with a heterogeneous echotexture. In severe cases, small, round, hypoechoic cystic structures within the testis are observed. The parenchyma has many dense echoic areas scattered through the testis, which may exhibit acoustic shadowing. Some of these areas could be foci of mineralization that occur in the chronic phase of orchitis. The mediastinum testis is unidentifiable. 1: Foci of mineralization within the mediastinum; 2: Acoustic shadow; 3: Testicular parenchyma.

Anomalies and Ultrasonographic Imaging of External and Internal Reproductive Organs

Testicular anomalies

Testicular anomalies include inflammatory disorders (orchitis and epididymitis), testicular and epididymal cysts, torsion, infarction, atrophy, trauma, and neoplasia. Disorders affecting the scrotum include accumulation of fluid (hydrocele and hematocele) and scrotal hernia. Inflammatory and traumatic anomalies can occur within the spermatic cord.

Orchitis

Orchitis is infrequently diagnosed in the bull and usually only one testis is affected. The opposite testis can undergo degeneration secondary to thermal injury from the inflamed testis. The infection may occur subsequent to hematogenous spread of organisms from infection in other parts of the body, including rumenitis, liver abscess, pododermatitis, and cystitis, or may be caused by trauma. The swelling associated with the inflammation leads to pressure necrosis of the testicular parenchyma due to the inelastic tunica albuginea. Often, history and physical examination are enough to establish a diagnosis of orchitis. The scrotum is painful, hot, and edematous in acute phase. However, as an adjunct, ultrasonography is highly sensitive for ruling out other painful conditions, such as testicular torsion, and for demonstrating inflammation of the testis or of the epididymis (Figure 9.15).

Testicular degeneration

Testicular degeneration is an acquired condition characterized by loss of testicular parenchymal integrity and, eventually, reduced size (Figure 9.16). It is an important cause of infertility in the bull and tends to be a progressive process that increases with age. Factors that modify scrotal thermal regulation (extremely hot or cold environmental temperatures, fat in scrotum, inflammation, etc.) may initiate testicular degeneration. Chronic exposure to certain drugs can also produce testicular degeneration. Laboratory species exposed to enrofloxacin (quinolone) developed testicular degeneration and associated adverse effects on spermatogenesis. No studies have been done in bovine species.

Testicular abscess

The testis with an abscess is usually larger than normal and is painful in the acute phase (Figure 9.17).

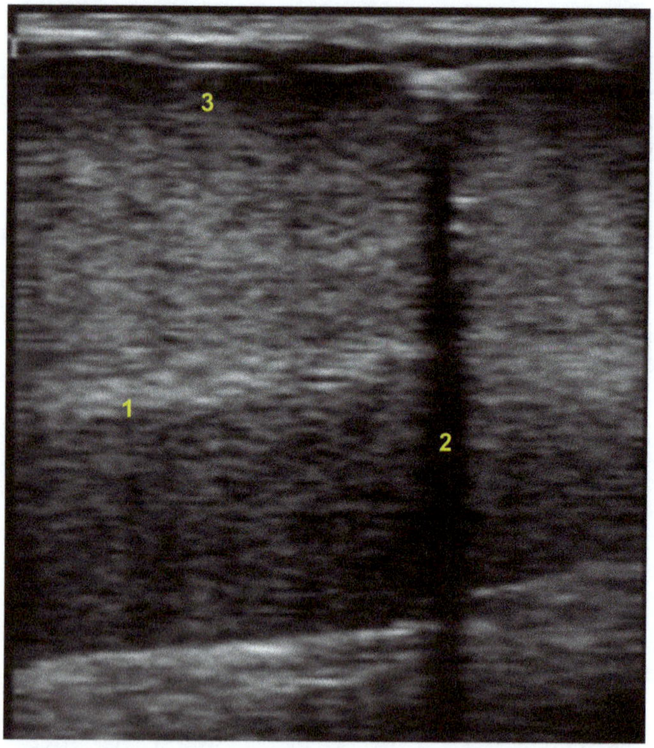

Figure 9.16. Sonogram of a longitudinal view of testicular degeneration (7.5 MHz probe; depth of 7 cm). With testicular degeneration, the testicular parenchyma loses its tissue architecture and becomes hyperechoic over time. Shadow artifacts are frequently seen with this condition. 1: Mediastinum; 2: Shadow artifact; 3: Loss of the homogenous appearance of the testicular parenchyma.

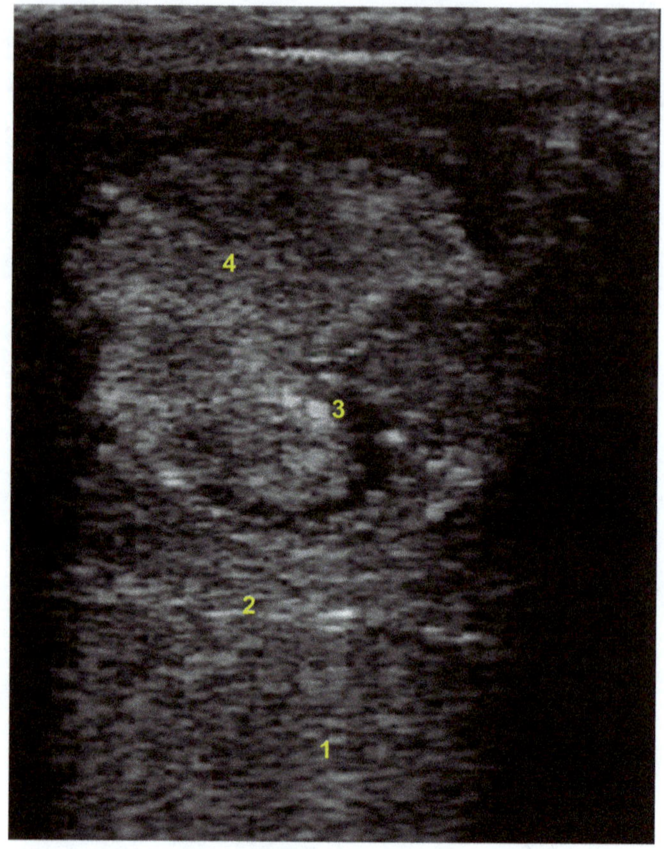

Figure 9.17. Testicular abscess in longitudinal view of a testis (5 MHz probe; depth of 7 cm). Courtesy of Dr. Denis Necchi. The abscess appears as a heterogeneous hypoechoic to anechoic mass, with no visible parenchyma, no distinct margin, and many small hypoechoic areas. Fibrinous debris may be observed in the anechoic fluid. The testicular tissue is displaced away from the abscess. 1: Normal testicular parenchyma; 2: Mediastinum; 3: Foci of mineralization in the abscess; 4: Degenerated tissues in the testis.

Testicular neoplasm

Testicular neoplasms have been reported in bulls and can be easily overlooked during a rapid evaluation. Interstitial cell tumors, Sertoli cell tumors, and seminomas are the main types of testicular tumors in bulls (Figure 9.18).

Epididymitis (head or tail)

Epididymitis is the most common abnormality of the epididymis and generally involves the tail (Figure 9.19).

Scrotal and testicular cord anomalies

Inguinal hernia

Inguinal hernias enlarge the neck of the scrotum (Figure 9.20). The intestinal loops are usually contained within the tunica vaginalis.

Hydrocele

Hydrocele is a fluid collection (more than 2 mm) within the tunica vaginalis surrounding the testis that causes painless scrotal swelling (Figure 9.21). The excessive fluid may be associated with many conditions: infection, neoplasm of the testis, torsion of the testis, systemic disease (heart or kidney), or idiopathic disease. It is a relatively rare condition in bulls.

Hematocele

A hematocele is blood within the tunica vaginalis. It is caused by direct trauma to the testis or by testicular torsion. In the early stage, the hematocele contains

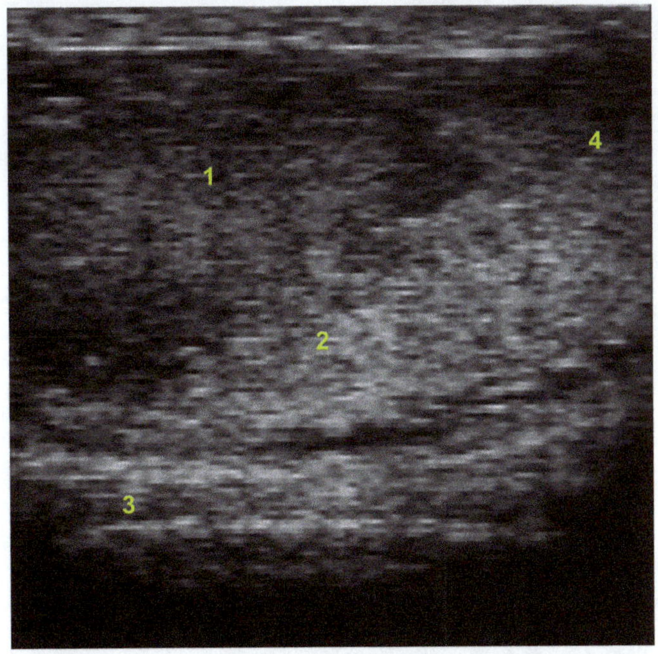

Figure 9.18. Neoplastic mass in the testis in transversal view (7.5 MHz probe; depth of 5.5 cm). Ultrasonographic images of testicular tumors are variable and range from circumscribed small nodules to large complex masses. Tumors may be hyperechoic, anechoic, or a mix of echogenicities and are usually distinguishable from the normal testicular parenchyma. 1: Neoplastic mass; 2: Mineralization; 3: Dartos muscle; 4: Degeneration of the testicular tissues.

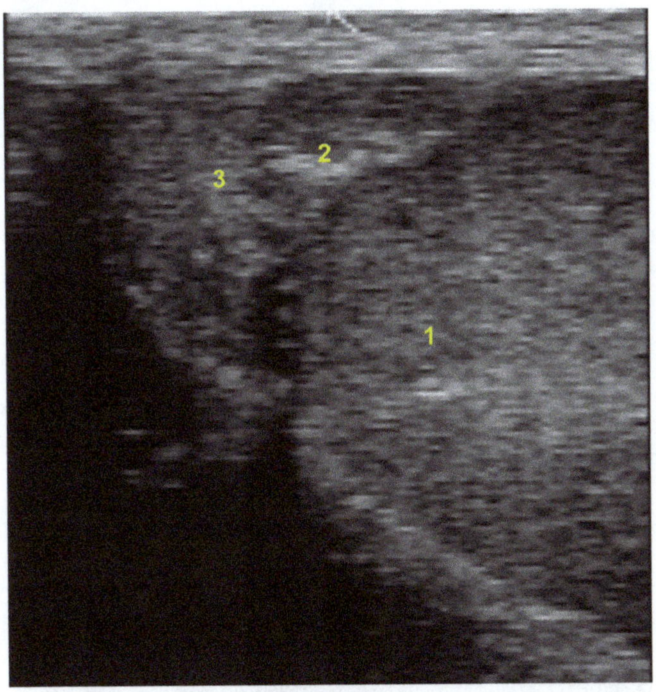

Figure 9.19. Chronic epididymitis of the tail in longitudinal view (7.5 MHz probe; depth of 6 cm). In the acute phase of epididymitis the epididymis is enlarged, less echogenic, and more coarse than normal. In the chronic stage the tissue becomes more heterogeneous and more hypoechoic, probably due to edema or the presence of a transudate. A few hyperechoic areas are seen in the affected tissues in the chronic phase. The lesions are surrounded by a distinct echoic line. Epididymitis is often accompanied by vesiculitis or orchitis. 1: Testis; 2: Mineralization; 3: Epididymis.

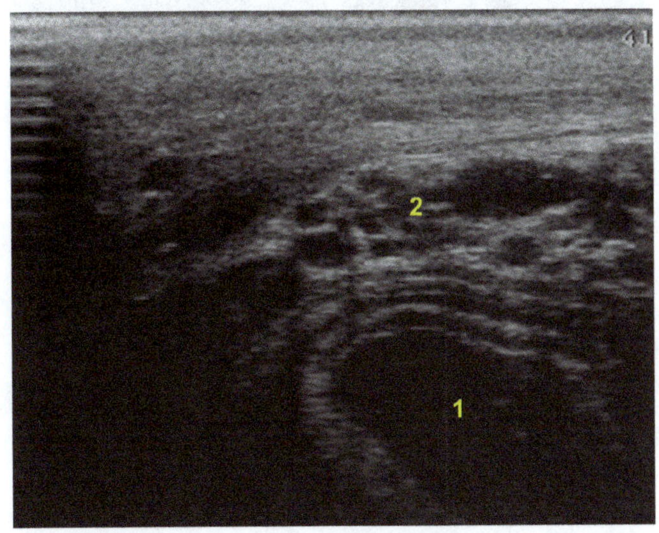

Figure 9.20. Ultrasonogram of an inguinal hernia in transverse view (5 MHz probe; depth of 8 cm). Courtesy of Dr André Desrochers (Université de Montréal). The echoic content of the intestinal loops can be observed in the inquinal hernia. In real-time scanning the movement of the contents is apparent. On rare occasions intraluminal gas is also observed. Note on this image the presence of an intestinal loop near the pampiniform plexux. 1: Intestinal loop; 2: Pampiniform plexus.

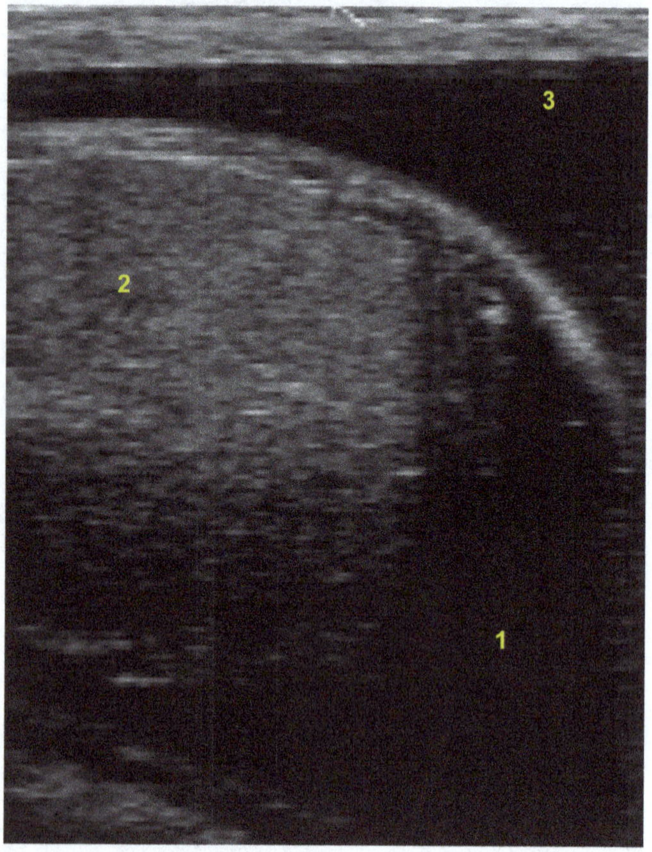

Figure 9.21. Ultrasonogram of a hydrocele (7.5 MHz probe; depth of 7 cm). The ultrasonographic scan usually shows a completely anechoic fluid-filled cavity. In an infectious process (for example, an incisional infection), adhesion of the tunica albuginea to the scrotal wall can be seen. Effusion within the peritoneal cavity is not always apparent on ultrasound. 1: Effusion within the vaginalis tunica; 2: Testis; 3: Effusion in the scrotum.

localized fluid with mixed echogenicity. Over time it becomes more hyperechoic.

Varicocele

This condition of varicosity and tortuosity of the testicular vascular cone is often associated with a reduction of the volume of the testis (Figure 9.22). It has been observed in the central portion of the scrotum of aged bulls, and vessels are subject to hemorrhage. Small varicoceles are normal in old bulls and are not associated with decreased fertility or poor semen quality[7].

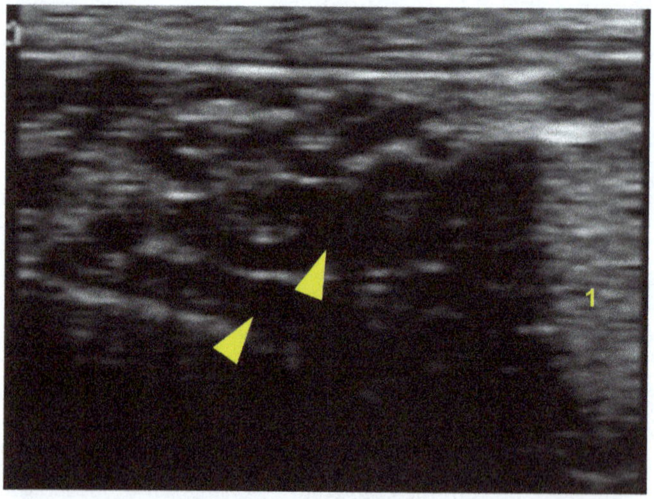

Figure 9.22. Sonogram of a varicocele on longitudinal view showing enlarged blood vessels (7.5 MHz probe; depth of 5 cm). Ultrasonographically, a varicocele appears as irregular hypoechoic areas, usually on the periphery of the spermatic cord, with no signs of pulsating blood flow. The size of the varicocele is variable. Sometimes, the central vein and its smaller branches can be dilated while the veins of the pampiniform plexus are moderately enlarged. Yellow arrowheads: Enlarged blood vessel; 1: Epididymis.

Penile abnormalities

Hematoma

The classical penile hematoma is the result of rupture of the dorsal surface of the tunica albuginea and subsequent escape of blood from the corpus cavernosum (Figure 9.23). The larger the hematoma, the larger the size of the tunica albuginea rupture. A symmetrical delineated swelling encompasses the penis and is

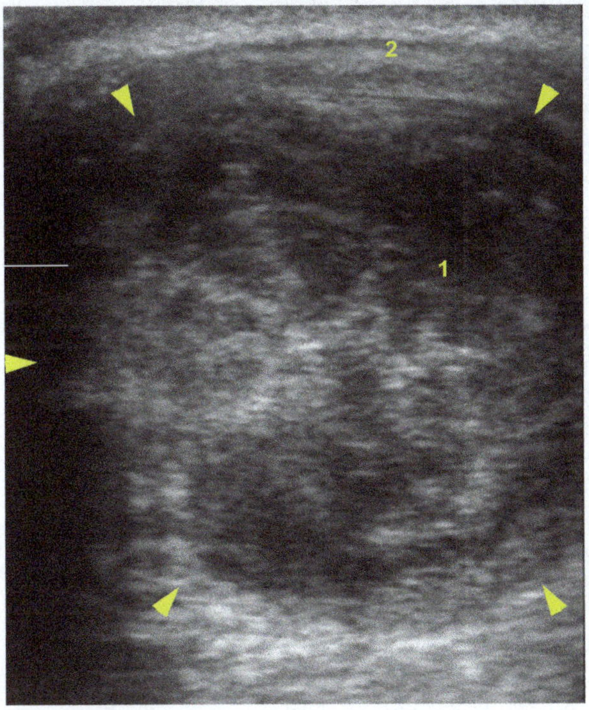

Figure 9.23. Ultrasound image of a penile hematoma (7.5 MHz probe; depth of 5 cm). Courtesy of Dr. André Desrochers (Université de Montréal). Ultrasonographic examination reveals a multilobed mass of mixed echogenicity and a well-delineated capsule on the dorsal aspect of the penis. 1: Hematoma (corpus cavernosum); 2: Tunica albuginea.

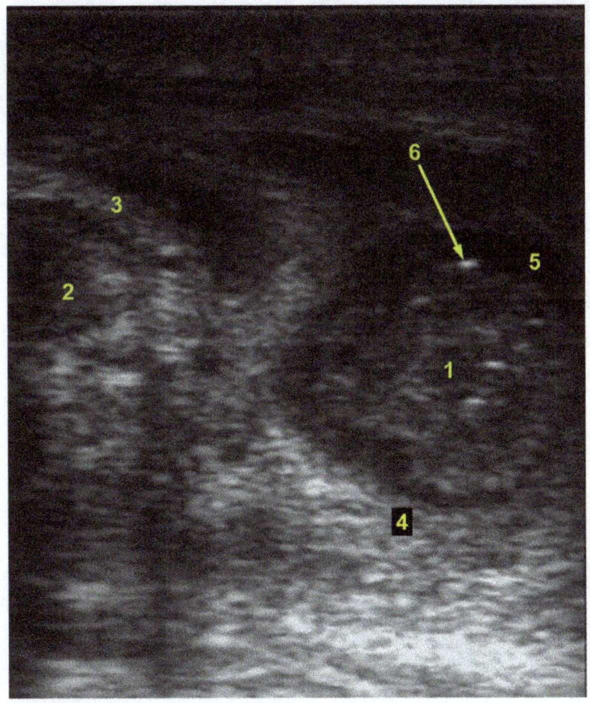

Figure 9.24. Ultrasound image in transverse section of a penile abscess (7.5 MHz probe; depth of 5 cm). Courtesy of Dr. André Desrochers (Université de Montréal). On ultrasonography, a thick-walled hyperechoic structure is seen in a well-organized and mature abscess. A mixture of multiple hypoechoic, hyperechoic, or anechoic areas is seen within the abscess. The ultrasonographic appearance changes with time. The older the abscess is, the more echoic it appears on ultrasonography. It generally forms a round structure very close to the penile body. 1: Abscess; 2: Penis; 3: Tunica albuginea; 4: Capsule of the abscess; 5: Anechoic area within the abscess; 6: Gas.

located cranial to the scrotum. A preputial prolapse frequently accompanies the condition and may be the reason for reproductive evaluation.

Abscess

The abscess is typically located midway between the prepuce and the scrotum and could be a complication of a penile hematoma (Figure 9.24). If the initial hematoma is over 15 cm in diameter, the risk of abscess formation is higher.

Vesiculitis

Even though the prevalence of vesiculitis is low (9%), it is the most common pathologic condition affecting the internal genitalia in bulls[1]. The etiology is not known; however the incidence of the condition appears to be much higher in some groups of young bulls where bacteria (*Brucella abortus, Arcanobacter pyogenes, Haemophilus somnus,* and *E. coli*) and virus (IBR) have been implicated. In the acute phase, vesiculitis is associated with pain, enlarged glands, and localized pelvic peritonitis (Figure 9.25). Chronic seminal vesiculitis is characterized by firm (fibrotic) and enlarged glands. Purulent exudate is consistently present in the semen. In young bulls managed in groups, the prevalence of seminal vesiculitis can be as high as 49%[2]. In old bulls (more than 10 years old), vesicular hypertrophy is observed and is generally normal.

Internal pelvic urethral hypertrophy

Figure 9.26 shows an ultrasonic image of an enlarged pelvic urethra.

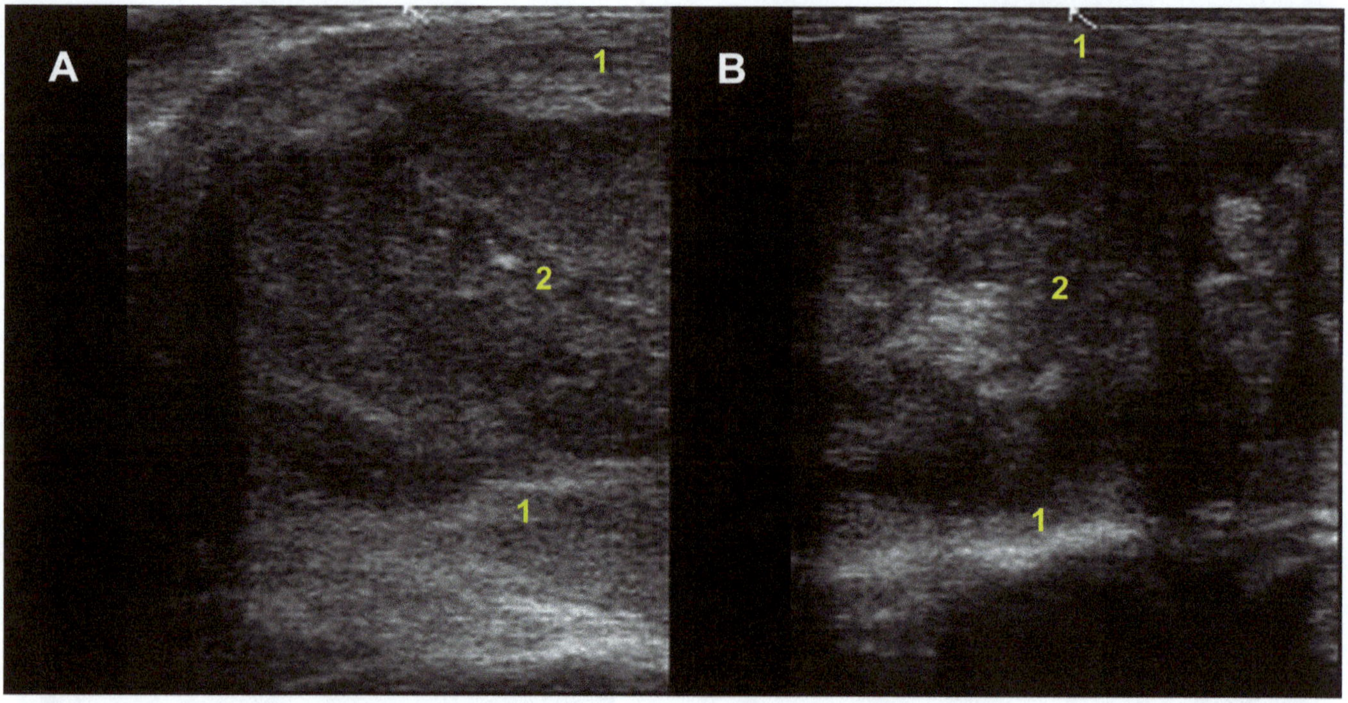

Figure 9.25. Ultrasonograms of vesiculitis (7.5 MHz probe; depth of 8 cm). Ultrasonographic findings of vesiculitis show an increase in overall size of the vesicular gland, a thickened wall, and increased echogenicity, when compared to the contralateral unaffected gland. See Figure 9.13 for comparison purposes. 1: Abscess capsule; 2: Pus.

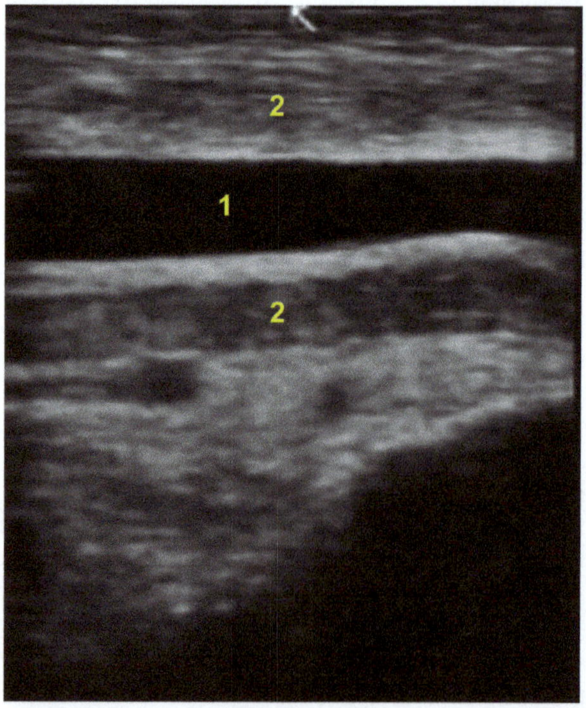

Figure 9.26. Ultrasound image of the hypertrophy of the pelvic urethra (7.5 MHz probe; depth of 8 cm). The urethra cannot normally be observed other than during micturition when it contains urine. Enlargement of the pelvic urethra is observed in cases of complete or partial urethral stenosis secondary to calculosis or urethritis. The lumen of the urethra appears enlarged and anechoic. 1: Lumen of the urethra; 2: Muscle of the urethra.

References

1. Bagshaw PA, Ladds PW (1974). A study of the accessory sex glands of bulls in abattoirs in northern Australia. Austral Vet J 50: 489–495.
2. Dargatz DA, Mortimer RG, Ball L (1987). Vesicular adenitis of bulls: A review. Theriogenology 28: 513–521.
3. Chandolia RK, Honaramooz A, Omeke BC, Pierson R, Beard AP, Rawlings NC (1997). Assessment of development of the testes and accessory glands by ultrasonography in bull calves and associated endocrine changes. Theriogenology 48: 119–132.
4. Evans ACO, Pierson RA, Garcia A, McDougall LM, Hrudka F, Rawlings (1996). Changes in circulating hormone concentrations, testes histology and testes ultrasonography during sexual maturation in beef bulls. Theriogenology 46: 345–357.
5. Gabor G, Szasz F, Sasser RG, Bozo S, Völgyi J, Barany I (1996). Using digitized video method for the measuring of testes sizes and prediction the testis volume in bulls. In: Proceedings of the 13th ICAR Congress, Sydney 2: 4–6.
6. Ginther O.J (1998). Ultrasonic Imaging and Animal Reproduction: Cattle. Chapitre 9, pp. 232–246.
7. Gnemmi G (2007). Place de l'échographie du taureau en pratique. Point Vétérinaire 275: 40–45.
8. Kh Abdel-Razed A, Ali A (2005). Development changes of bull (*Bos Taurus*) genitalia as evaluated by calliper and ultrasonography. Reprod Dom Anim 40: 23–27.
9. Miller D.L (1991). Update on safety of diagnostic ultrasonography. J Clin Ultrasound 19: 531–540.
10. Pierson RA, Kastelic JP, Ginther OJ (1988). Basic principles and techniques for transrectal ultrasonography in cattle and horses. Theriogenology 29: 3–20.
11. Pursley JR. Practical OvSynch programs (2007). Proceedings of the 40th annual convention of American Association of Bovine Practitioners 40: 44–49.
12. Rault P, Gérard, O (2006). Examen échographique génital du taureau. Point Vétérinaire 37 (numéro spécial): 32–39.
13. Trenkle A, William RL (1977). Beef production efficiency. Science 198: 1009–1015.
14. Weber JA, Hilt CJ, Woods GL (1988). Ultrasonographic appearance of bull accessory sex glands. Theriogenology 29: 1347–1355.
15. Zemjanis, R (1970). Diagnostic and Therapeutic Techniques in Animal Reproduction, 2ième éd., William and Wilkins Company, Baltimore, pp. 55–77.

Points to Remember

- The ultrasonographical examination of the male reproductive tract should always be preceded by, at least, a partial BSE and is not mandatory with a satisfactory BSE.
- In older animals with normal testes, small hyperechoic foci representing testicular septa are occasionally visible. Hyperechoic dots may appear and could represent fibrosis or mineralization, secondary to insults.
- Epididymitis is the most common abnormality of the epididymis and generally involves the tail.
- Even though the prevalence of vesiculitis is low, it is the most common pathologic condition affecting the internal genitalia in bulls.
- Ultrasonographic findings of vesiculitis show an increase in overall size of the seminal vesicular gland, a thickened wall, and increased echogenicity when compared to the contralateral unaffected gland.
- Ultrasonography is a useful tool for the diagnosis of reproductive pathologies in the bull.

Summary Questions

1. What characteristic of ultrasonography enhances the breeding soundness evaluation (BSE) in bulls?
   a. Ultrasonographic imaging allows better clinical assessment of the structures and functions of the reproductive tract.
   b. Ultrasonographic imaging allows better clinical assessments of only the functions of the reproductive tract.
   c. When the initial BSE is normal, ultrasonography is essential and adds more details to the description of the tissue structure.

2. Epididymitis is the most common unilateral condition affecting the scrotal reproductive organs. Describe the ultrasonographic evolution of the condition.

a. In the acute phase, a few hyperechoic areas are seen in the affected tissues and the epididymis gets smaller. In the chronic phase, the epididymis is enlarged, less echogenic, and coarser than normal; the tissue becomes more heterogeneous with diffuse lucency, probably due to edema.
b. In the acute phase, the epididymis is enlarged, less echogenic, and coarser than normal; the tissue becomes more heterogeneous with diffuse lucency, probably due to edema. In the chronic phase, a few hyperechoic areas are seen in the affected tissues and the epididymis gets smaller.
c. In chronic and acute epididymitis, the ultrasonographic appearances of the lesions are similar.

3. Young bulls are the most affected by the following condition even though its prevalence is relatively low in the general population of bulls (about 9%):

a. Testicular degeneration
b. Epididymitis
c. Vesiculitis

4. What is the most cranial accessory gland in bulls and what are the ultrasonographic characteristics of the organ?

a. Ampullae are the most cranial accessory glands and have a tube shape with thick walls. The lumens of ampullae appear irregular and homogeneously anechoic, if filled with sperm, and they represent 10 to 60% of the whole ampullae diameter. Sometimes, valves are seen within the lumen.
b. The vesicular glands are the most cranial accessory glands. The lumens of vesicular glands appear irregular and always homogeneously hyperechoic. Sometimes, valves are seen within the lumen.
c. Ampullae are the most cranial accessory glands and have a tube shape with thin walls. The lumens of ampullae appear regular and heterogeneously hyperechoic because of the presence of sperm.

5. For biosecurity reasons, what can be done to prevent disease transmission during the transrectal examination of the internal reproductive organs of the bull?

a. There is no reason to worry because there is no disease that can be transmitted during transrectal examination in bulls.
b. There is no biosecurity concern during the transrectal examination of bulls. However, a plastic sleeve will prolong the functional life of the transducer.
c. For biosecurity reasons (Johne's disease, leukosis, BVD/MD) and to protect the transducer for a prolonged functional life, the transducer can be introduced in a plastic sleeve with coupling medium (ultrasound gel) and an appropriate amount of lubricant in the rectum.

6. What is seen in this ultrasound image of the testis (7.5 MHz probe; depth 6 cm)?

a. Normal testicular parenchyma
b. Abnormal testicular parenchyma
c. Normal testicular parenchyma but the ultrasound unit was incorrectly set

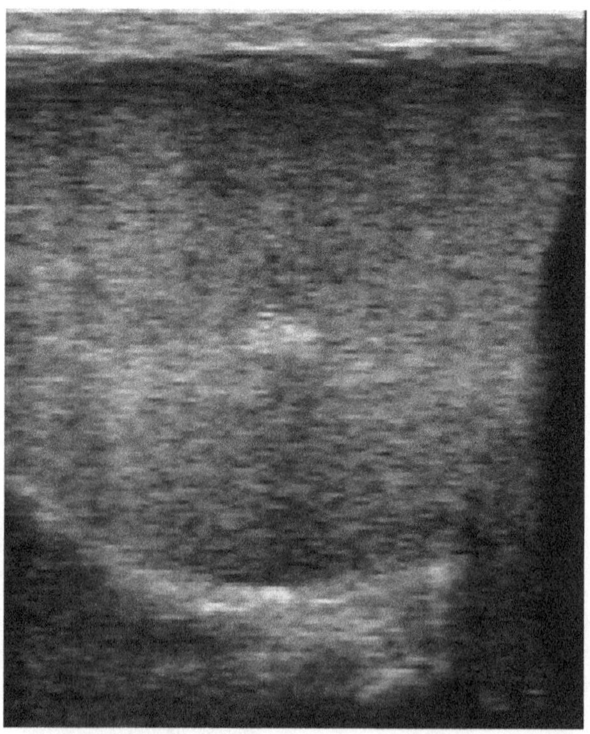

7. Which type of probe is better for scanning the male reproduction tract?
   a. Linear 5.0–7.5 MHz
   b. Convex or curvilinear 2.5–5 MHz
   c. Sector 5.0 MHz

8. What is seen in this ultrasonogram of the testis (7.5 MHz probe; depth 6 cm)?
   a. Abscess in the testis
   b. Testicular fibrosis
   c. The rete testis

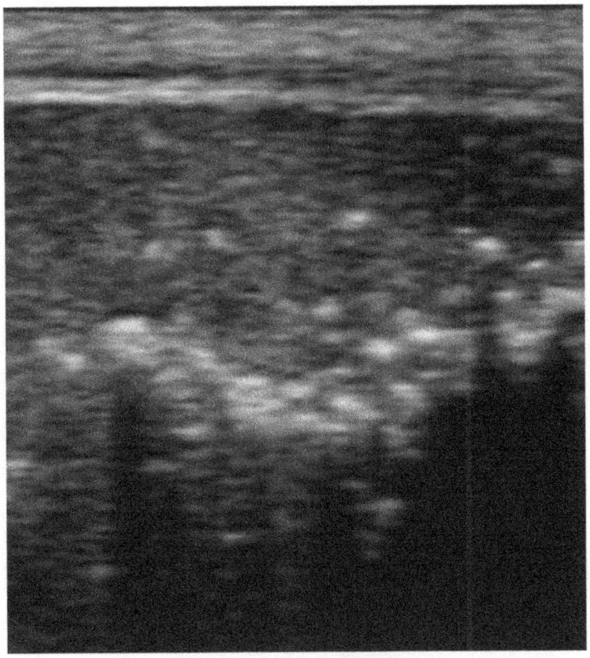

9. What do you see in this ultrasound image of the bull's external genital organs (7.5 MHz probe; depth 5 cm)?
   a. Pampiniform plexus
   b. Head of the epididymis
   c. Tail of the epididymis

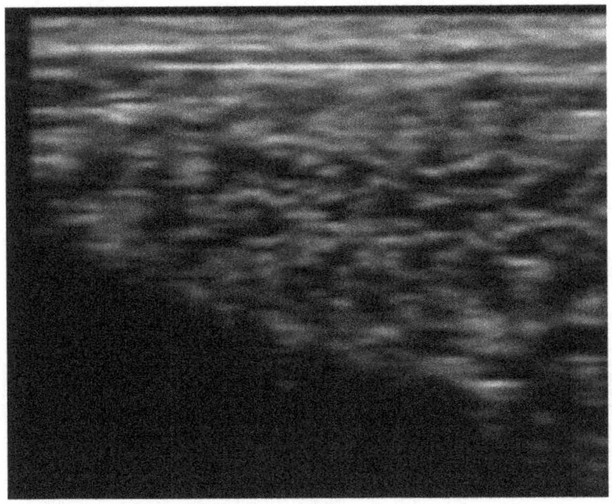

10. When is it useful to do an ultrasound examination of the male genital tract?
   a. In all bulls over 5 years of age
   b. Whenever semen quality or quantity is poor
   c. Whenever fertility of the bull is poor

11. What do you see in this ultrasound image of the bull's internal genital organs (7.5 MHz probe; depth 6 cm)?
   a. Normal vesicular gland
   b. Bulbourethral gland with an abscess
   c. Longitudinal section of the urethra

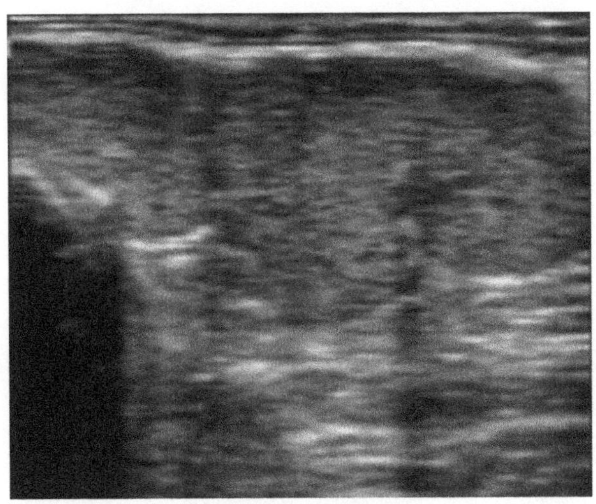

Answers

1. a
2. b
3. c
4. a
5. c
6. b
7. a
8. b
9. a
10. c
11. a

CHAPTER TEN

Buffalo and Zebu Cattle

Giovanni Gnemmi and Heraldo Marcus Rosi Cruvinel

This chapter describes the practical use of ultrasonography in water buffalo and zebu cattle. Ultrasound is an integral component of a reproductive management program. Early pregnancy diagnosis, early embryonic death diagnosis, follicular dynamic control (and application of synchronization programs), fetal sex diagnosis, and ovarian and uterine physiopathology monitoring are economically valuable in these two species.

Introduction

In the order Artiodactyla, the cloven-hoofed mammals, cattle belong to the genus *Bos* within the Family Bovidae. All modern bovidae have developed by natural selection into many distinct species, including *Bubalus bubalis*, the domesticated water buffalo; *Bos taurus*, the domesticated cow of Europe; and *Bos indicus*, the domesticated zebu of India, Asia, and Africa[2].

The buffalo (Figure 10.1) is present on every continent. According to the United Nations Food and Agriculture Organization (FAO) in 2002 the world buffalo population was estimated at 168 million head with the majority of the population in Asia (96%), where buffalo supply 40% of the milk and 3.32% of the meat. The buffalo population is increasing every year in every part of the world[33].

Buffalo husbandry has been recognized throughout the world as a viable solution for food production in many areas within the tropical countries. Besides economic benefits buffalo have many other advantages, such as their excellent adaptability to different ecosystems, good fertility and longevity, and ability to learn quickly to respect electrical fencing. These benefits lead to more income for farmers[30].

Bubalus bubalis is a domestic species distributed in every continent and used mostly for milk and meat production and for work. Meat buffalo are found mostly in South America (Argentina, Brazil, Colombia, Venezuela), Asia, and Oceania (Australia). Milk buffalo are mostly concentrated in Asia and Mediterranean areas, particularly Italy[5].

The zebu (Figure 10.2) was introduced to South America in the beginning of the 20th century and is the most important species of the genus *Bos*. In Brazil, there are 206 million head of cattle and about 80% of them are zebu or zebu/*Bos taurus* crosses. Because of good adaptability to tropical temperatures and tick resistance, zebu are the primary source of meat cattle in Brazil and are crossbred with Holstein for dairy

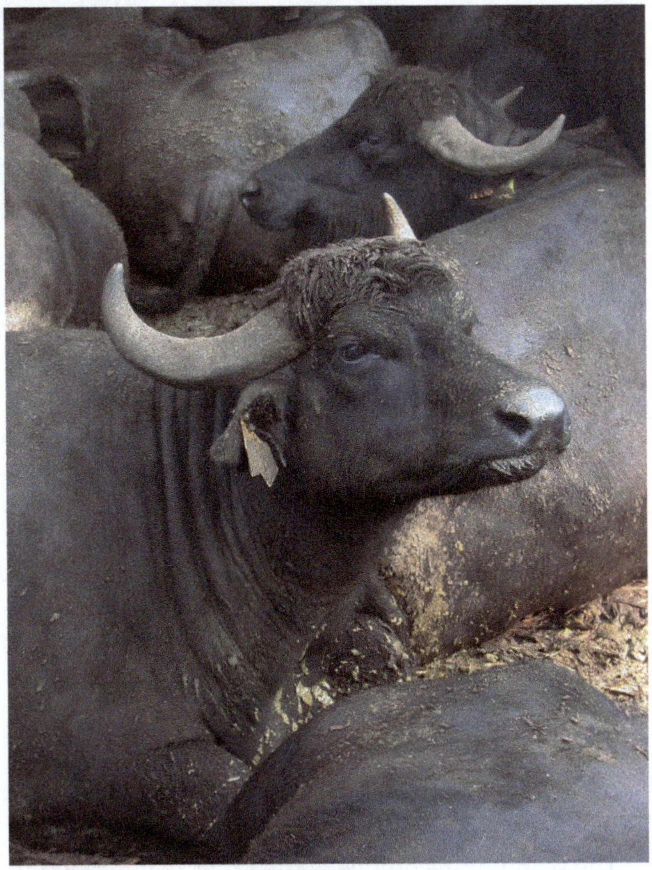

Figure 10.1. *Bubalus bubalis* is present on every continent.

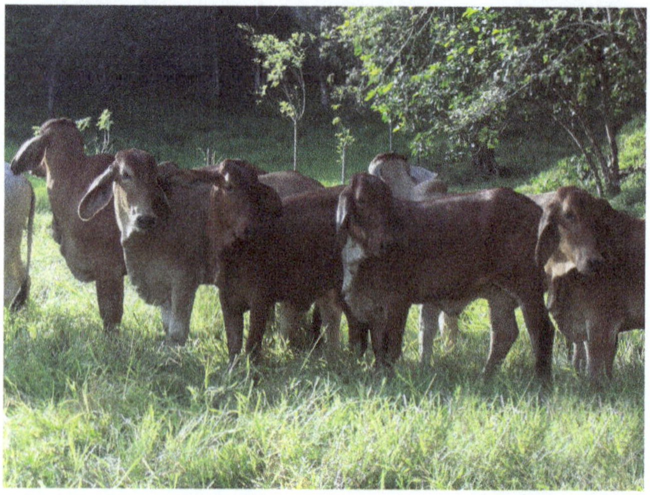

Figure 10.2. The zebu is the most important species of the genus *Bos* in South America. The Nelore is the most popular zebu breed chosen for meat production.

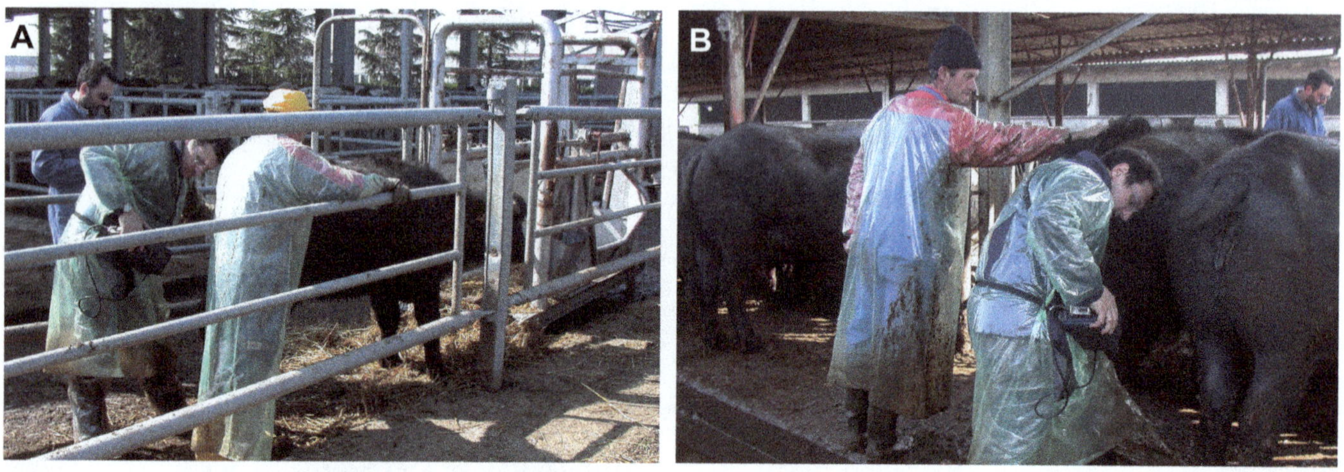

Figure 10.3. Ultrasound examination of a water buffalo with or without a chute. The veterinarian is behind the animal with an assistant to hold the tail to avoid strong pressure on the arm of the veterinarian and movement of the dangerous tail.

production. Nelore is the chosen breed for meat production due to its good rate of gain on pasture, with 80% of the cattle registered in the zebu association (ABCZ). Gir is the zebu dairy breed.

Equipment and Scanning Techniques

Portable ultrasound units with self-contained power sources are preferable over cart-based units. Buffalo and zebu are normally very quiet, but field conditions and management situations are often very difficult.

The scanning technique is the same as described in Chapter 2. The probe may be held with the fingers or it may be rested in the palm with fingers free. The second method has the advantage of allowing the operator to retract the uterus while scanning, if necessary.

The probes normally used are 5 to 7.5 MHz linear or sector probes. When working with smaller ovaries it may be preferable to use a 7.5 MHz linear or sector probe.

The examination can be done from behind the animal in an appropriate chute (Figure 10.3). Domestic buffalo are very quiet animals in spite of their great size. However, the rectal contractions are very strong. Thus, it may be helpful to have an assistant hold the tail. Under field conditions an experienced veterinarian with assistance can perform between 30–50 ultrasound examinations per hour.

Table 10.1.
Dimensions of the reproductive tract in female buffalo, cows, and zebu (adapted data from Aboul-Fadle et al. 1974; Luktuke and Rao 1962; Mobarak 1969)

	Buffalo	Cow	Zebu
Adult body weight (kg)	600–1,100	500–700	340–589
Adult withers height (cm)	125	137–138	
Ovary length (cm)	2.2–2.9	2.8–3.8	
Diameter of ovulatory follicle (cm)	1.32–1.50	1.9–2.2	1.1–1.3
Diameter of mature corpus luteum (cm)	1.3–1.6	1.7–3.0	1.3–2.8
Oviduct length (cm)	19–23	25–26	
Uterus length (cm)	30–38	35–45	
Uterine body diameter (cm)	2.1–2.8	2.5–5.0	
Puberty (months)	16–22	10–14	16–32
Length of the cycle (days)	20–22 River buffalo 19–20 Swamp buffalo	18–24	20–22
Duration of estrus (hours)	12–28	18–24	11
Ovulation	10 hours after the onset of heat	28–31 hours after the onset of heat	24–26 hours after the onset of heat
Pregnancy duration (days)	310–330	270–282	292

Major Differences Between Bovine and Bubaline Species

Anatomy

There is considerable similarity in the anatomy of the reproductive tracts of buffalo, cows, and zebu. The smaller total size of *Bubalus bubalis* and *Bos indicus* reflects the smaller size of their organs compared to *Bos taurus*[1] (Table 10.1; Figures 10.4, 10.5). There are insufficient data for the zebu for some measurements to complete Table 10.1.[1]

Physiology

Seasonality

Buffalo and zebu are generally seasonally polyestrous short-day breeders. Thus, their reproductive efficiency (displaying estrous behavior, conception rate, calving rate, days postpartum to cyclicity) changes throughout the year. The female is usually sexually inactive from March to the end of June. Hours of daylight are important in controlling seasonality in buffalo and zebu, but other correlated environmental factors such as temperature (buffalo have lower plasma progesterone values and a lowered LH response to GnRH during the hotter months[1]), rainfall, and food supply appear to be of overriding importance[1]. This is one of the reasons for the prolonged intercalving period during the off season[39]. For *river buffalo*, the female is active from July until the end of February. The peak of first mating occurs during autumn and winter. *Swamp buffalo* cycle throughout the year, but a nutritional seasonal pattern is observed.

Breeding during the rainy period and the winter appears to be most favorable while summer appears to be least favorable for buffalo reproduction[37]. Buffalo and zebu have a tendency to seasonality that depends in part upon the environmental characteristics of their place of origin. In the subtropical zones, north of the equator, forage availability and nutritional management vary considerably throughout the year[37] leading to seasonality of the estrous cycle. This condition is absent in Italy where intensive breeding of buffalo occurs throughout the year. Climate and photoperiod (melatonin secretion!) are also important in buffalo and zebu seasonality. The proportion of buffalo exhibiting estrus during the period of short-day length is significantly higher than during the period of long-day length, indicating that decreasing daylight is a strong determinant for the resumption of ovarian activity[39].

In Brazil, below the equator where the average temperature varies between 10 °C and 15 °C, there is a period of good quality pasture during the rainy

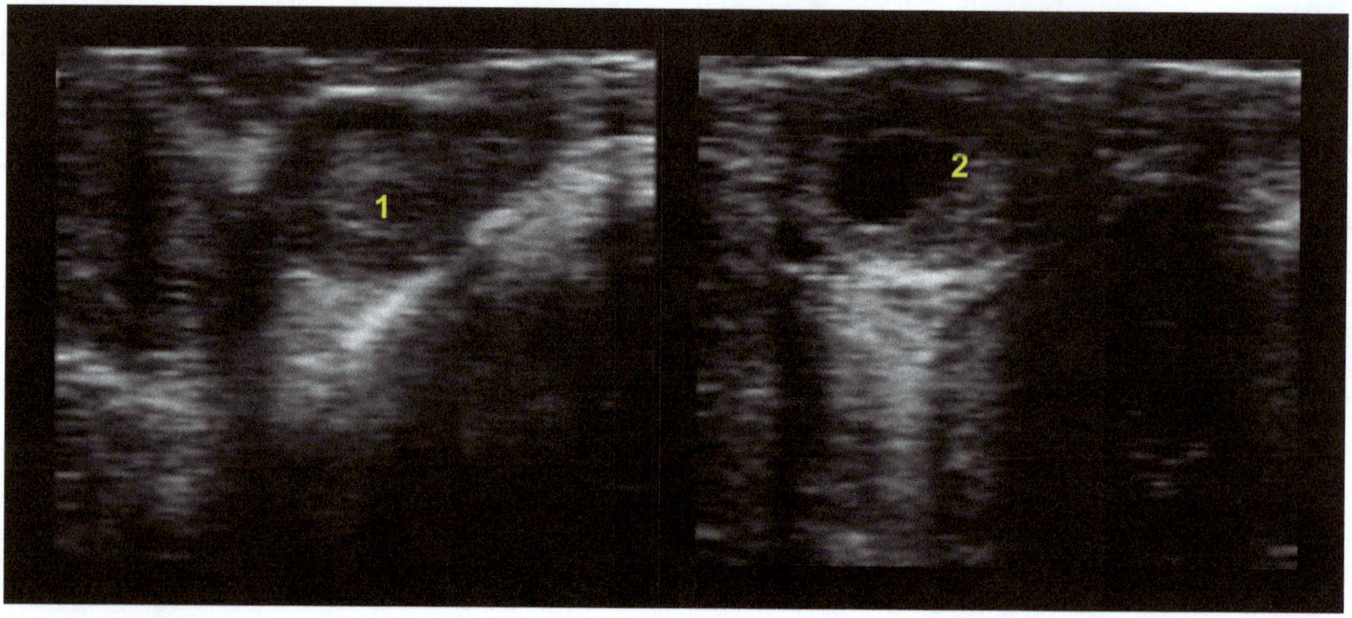

Figure 10.4. Ultrasonographic image of a compact and cavitary corpus luteum (CL) in a water buffalo (7.5 MHz linear probe; depth 5 cm). The size of the CL is smaller compared to *Bos taurus*. 1: Compact CL; 2: Cavitary CL.

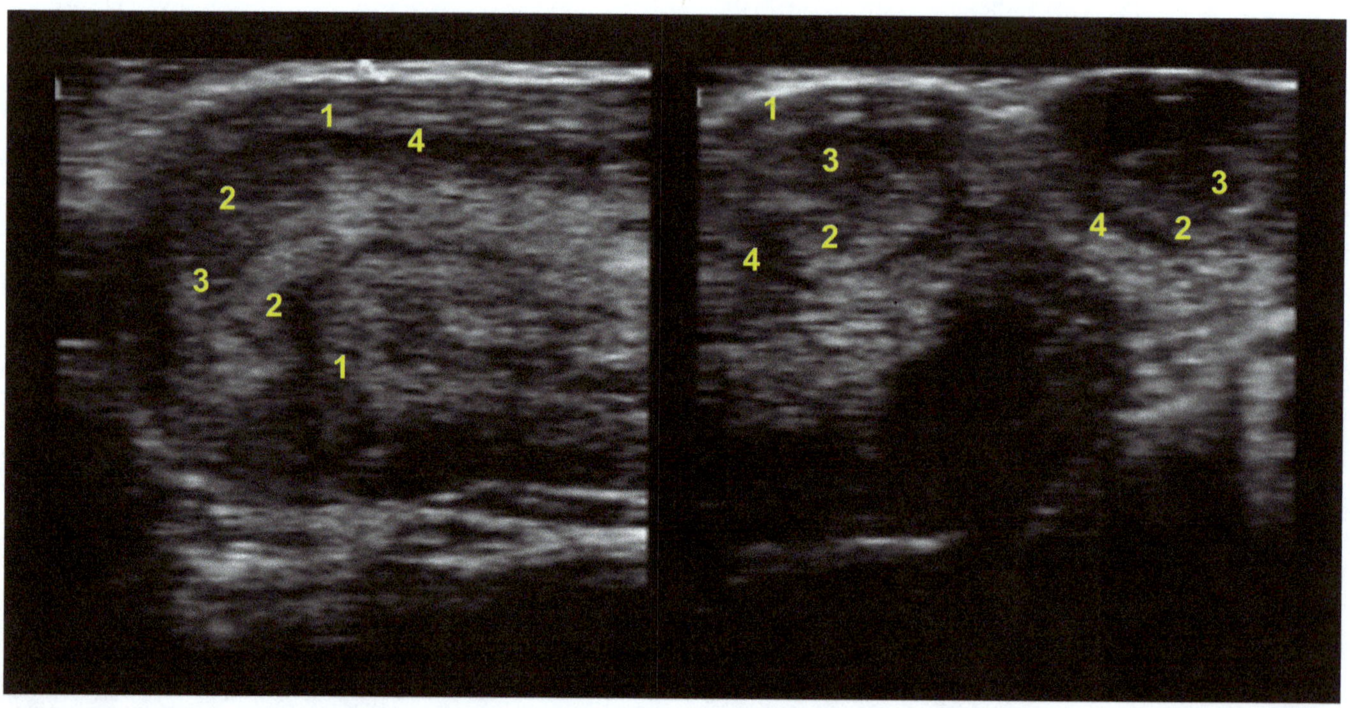

Figure 10.5. Ultrasonographic images of longitudinal (A) and transverse sections (B) of the uterus in a zebu (7.5 MHz linear probe; depth 6 cm). B: Note the presence of two uterine sections in this image; 1: Myometrium; 2: Endometrium; 3: Uterine lumen; 4: Vascular portion of the uterus.

Table 10.2.
Detection of the first postpartum estrus of dairy Gir after calving according to season (Ferreira et al. 2005)

	First Postpartum Estrus	
Season	n	1st postpartum estrus (days)
Summer	31	98.6
Winter	17	85.5

summer season from October to March. Between April and September the temperature is lower, it is less humid, and the length of day is shorter. The onset of estrus is delayed during this colder, dry period, and it is also the same time as the lower growing rate of the forage. There are many strategies to minimize the effects on ovarian activity. One of them is to restrict the breeding season to October through March. This method is used mainly for beef cattle at pasture. For dairy cattle, breeding occurs throughout the year but nutritional supplementation with silage, grass, hay, and other crops is provided during the colder dry months. Because of this supplementation, the nutritional status of the dairy cattle during the dry season becomes better than during the rainy season, which translates into a more rapid onset of follicular development. Table 10.2 presents the average first detection of estrus after parturition of dairy Gir according to season.

Puberty

The attainment of puberty depends largely on body weight and nutritional management. In well-nourished buffalo the first signs of estrus occur at 15–18 months of age, although under some field conditions the onset of puberty has been reported at 24–36 months.

Puberty occurs at a later age (16–24 months) and higher percentage of adult body weight[1] in the zebu. There is much difference among the zebu breeds. The dairy Gir is the slowest, beginning puberty at over 20 months for a first calving between 30 and 42 months. On the Getulio Vargas Experimental Farm (Uberaba MG, Brazil), the age average at first calving for Gir was 39 months, with 392 Kg of live weight[26]. For beef breeds of zebu (Nelore, Tabapuã, Guzera, Brahman) the onset of puberty occurs earlier but their nutritional management is significantly better. To participate in the Brazilian zebu show (Expozebu), the beef breed heifers must be pregnant at 20 months (www.expozebu.com.br/2008/downloads/regulamento). The body weight generally determines when it is time to breed. For Gir and Sindi the accepted breeding weight is 250–270 kg, and for the others it is over 300 kg.

Table 10.3.
Characteristics of follicular turnover during an estrous cycle in buffalo having two or three follicular wave patterns (adapted from Baruselli 1997)

	N° Waves	
	2	3
Percent of buffalo (%)	66.6	33.3
Duration of estrous cycle (days)	22.3 ± 0.9	24.5 ± 1.9
Emergence of first wave (days)	1.2 ± 0.5	1.1 ± 0.3
Emergence of second wave (days)	10.8 ± 1.1	9.3 ± 1.2
Emergence of third wave (days)		18.8 ± 1.2

Table 10.4.
Characteristics of estrous cycle in dairy Gir (zebu breed) having two to five follicular wave patterns

	N° Waves			
	2	3	4	5
Percent of dairy Gir (%)	36	41	14	9
Duration of estrous cycle (days)	20.2 ± 1.0	20.3 ± 1.2	20.5 ± 0.7	19.5 ± 0.7

Table 10.5.
Characteristics of follicular waves in Gir dairy cows with three follicular waves (Ferreira et al. 2005)

Characteristics	First Wave	Second Wave	Third Wave
Wave onset (days)	0.8 ± 0.4	7.1 ± 1.0	13.2 ± 2.4
Wave length (days)	13.0 ± 1.6	11.4 ± 2.2	7.7 ± 1.8

Follicular dynamics

Ovarian follicular growth in buffalo is similar to that observed in cattle and is characterized by follicular waves[9,10]. It has been demonstrated that buffalo typically have two follicular waves (66.6%) or three follicular waves (33.3%) during an estrous cycle[9,10] (Table 10.3). In dairy zebu breeds, most of the cows have two to three follicular waves, although 23% of them have more than three follicular waves (Table 10.4). The characteristics of the follicular waves of Gir dairy cows with two to five follicular waves are presented in Tables 10.4 and 10.5.

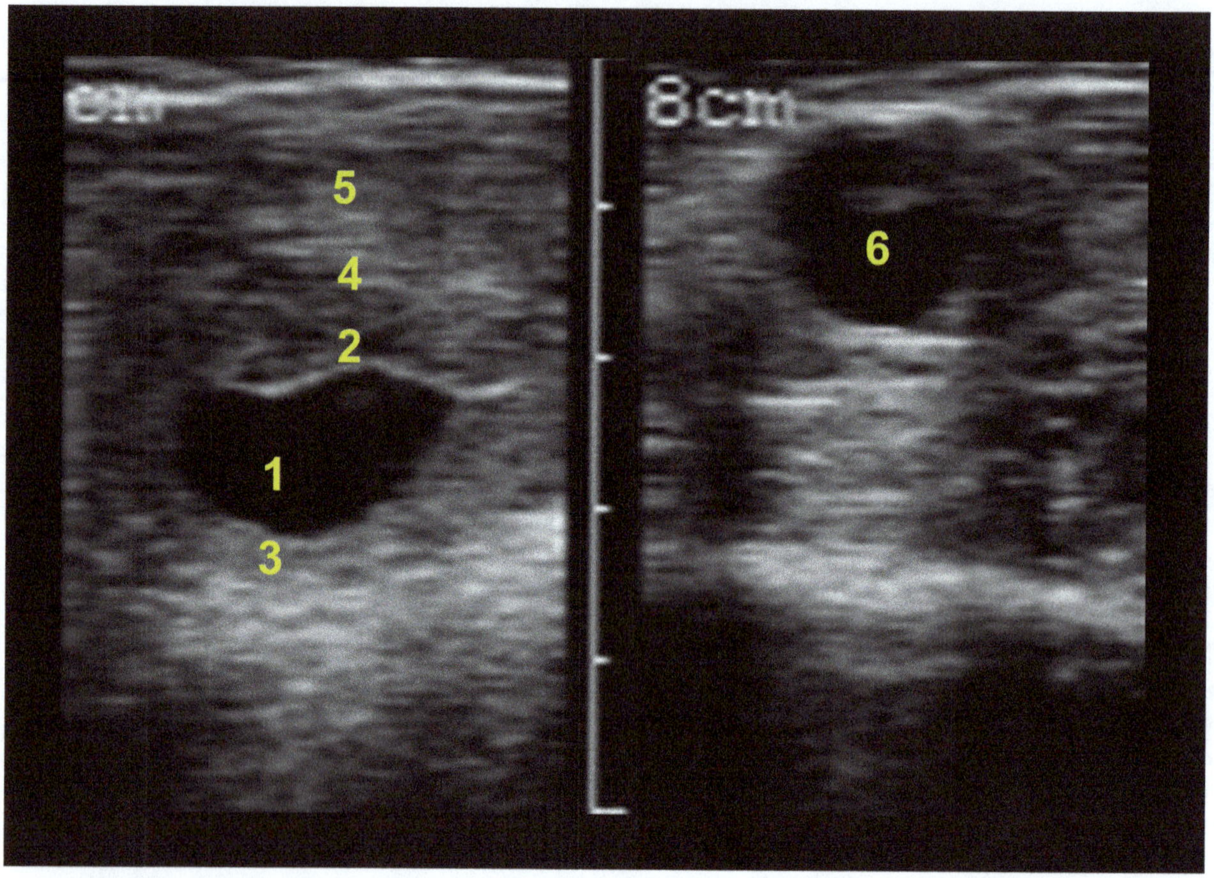

Figure 10.6. Ultrasonogram of the uterus of a water buffalo in heat (7.5 MHz linear probe; depth 5 cm). 1: Uterine lumen with fluid; 2: Specular reflection; 3: Endometrium; 4: Vascular portion of the uterus; 5: Myometrium; 6: Follicle.

The length of the estrous cycle is similar in each species. Buffalo have a mean cycle length of 21.6 ± 0.2 days. Zebu values of 21.3 ± 0.1 days have been reported, with 85% in estrus between 18–22 days[15]. Figure 10.6 presents an ultrasonogram of the uterus of a water buffalo in heat.

The changes in the ovarian steroids and gonadotrophin blood concentrations during the estrous cycle in buffalo cows are considered to be comparable to those of *Bos taurus* cows[25]. The statement is generally correct, but during the hottest months in warmer countries these values are depressed[28].

Estrous behavior

Homosexual activity in buffalo and in zebu is not as pronounced as in the cow[23,30]. The duration of estrous signs ranges from 11 to 30 hours, but the intensity of signs is lower in buffalo[15]. Ovulation occurs spontaneously about 10 hours after the end of the estrus[15]. Silent heat is common in buffalo. Although the estrous cycle is present, the external symptoms of heat are absent or much reduced. This is due to the deficiency of LH as well as estrogen or progesterone[39]. The duration of estrus in buffalo during early summer is shorter, and this may be mistaken for anestrus[15]. Detection of estrus to determine the proper time of AI can be difficult[11]. This is the principal reason for the development of the synchronization programs in buffalo.

Postpartum return to cyclicity, nutrition, and body condition score

Buffalo and zebu calving in the cooler winter months have shorter intervals from calving to first estrus[2]. Table 10.6 presents physiologic reproductive characteristics of Gir dairy cows after calving according to the type of nutrition programs. Gir cows show low repro-

Table 10.6.
Physiologic reproductive characteristics of dairy Gir cows after calving, according to the type of nutrition programs (Ferreira et al. 2005)

	Calving to 1st Ovulation Interval (Days)	1st Ovulation to 1st Estrous Interval (Days)	Calving to 1st Physiological Cycle Interval (Days)	Calving to 1st Detected Heat (Days)	Length of Estrous Cycle (Days)	N° of Follicular Waves per Cycle
Supplementation	58.7	9.2	66	83.8	20.7	2.9
Pasture only	68.8	7.6	75	76.7	20.9	2.7
Overall averages (Std deviations)	63.8 (21.3)	8.7 (1.7)	71.3 (23.3)	80.3 (26.6)	20.8	2.8

ductive efficiency due to the long period between calving and rebreeding, normally over 100 days in pasture conditions[20]. This long postpartum anestrus is the main reason for the economic loss in production systems of the tropical countries. The length of this period is affected by many factors in the zebu breeds, by nutritional variations due to the seasonal production of forages, and by the suckling effect, the most important reason for the delay to first estrus[40]. Suckling management increases the LH pulse frequency and can promote the beginning of ovarian activity. In addition, many progesterone, estradiol, and equine chorionic gonadotropin (eCG) programs have been used to promote estrus and ovulation on anestrous dairy cows[41].

Poor body condition can invalidate any positive effect of suckling management on the ovarian activity in zebu cows[19]. Many authors emphasize the importance of body condition score (BCS) to improve the interval between calving and first breeding[3,31,32,38]. Others assert that a good BCS at calving allows a modest body weight loss during the beginning of the lactation without delaying the postpartum estrus[13,16,21,38,42]. Long postpartum anestrus is mainly caused by low BCS at calving or by excessive body weight loss in the first 2 or 3 months of lactation even if the initial BCS was good. For this reason, BCS has been proposed as an auxiliary method to evaluate nutritional and reproductive herd management[22]. More studies are needed about the relationship between body condition and the onset of the postpartum ovarian activity in *Bos indicus*. Similarities to *Bos taurus* cannot be assumed because there are differences in reproductive physiology (length and intensity of estrus, follicular development, corpus luteum volume, etc.) and fat deposition (internal versus external) between these two species[6,7,17]. In general, however, lower BCS at calving appears to lead to a longer interval to the first postpartum estrus in *Bos indicus* females.

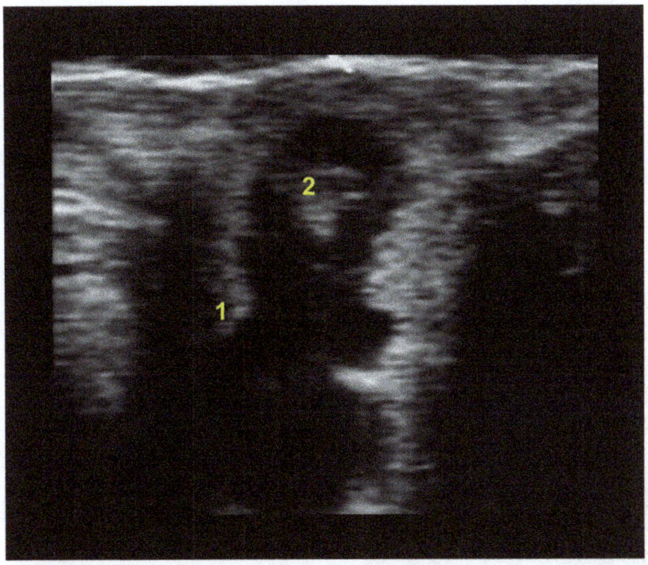

Figure 10.7. Ultrasonographic image of a 28-day pregnancy in a buffalo (7.5 MHz probe; depth 5 cm). 1: Endometrium; 2: Embryo (0.8–1.0 cm).

Pregnancy

The gestation period of buffalo is between 310–330 days; pregnancy in the zebu lasts 292 days[1]. The total number of placentomes in the pregnant zebu uterus is about 69, lower than the 70–142 reported for cows[1].

Figures 10.7 to 10.13 present ultrasonographic images of pregnancy from 28 to 56 days in water buffalo.

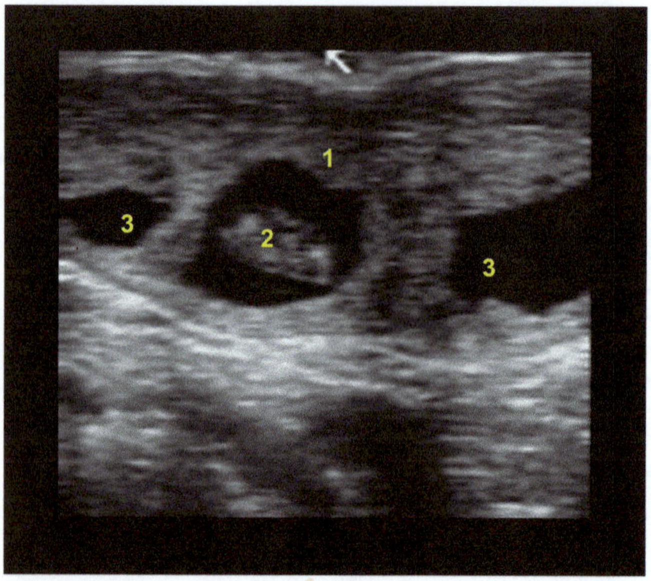

Figure 10.8. Ultrasonographic image of a 32-day pregnancy in a buffalo (7.5 MHz probe; depth 5 cm). 1: Uterus; 2: Embryo (1.5 cm); 3: Gestational pockets.

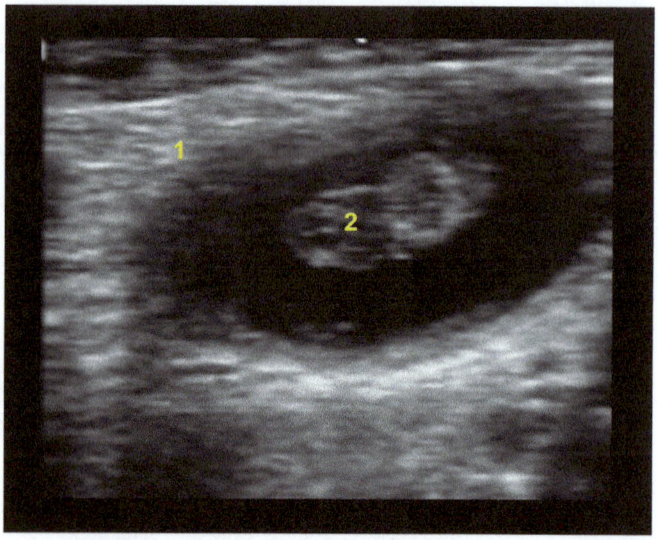

Figure 10.10. Ultrasonographic image of a 36-day pregnancy in a buffalo (7.5 MHz probe; depth 5 cm). 1: Endometrium; 2: Embryo (2.5 cm).

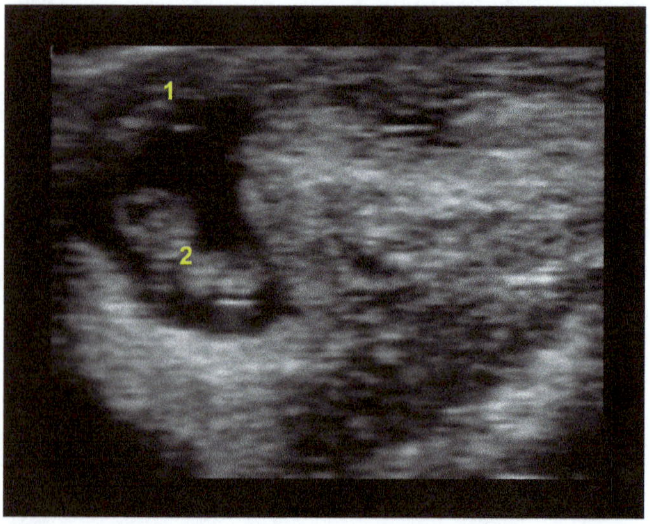

Figure 10.9. Ultrasonographic image of a 34-day pregnancy in a buffalo (7.5 MHz probe; depth 5 cm). 1: Endometrium; 2: Embryo (2 cm).

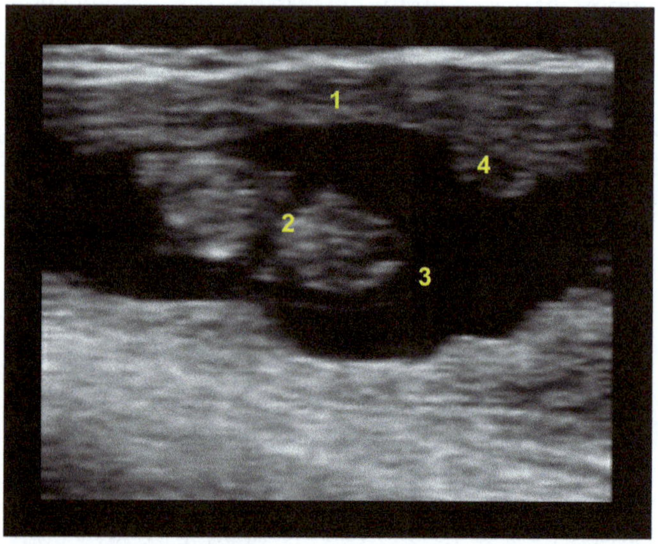

Figure 10.11. Ultrasonographic image of a 40-day pregnancy in a buffalo (7.5 MHz probe; depth 5 cm). 1: Endometrium; 2: Embryo (3.0 cm); 3: Amniotic membrane; 4: Placentome.

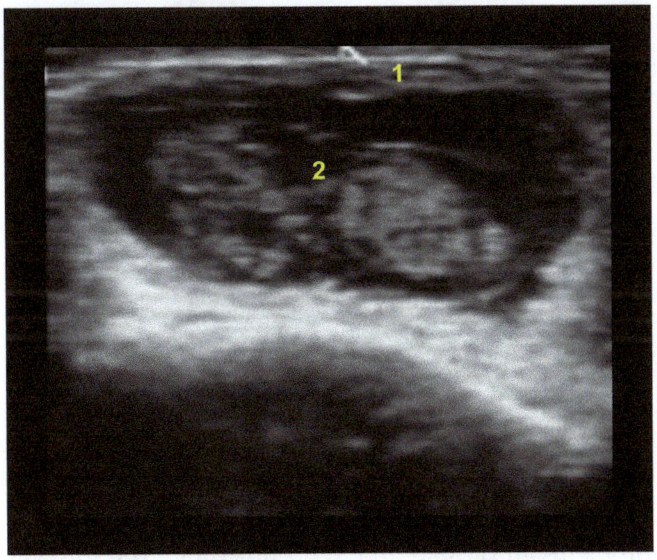

Figure 10.12. Ultrasonographic image of a 48-day pregnancy in a buffalo (7.5 MHz probe; depth 5 cm). 1: Endometrium; 2: Embryo (4.0 cm).

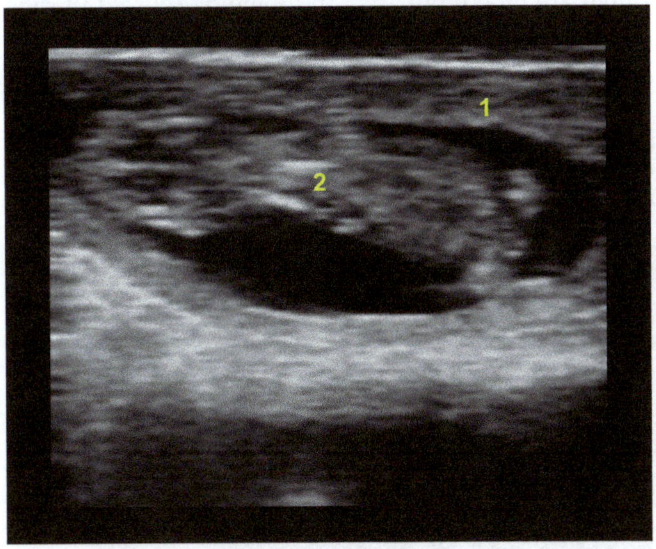

Figure 10.13. Ultrasonographic image of a 56-day pregnancy in a buffalo (7.5 MHz probe; depth 5 cm). 1: Endometrium; 2: Embryo (5.0 cm).

Pathology

Vulvar lesions[34,35]

Laceration of the vagina and vulva can occur during parturition mainly in heifers or during forceful manipulation in cases of dystocia (Figure 10.14).

Cervicitis and vaginitis[34,35]

These pathological conditions are very common in female buffalo (Figure 10.15). Usually they originate from rough manipulation during parturition or from uterine prolapse.

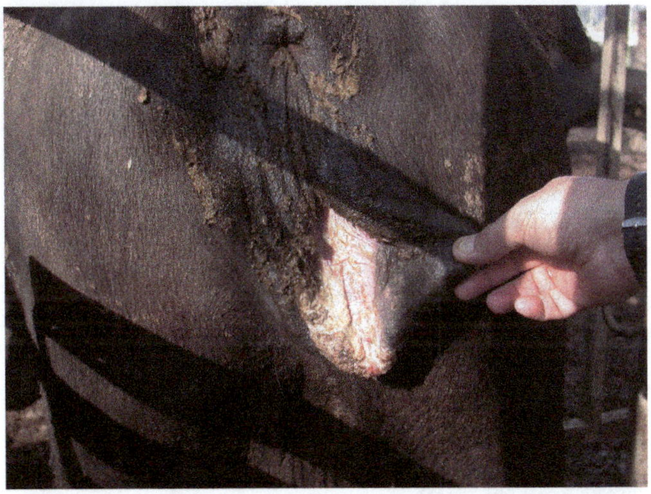

Figure 10.14. Vulvar traumatic lesion in a *Bubalus bubalis*. This type of lesion is very frequent and is always the consequence of forceful manipulations during calving assistance.

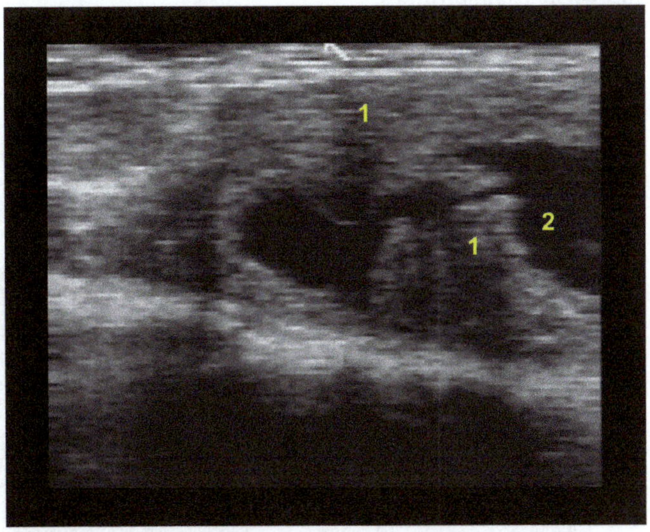

Figure 10.15. Ultrasonographic images of cervicitis in buffalo (7.5 MHz linear probe; depth 5 cm). 1: Internal cervix ring; 2: Fluid in the vagina.

Uterus

Uterine involution is more rapid in buffalo than in cows after normal parturition. Puerperal infection is the most important cause of reproductive failure in buffalo[39]. There is a 20–30% incidence of postpartum clinical metritis/endometritis in buffalo and zebu[15] (Figure 10.16).

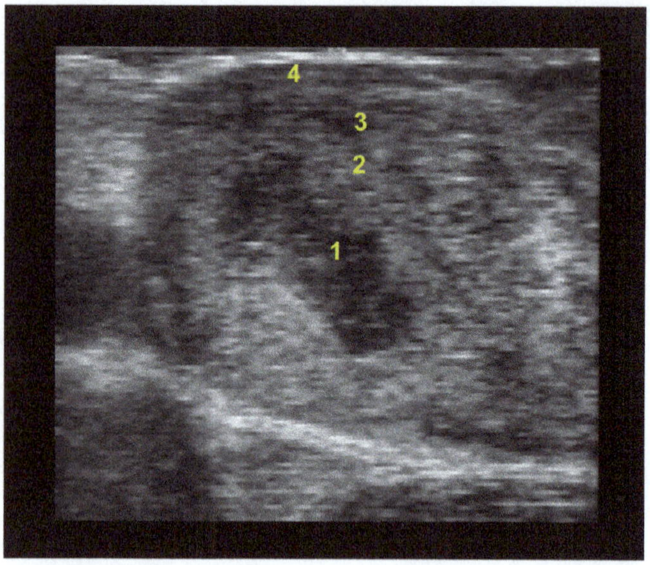

Figure 10.16. Ultrasonogram of endometritis in a zebu (7.5 MHz probe; depth 5 cm). 1: Purulent material in the uterine lumen; 2: Endometrium; 3: Vascular portion of the uterus; 4: Myometrium.

Bursal adhesions, hydrosalpinx, and bursal cyst

Pathological conditions of the ovarian bursa and oviduct are also common abnormalities observed as causes of infertility in female buffalo (Figure 10.17). These conditions originate from a primary infection in another segment of the tubular genital system, such as vaginitis, cervicitis, or endometritis[36,37].

Ovarian abnormalities

The most common ovarian abnormalities in buffalo are ovarian inactivity, ovarian cysts, and infantile ovaries (particularly in buffalo heifers).

The long intercalving period is one of the major problems in buffalo and zebu breeding. The interval from calving to resumption of ovarian function is longer in buffalo and zebu compared with dairy cattle. The reasons for this delay are numerous; the most frequent are breed, nutrition, milk yield, delayed uterine

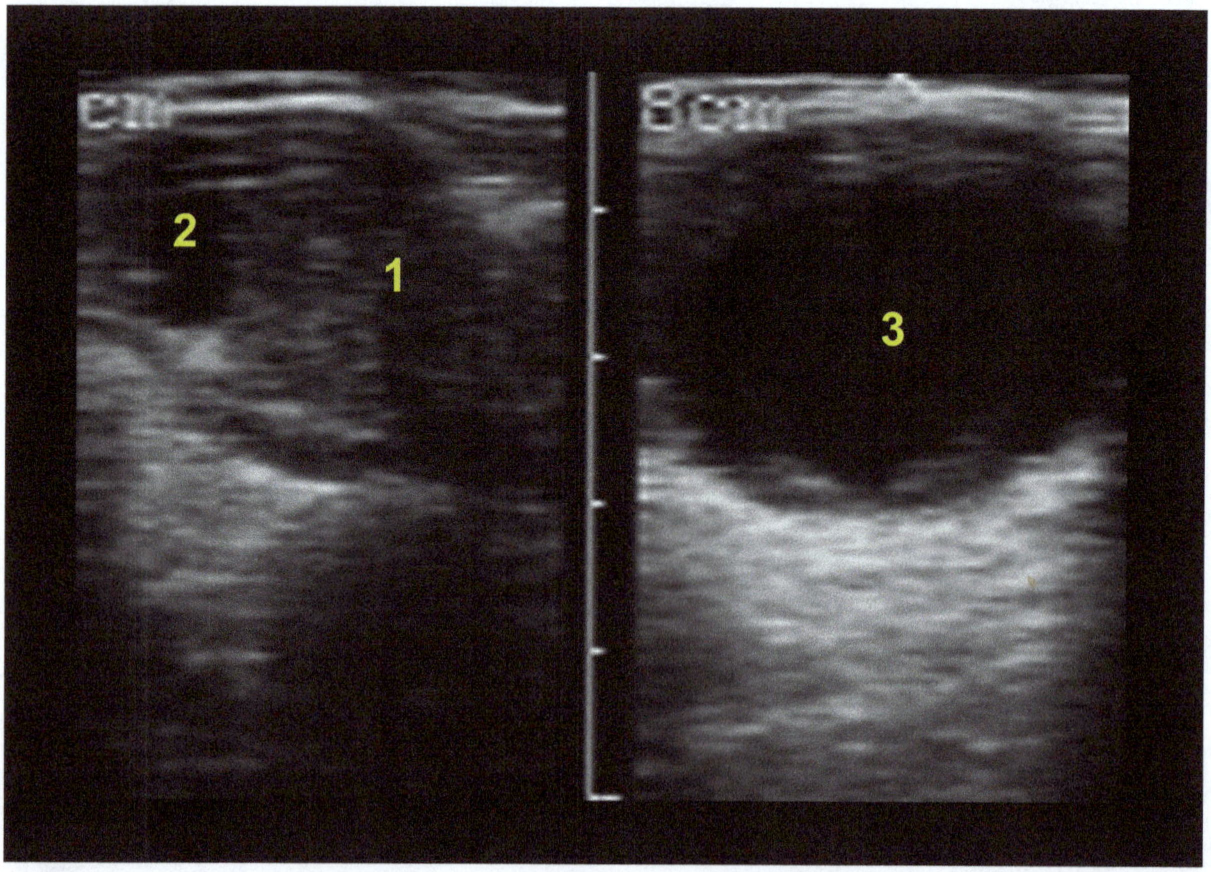

Figure 10.17. Ultrasonogram of hydrosalpinx in a female buffalo (7.5 MHz linear probe; depth 5 cm). This is a rare pathologic condition in *Bubalus bubalis*, as in *Bos indicus* and *Bos taurus*. 1: CL; 2: Follicle; 3: Transversal section of the dilated salpinx.

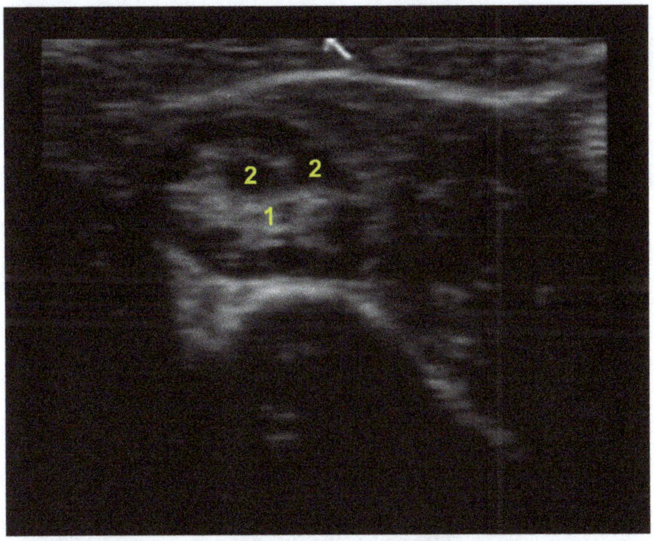

Figure 10.18. Ultrasound image of ovarian inactivity in a buffalo (7.5 MHz linear probe; depth 5 cm). This is a very common condition in *Bubalus bubalis* and *Bos indicus*. 1: Ovarian stroma; 2: Small follicles of less than 3 mm.

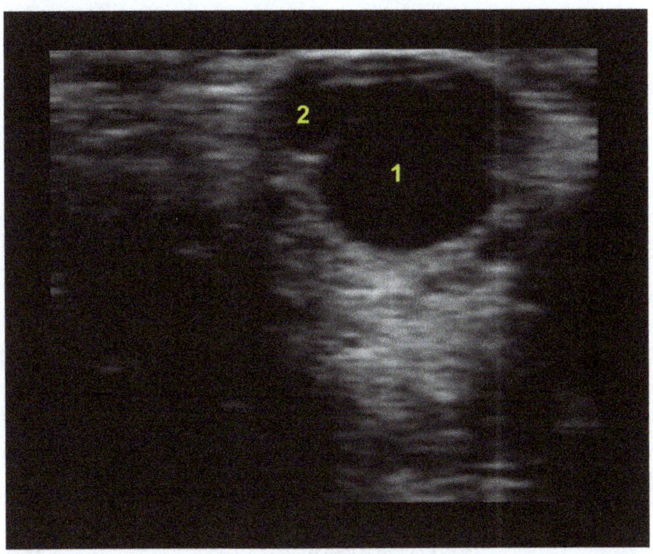

Figure 10.19. Ultrasonogram of a cystic follicular degeneration in a Mediterranean water buffalo (7.5 MHz linear probe; depth 5 cm). This is a common condition in *Bubalus bubalis* and *Bos indicus*. 1: Cystic follicular degeneration (2 cm); 2: Follicle.

involution, suckling, and seasonality[5]. Ovarian inactivity (Figure 10.18) is correlated with all these factors.

Cystic follicular degeneration (Figure 10.19) is more common in high-producing milk buffalo (Mediterranean water buffalo). There is no difference in the rate of cystic follicular degeneration in buffalo compared to cows. However, nymphomania associated with this condition in buffalo is not a common observation, as it is in cows[39].

Congenital and Hereditary Defects

Congenital problems such as imperforate hymen or hymenal bands have been described and are generally associated with morphological disturbances of genetic origin.

Intersexes such as true or pseudohermaphrodites and freemartinism are rare conditions in buffalo. Other abnormalities commonly observed are uterus unicornis segmental aplasia of one segment of the uterine horn, underdevelopment of genitalia, absence or double cervix, and atresia of the vagina[34,35].

Ultrasound Services in Buffalo and Zebu

The following ultrasound services are available for buffalo and zebu:

1. Uterine, ovarian, and follicular activity monitoring
2. Early pregnancy determination
3. Fetal viability determination
4. Embryo and fetal age determination
5. Fetal sex determination
6. Improvement of synchronization programs

The techniques for these examinations are similar to those in the bovine with only minor differences.

Determination of the age of embryos or fetuses

Determining the age of an embryo or fetus may be useful to determine the paternity of each pregnancy because in buffalo herds it is very common to use more that one bull in different time periods. It is possible to use the same parameters used in *Bos taurus* to determine the age of embryos or fetuses (see Chapters 6 and 7 for more details).

Fetal gender determination

Fetal sex determination is possible and advisable after day 60 of pregnancy. See Chapter 7 to review the fetal

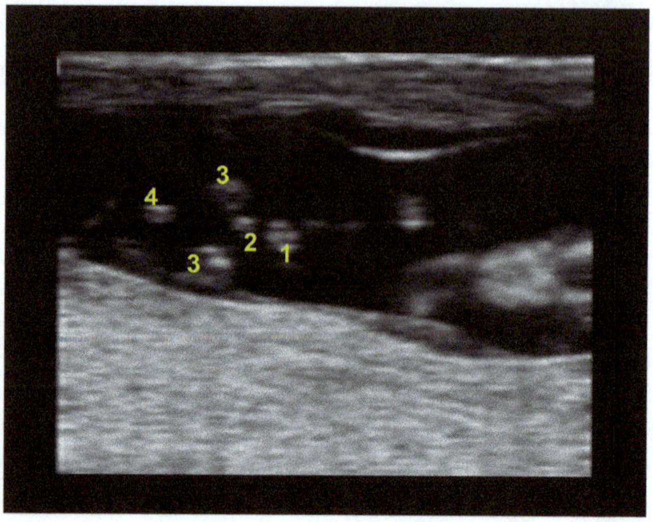

Figure 10.20. Male buffalo fetus at 62 days (7.5 MHz linear probe; depth 5 cm). 1: Umbilicus; 2: Male genital tubercle; 3: Posterior limb; 4: Tail.

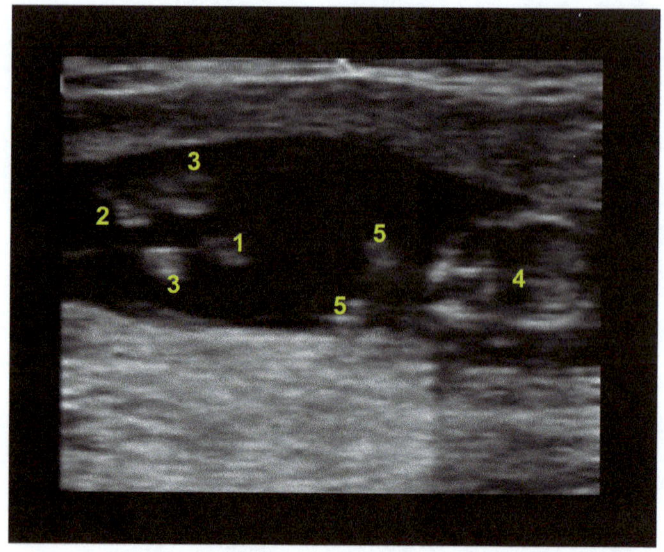

Figure 10.21. Female buffalo fetus at 60 days (7.5 MHz linear probe; depth 5 cm). 1: Umbilicus; 2: Female genital tubercle; 3: Posterior limb; 4: Head; 5: Anterior limb.

sexing techniques. It is possible to extend this exam until 110–120 days of pregnancy (Figures 10.20 and 10.21).

Synchronization programs and usefulness of the ultrasonographic examinations

Poor heat detection, long periods of anestrus, seasonality, and the growing interest in artificial insemination in *Bubalus bubalis* and *Bos indicus* have led to the increase in the importance of synchronization programs in these species.

The success of synchronization protocols can be improved by choosing the most appropriate protocol based on ovarian structures. Because the ovaries and ovarian structures in these species are smaller than in *Bos taurus*, ultrasound improves diagnostic accuracy considerably over palpation.

Buffalo cows with the presence of CL[11,14]

In buffalo and zebu with a CL, two methods of synchronization can be used: Target Breeding and OvSynch. In the first case prostaglandins injections are given twice at an interval of 11–14 days and the animal is inseminated 80 hours after the second injection.

There is a commonly held opinion that prostaglandins are less effective in zebu cows. This is not true because the efficacy of the commercial products in terms of luteolysis is absolutely comparable in cows of both genetic types.

The OvSynch protocol is widely used for synchronization for the bovine species and is now applied successfully in the reproductive management of buffalo. The protocol used is the same as for cows.

The downside of this program is the need to restrain the cow four times for injections and insemination. Some buffalo farms do not have adequate facilities to restrain individual cows. On these farms the drugs can be administered in the milking room during milking and there may be a need to reprogram milking times to accommodate the protocol.

The conception/pregnancy rate achievable with the OvSynch protocol varies according to the factors discussed in the physiology section of this chapter. In one author's experience, a yearly average conception rate of 35% can be expected. Although nonseasonal, buffalo cows have better conception rates when inseminated during autumn and winter.

In the near future, practitioners will be able to introduce synchronization programs such as PreSynch, CoSynch 48, and CoSynch 72 for these species. The latter two would require fewer times for restraint. However, conception rates may lower when we assume that zebu and buffalo will respond similarly to these protocols as do dairy cows.

Table 10.7.
Follicular parameters of Gir and Nelore cows synchronized with prostaglandin $F_{2\alpha}$ (Borges et al. 2003)

Characteristics	Gir	Nelore
Growth rate before $PGF_{2\alpha}$ (mm/day)	1.3 ± 0.8^a	1.1 ± 0.6^a
Growth rate after $PGF_{2\alpha}$ (mm/day)	1.6 ± 0.3^a	1.2 ± 0.2^b
Number of growth days before $PGF_{2\alpha}$	2.7 ± 2.3^a	2.2 ± 1.6^a
Number of growth days after $PGF_{2\alpha}$	3.2 ± 1.6^a	3.7 ± 1.4^a

Values with different superscript letters within rows differ ($P < 0.05$) by F-test.

Table 10.8.
Means and standard errors for the intervals (hours) between prostaglandin $F_{2\alpha}$ treatment to beginning of estrus and to ovulation in Gir and Nelore cows (Borges et al. 2003)

Breed	$PGF_{2\alpha}$ to Estrus (Hours)	$PGF_{2\alpha}$ to Ovulation (Hours)
	Mean ± sd	Mean ± sd
Gir (n = 11)	91.6 ± 28.0^a	113.1 ± 30.2^b
Nelore (n = 7)	88.7 ± 26.1^b	119.5 ± 31.9^b

Values with different superscript letters within columns differ $P < 0.05$) by F-test.

Buffalo cows without the presence of CL[4,8,11]

In the absence of a CL the situation is much more complicated. The success rates are lower and the management costs of these animals increase significantly. There are essentially two reasons for the absence of CL: 1) cystic follicular degeneration and 2) ovarian inactivity.

For both conditions the same pathophysiological considerations are valid. In cases of cystic degeneration, the preovulatory LH peak is missing. In the case of ovarian hypoplasia, the LH pulse, which is indispensable for the growth of the dominant follicle and for a normal course of follicular dynamics, is missing.

These situations can be addressed by improvement of nutritional and environmental management, but also by using slow progesterone releasing devices as part of a synchronization protocol. Intravaginal devices for slow release of natural progesterone offer the advantages of easier insertion and removal compared to those introduced under the skin of the ear or under the tail. The animal still must be restrained. but device removal is much easier. Limits to the use of these devices are changes to the vestibule, not infrequent conditions in a species in which prolapse of the uterus and Bühner sutures are very common. Fibrosis of the vaginal vestibule makes the real absorption of progesterone difficult to predict.

The availability and legality of the various drugs and implants needed for these protocols varies geographically; hence, detailed explanations of reproduction synchronization programs are not discussed in this chapter.

Tables 10.7 and 10.8 present follicular characteristics and intervals between the injection of prostaglandin and estrus or ovulation for Gir and Nelore cows synchronized with prostaglandin $F_{2\alpha}$.

References

1. Aboul-Fadle SW, Fahmy FE, El-Shafey SM (1974). Histological studies on the ovaries of the Egyptian buffalo with special reference to the corpus luteum. Zentbl VetMed A21: 581–591.
2. Ahmed N, Chaundry RA, Khan BB (1981). Effect of month and season of calving on the length of subsequent calving interval in Nili-Ravi buffaloes. Anim Reprod Sci 3: 301–306.
3. Bakke M (1995). Rotina das vacas define manejo. Balde Branco, São Paulo 349: 9–11.
4. Barile VL, De Santis G, Malfatti A, Barbato O, Borghese A (2003). Atti II Congresso Nazionale sull'Allevamento del Bufalo. Monterotondo Roma.
5. Barile VL (2005). Reproductive Efficiency in Female Buffaloes. Buffalo Production and Research. FAO Regional Office for Europe. Rome 67: 87–107.
6. Barros CM, Figueiredo RA, Pinheiro OL (1995). Estro, ovulação e dinâmica folicular em zebuínos. Revista Brasileira de Reprodução Animal. Belo Horizonte 19(1/2): 9–22.
7. Barros CM, Moreira MBP, Fernandes P (1998). Pharmacological manipulation of the estrous cycle to improve artificial insemination or embryo transfer programs. Arquivo da Faculdade de Veterinária da UFRGS, Porto Alegre 26(1): 179–198.
8. Bartolomeu CC, Del Rei AJ, Alvares CTG, Vilar GD (2007). Follicular dynamics during synchronization of ovulation of nulliparous buffalo cows during unfavourable reproductive status. VIII World Buffalo Congress, Suppl. 2, Part 1, Caserta.
9. Baruselli PS (1997). Folliculogenesis in buffalo. Bubalus bubalis, Suppl. 4: 79–92.
10. Baruselli PS, Mucciolo RG, Visintin JA, Viana WG, Arruda RP, Madureira EH, Oliveira CA, Molero-Filho (1997). Ovarian follicular dynamics during the oestrus cycle in buffalo (*Bubalus bubalis*). Theriogenology 47(8): 1531–1547.

11. Baruselli PS (2003). Artificial Insemination in the Developing Countries. Atti II Congresso Nazionale sull'Allevamento del Bufalo. Monterotondo Roma.
12. Borges AM, Torres AA, Ruas JRM, Rpcha Junior VR, Carvalho GR, Fonseca JF, Marcatti Neto A, Assis AJ (2003). Características da Dinâmica Folicular e Regressão Luteal de Vacas das Raças Gir e Nelore após Tratamento com Cloprostenol Sódico. R Bras Zootec 132(1): 85–92.
13. Boyd GW; Kiser TE, Cowrey RS (1987). Effects of prepartum energy intake on steroid during late gestation on cow and calf performance. J Anim Sci 64: 1703–1709.
14. De Rensis F, Ronci G, Guarneri P, Ubaldi A, Nguyen BX, Presicce GA (2003). Atti II Congresso Nazionale sull'Allevamento del Bufalo. Monterotondo Roma.
15. Dobson H, Kamonpatana M (1986). A review of female cattle reproduction with special reference to a comparison between buffaloes, cows and zebu. J Reprod Fert 77: 1–36.
16. Ferguson JD (1996). Diet, production and reproduction in dairy cows. Anim Feed Sci Technol, Amsterdam 59: 173–184.
17. Ferguson JD, Otto KA (1989). Managing body condition in dairy cows. Proceedings, Cornell nutrition conference for feed manufacturers, Ithaca, NY. Cornell University, pp. 75–87.
18. Ferreira MBD, Lopes BC, Azevedo NA, Ledic IL (2005). Escore corporal e manejo reprodutivo de vacas Gir leiteiro. Revista Gir Leiteiro. ISNN 1679-6659 5: 46–54.
19. Fonseca VO, Andrade VJ, Chow LA et al. (1987). Efeito de diferentes métodos de amamentação sobre as eficiências produtiva e reprodutivas de um rebanho bovino de corte. Arq Bras Med Vet Zoot 39(2): 233–240.
20. Galina CS, Arthur GH (1989). Review of cattle reproduction in the tropics. 2. Parturition and calving intervals. Anim Breed Abstr 57: 679–686.
21. Garnsworthy PC, Jones GP (1987). The influence of body condition at calving and dietary protein supply and voluntary food intake and performance in cows. Anim Prod Edinburgh 44(3): 347–353.
22. Hady PJ, Domeco JJ, Kaneene JB (1994). Frequency and precision of body condition scoring in dairy cattle. J Dairy Sci 77(6): 1543–1547.
23. Hafez ESE (1954). Oestrus and some related phenomena in buffalo. J Agric Sci Camb 44: 165–172.
24. Harris Junior B (1993). Feeding for maximum reproductive performance. Agropractice 14(3): 39–41.
25. Jainudeen MR, Hafez ESE (2000). Cattle and Buffalo in Reproduction in Farm Animals, 7th ed. Hafez ESE, Hafez B (Eds.). Lippincott Williams & Wilkins, Baltimore MD.
26. Ledic IL, Fernandes LO, Verneque RS, Faria RS, Ferreira MB, Silva FF, Xavier FT, Fernandes AR (2004). O Gir Leiterio da Fazenda Experimenteal Getúlio Vargas. Series Documentos n° 40 ISSN 0102-2164 EPAMIG, Belo Horizonte, p.21.
27. Luktuke SN, Rao ASP (1962). Studies of biometry of the reproductive tract of the buffalo cow. Indian J Vet Sci 32: 106–111.
28. Malfatti A (2003). Recent Advances in Buffalo Endocrinology. Atti II Congresso Nazionale sull' Allevamento del Bufalo. Monterotondo Roma.
29. Mobarak AM (1969). Anatomical studies of the female genitalia of buffaloes. Vet Med J Guza (Egypt) 16: 91–118.
30. Rahka AM, Igboeli G, Hale D (1970). The oestrous cycle of Zebu and Sanga breeds of cattle in Central Africa. J Reprod Fert 23: 411–414.
31. Richards MW, Wetteman RP, Schoenemann HM (1989). Nutritional anestrus in beef cows: body weight change, body condition, luteinizing hormone in serum and ovarian activity. J Anim Sci 67(6): 1520–1526.
32. Selk GE, Wettemann RP, Lusby KS, Oltjen JW, Mobley SL, Rasby RT, Garmendia JC (1988). Relationships among weight change, body condition, ovarian activity and estrus behaviour. J Anim Sci 66(12): 3153–3159.
33. Tonhati H, Ferriera Lima AL (2003). Buffalo Meat: Production and Quality. Atti II Congresso Nazionale sull'Allevamento del Bufalo. Monterotondo, Roma.
34. Vale WG, Sousa JS, Ohashi OM, Samapaio MIC (1979). Utero unicorno gestante associado a agenesia ovariana em bufalo (*Bubalus bubalis*). Desrcicao de um caso. Ver Bras Reprod Anim 3: 17–22.
35. Vale WG, Sousa JS, Ohashi OM, Ribeiro HFL (1981). Anomalias do desenvolvimento do sistema genital de bufalas (*Bubalus bubalis*) abatidas em matadúro. Pesq Vet Bras 3: 101–104.
36. Vale WG, Ohashi OM (1994). Problems of reproduction in buffaloes. Buffalo J, Suppl. 2: 103–122.
37. Vale WG (1994). Reproductive management of water buffalo under Amazon conditions. Buffalo J 10(2): 85–90.
38. Villa-Godoy A, Hughes TL, Emery, RS, Chapin CT, Fogwell RL (1988). Association between energy balance and luteal function in lactating dairy cows. J Dairy Sci 71(4): 1063–1072.
39. William G, Vale WG (2003). Path-Physiology of Buffalo Female Genital System. Atti II Congresso Nazionale sull'Allevamento del Bufalo. Monterotondo Roma.
40. William GL (1990). Suckling as a regulator of postpartum rebreeding in cattle: A review. J Anim Sci 68: 831–852.
41. Xu ZZ, Verkerk GA, Mee JF et al. (2000). Progesterone and follicular changes in postpartum noncyclic dairy cows after treatment with progesterone and estradiol or with progesterone, GnRH, PGF_2 and estradiol. Theriogenology 54: 273–282.
42. Yoshimeki S, Nakao T, Moryochi N, Kawata K (1986). Effect of energy and protein intake on ovarian activity in postpartum high-producing Holstein cows. Japanese J Zootech Sci, Tokyo 57(7): 553–560.

Points to Remember

- Buffalo and zebu are generally seasonally polyestrus short-day breeders. Thus, their reproductive efficiency (displaying estrus, conception rate, calving rate, days postpartum to cyclicity) changes throughout the year.
- Breeding during the rainy period and the winter appears to be most favorable while summer appears to be least favorable.
- The length of the estrous cycle is very similar in each species (21.6 ± 0.2 days) with 85% in estrus between 18–22 days.
- The duration of estrus signs ranges from 11 to 30 hours, but the intensity of signs is lower in buffalo. Ovulation occurs spontaneously about 10 hours after the end of the estrus. Silent heat is common in buffalo. Although the estrous cycle is present, the external symptoms of heat are absent or much reduced.
- The smaller total size of *Bubalus bubalis* and *Bos indicus* reflects the smaller size of their organs compared to *Bos taurus*.
- The gestation period of buffalo is 310–330 days; pregnancy lasts 292 days in the zebu.
- The long intercalving period is one of the major problems in buffalo and zebu breeding. The interval from calving to resumption of ovarian function is longer in buffalo and zebu compared with dairy cattle. The reasons for this delay are numerous; the most frequent reasons are breed, nutrition, milk yield, delayed uterine involution, suckling, and seasonality.
- The incidence of puerperal infection (metritis-endometritis) is 20–30%. These infections are the most important cause of reproductive failure in buffalo and zebu and are generally associated with rough manipulations during parturition or from uterine prolapse.
- The most common ovarian abnormalities in buffalo are ovarian inactivity, ovarian cysts, and infantile ovaries (particularly in buffalo heifers).
- Poor heat detection, long periods of anestrus, seasonality, and the growing interest in artificial insemination in *Bubalus bubalis* and *Bos indicus* have led to the increased importance of synchronization programs in these species.
- The success of synchronization protocols can be improved by choosing the most appropriate protocol based on ovarian structures. Because the ovaries and ovarian structures in these species are smaller than in *Bos taurus*, ultrasound improves diagnostic accuracy considerably over transrectal palpation.

Summary Questions

1. Why is it particularly important to use ultrasound for the examination of *Bos indicus* and *Bubalus bubalis*?
   a. Because they are very aggressive and do not tolerate manual examination of the reproductive tract
   b. Because ovarian structures (CL and follicles) are smaller than in *Bos taurus*
   c. Because the anatomy of the reproductive tract does not permit manual examination

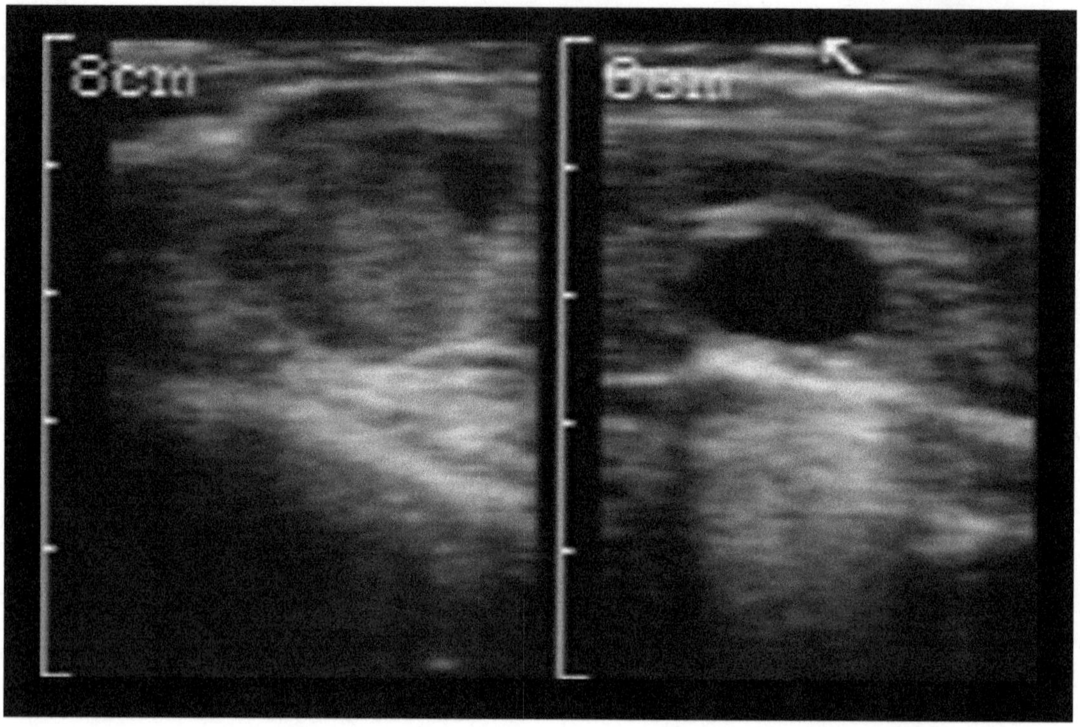

2. What is the above ultrasound image, which was taken from a *Bos indicus* in BB-mode?
   a. Left: A compact CL with a small follicle; Right: A large dominant follicle with two smaller ones
   b. Left: Ovarian stroma; Right: Cystic follicular degeneration
   c. Left: Ovarian stroma; Right: 28-day pregnancy in cross section

3. What are the following ultrasound images, which were taken from a *Bos indicus*?
   a. A: 23-day pregnancy; B: Cavitary CL
   b. A: Cavitary CL; B: Uterus in estrus in cross section
   c. A: Cavitary CL; B Endometritis in cross section

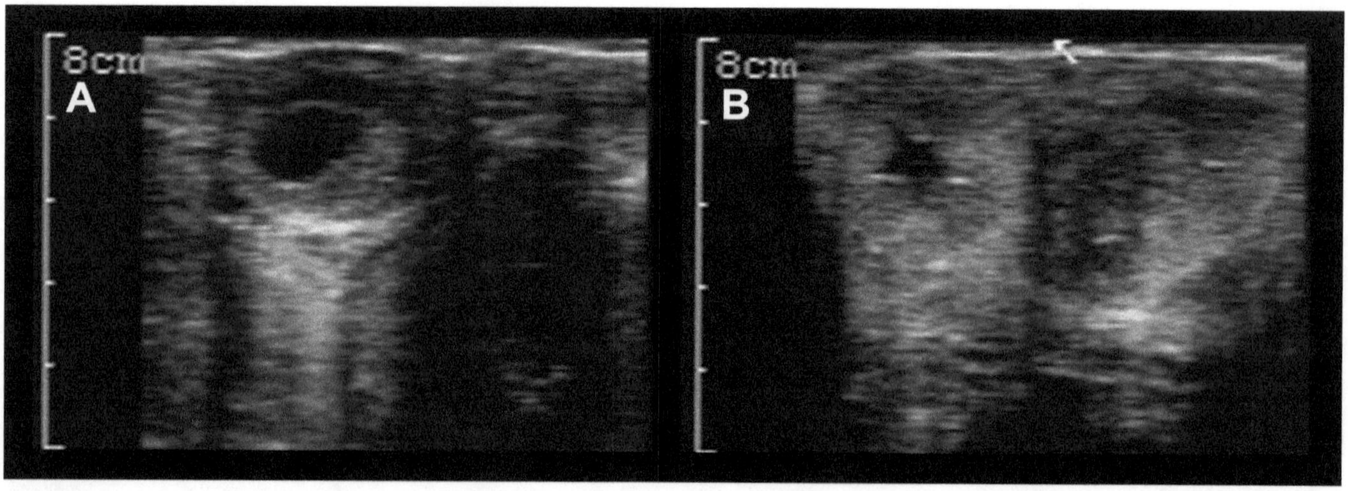

4. What is the following ultrasound image, which was taken from a *Bubalus bubalis* in BB-mode?
   a. Left: 24-day pregnancy in cross section; Right: 24-day pregnancy showing the embryo
   b. Left: Endometritis; Right: 24-day pregnancy
   c. Left: Uterus in estrus in cross section; Right: Follicle

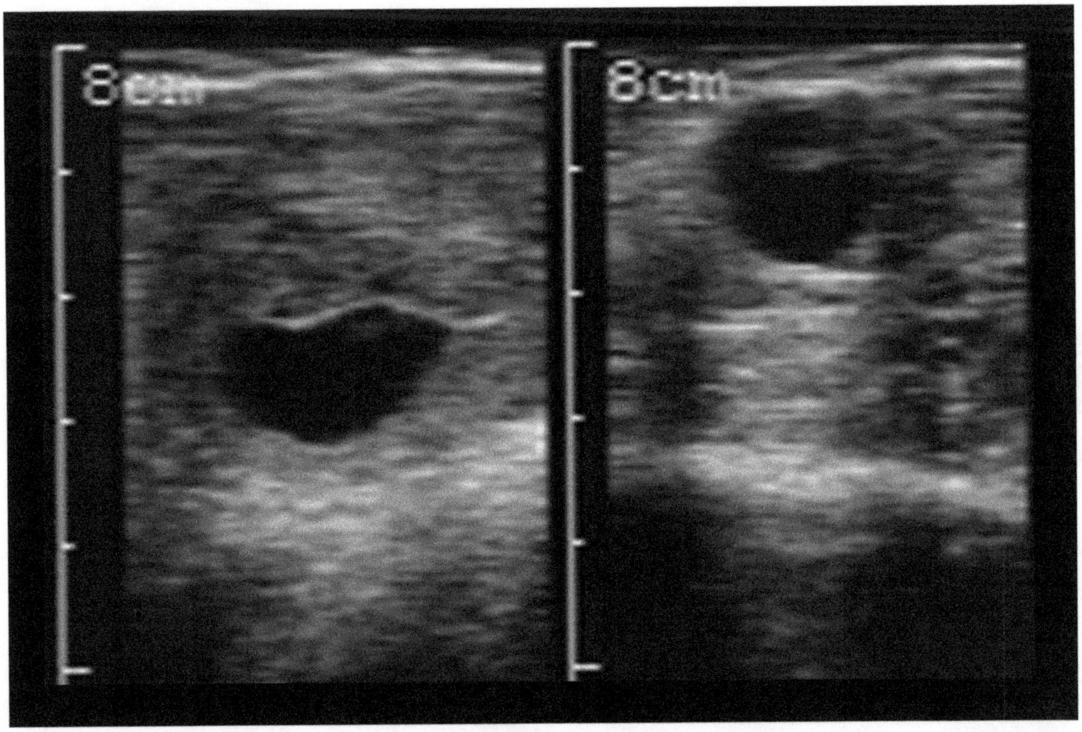

5. Which is the most frequent ovarian problem in *Bos indicus* and *Bubalus bubalis*?
   a. Persistent CL
   b. Ovary inactivity
   c. Ovarian neoplasia

6. What is the following ultrasound image, which was taken from a *Bubalus bubalis*?
   a. A compact CL
   b. The ovarian stroma immediately after ovulation
   c. A placentome

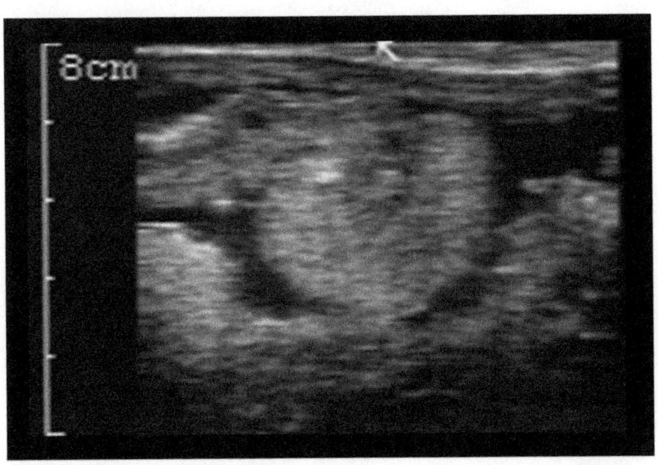

Answers

1. b
2. a
3. b
4. c
5. b
6. c

CHAPTER ELEVEN

Sheep and Goats

Carolina Viñoles-Gil, Antonio Gonzalez-Bulnes, Graeme B. Martin, Francisco Sales Zlatar, and Sebastiano Sale

Usefulness of Ultrasonography in Small Ruminants

Many of us can remember the first Doppler machines that were used for pregnancy diagnosis in sheep. The relatively poor performance of this technology led to a degree of skepticism that probably inhibited widespread acceptance of B-mode ultrasound when it arrived in the mid-1980s. However, within a few years of demonstrations by Ginther and colleagues of the power of the new generation of machines, a wide range of applications was developed. This led to several breakthroughs in research into, and management of, the reproductive performance of small ruminants. There were technical developments on two fronts: the ultrasound probes and the software used to interpret the reflections. This development continues apace as we explore the possibilities of both three-dimensional imaging for studies of structural details and color Doppler ultrasound for real-time studies of physiological functions such as blood flow.

In females, ultrasound is now used routinely for observing follicular development and atresia (follicular "waves"), ovulation, and ovulation rate. Indeed, the study of follicular waves would never have been feasible without the use of ultrasound because it requires serial, daily observations of the interior of the ovary. The corpus luteum (CL) posed some initial difficulties, but ultrasound operators are now so confident at identifying corpora lutea that this technology is effectively replacing the more invasive "gold standard" of laparoscopy. This revolution in the study of ovarian function became feasible only with the advent of internal transrectal probes. These same probes are also useful for very early detection of pregnancy in the first 4 weeks after conception. External probes are essential for later stages of pregnancy, including measurement of litter size and fetal age. At first, fetal aging seemed to be of limited use, but as we move toward sophisticated systems for managing reproduction in farm animals precise determination of fetal age will be important to plan for parturition, including feeding for colostrum production and early postnatal care[10]. Finally, ultrasound can be used to detect pathological conditions and abnormalities in both sexes, where it has replaced very invasive techniques such as biopsy.

In this chapter the authors present a guide for the use of ultrasonography in small ruminants. They describe the relevant equipment and techniques for ultrasound scanning, the anatomy of the reproductive tract in parallel with descriptions of the images generated by the different structures, the endocrine and ovarian processes that comprise the normal cycle, the embryonic and fetal development, and uses of ultrasonography during pregnancy (age, sex, and number of fetuses, and pathological conditions of the tract). Finally, the anatomy of the male reproductive tract and the use of ultrasound to evaluate the testis, epididymis, and accessory sex glands are presented.

Equipment and Scanning Techniques

A very important step is the selection of the most suitable machine. This is based on the principal use (research versus private practice) and whether the work will be restricted to small ruminants or will also include large animals. In the marketplace there are nontransportable hospital-type units, transportable machines, and portable machines (see Chapter 1, Figure 1.2).

Table 11.1.
Characteristics of the probes most frequently used for obstetrics and gynecology in small ruminants

Frequency	Type	Penetration (cm)	Uses
7.5 MHz	Linear, convex	5–7	Ovarian structures and early-pregnancy diagnosis
5.0 MHz	Linear, convex, sector	10–17	Corpora lutea and early- to mid-pregnancy diagnosis
3.5 MHz	Linear, convex, sector	17–20	Mid- to late-pregnancy diagnosis

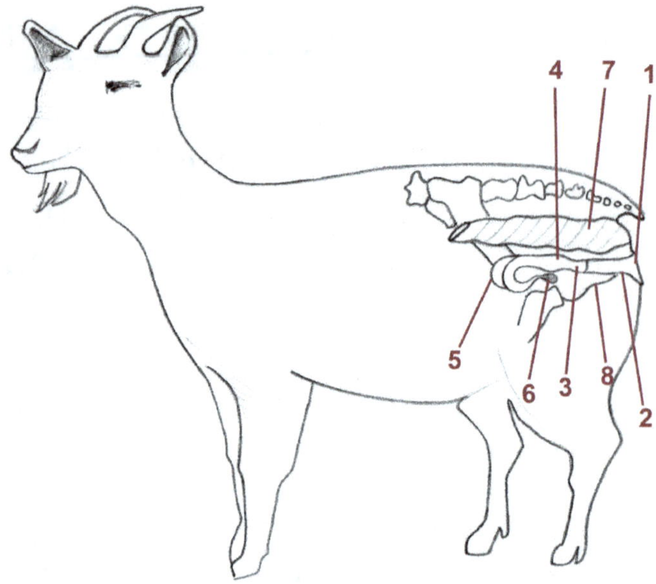

Figure 11.1. Anatomy of the female reproductive tract. 1: Vulva; 2: Vagina; 3: Cervix; 4: Body of the uterus; 5: Uterine horn; 6: Ovary; 7: Rectum; 8: Pelvic bone (cut).

Nontransportable instruments produce very high-quality images, and there is a great variety of machines and probes (Table 11.1). Their disadvantages are expense, weight, and large size, which make them difficult to transport. They are useful in research centers for accurate examinations using a range of external and internal probes.

Transportable units are light (6–20 kg) and can function with batteries or main power, so they are easily carried to field sites and used in research. Several options are available on the market (Figure 1.2). It is important to evaluate their quality and robustness before buying a machine.

Portable ultrasound units are a great choice for field practitioners because they are very light (<3 kg) and they function with a battery that allows for 2.5 to 7.0 hours of continuous work, depending on the manufacturer, the type of viewing device and the environmental temperature. In small ruminant practice the selection of the probe is crucial (Table 11.1). Ultrasound units that allow the use of both linear and sectorial probes are preferable (see Chapter 1, Figure 1.3). Sectorial probes have an advantage because they require less contact with the surface of the skin, which reduces the time required per ewe and avoids the need to clip the wool in front of the udder.

For gynecological examination of the reproductive tract the practitioner can use transrectal, transvaginal, and transabdominal techniques. The choice depends on what one wants to study, so it is important to understand the advantages and limitations of each technique. For all techniques, however, the first step is to become familiar with the equipment in order to adjust all the settings properly (see Chapter 1 for more details).

Ultrasonographic Imaging of the Female Reproductive Tract

An ultrasound examination of the female reproductive tract requires knowledge of its spatial anatomy as well as real familiarity with the ultrasound image created by each structure. The reproductive tract is located in the pelvic cavity, delimited by the pelvic bone (Figure 11.1). Due to the close proximity of the rectum to the reproductive tract, the transrectal route is ideal for ultrasonographic evaluation of the ovaries. This technique can be performed with the animal standing or in dorsal recumbency, as depicted in Figures 11.2–11.4.

Irrespective of the technique, the urinary bladder is the major reference structure for identifying the reproductive tract. The urinary bladder is readily visualized as a nonechogenic structure (Figure 11.5) of a size that depends on the volume of urine that it contains.

The vagina generates an image that appears as gray shadows over the bladder. At the internal end of the

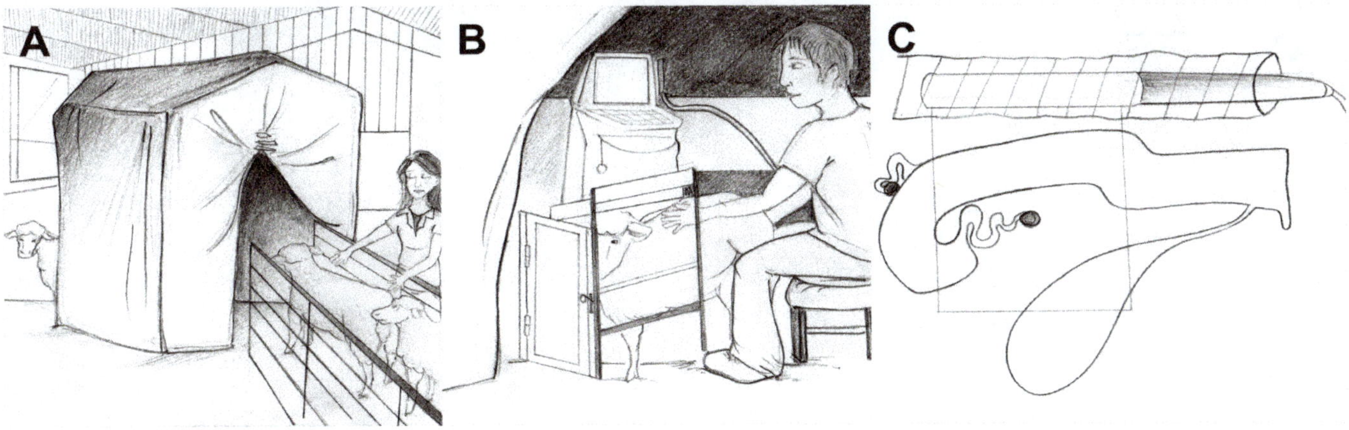

Figure 11.2. Illustration of the transrectal technique for ultrasonographic examination of the reproductive tract with the animal in the standing position. A: It is crucial to have a darkened workplace (e.g., a tent) for viewing the ovaries; B: Once the ewe enters the crate, approximately 20 ml of lubricant is injected into the rectum and the abdomen is pushed up by the left knee of the operator; C: The 7.5 MHz rigid linear probe is introduced into the rectum and rotated clockwise and counterclockwise to locate the left and right ovaries.

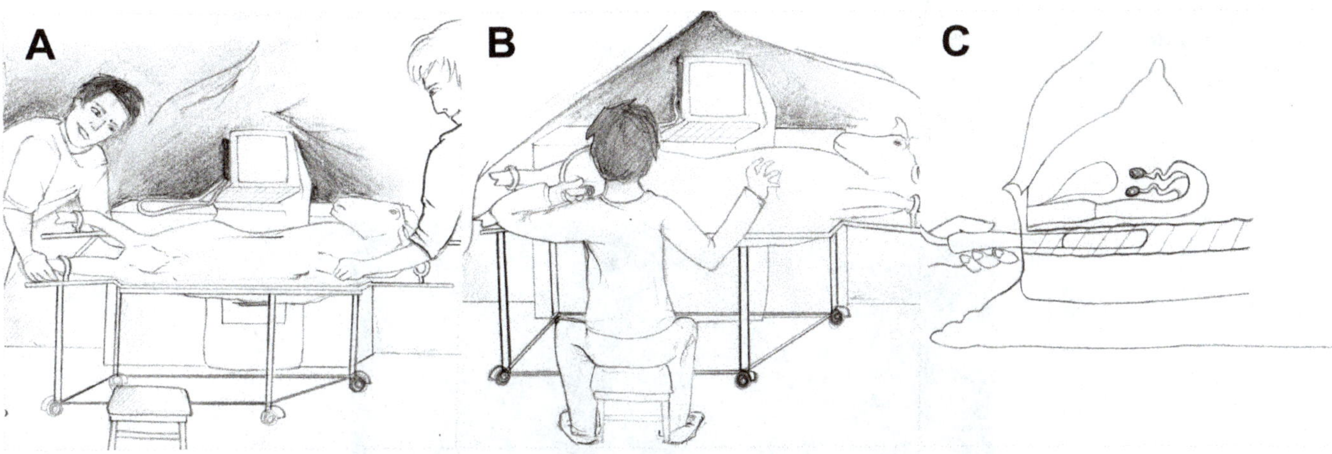

Figure 11.3. Illustration of the transrectal technique for ultrasonographic examination of the reproductive tract with the animal in dorsal recumbency. A: The ewe is restrained in dorsal recumbency in an insemination crate; B: Lubricant is added and feces are removed if necessary; C: The 7.5 MHz rigid probe is inserted into the rectum and rotated clockwise and counterclockwise to locate the left and right ovaries.

vagina is the cervix. Due to its fibrous composition, the cervix is a more echogenic structure than the vagina.

The uterus is a muscular structure that generates a gray echogenic image (Figure 11.6). The echogenic properties of the uterus depend on uterine tone, so it is affected by hormonal changes during the estrous cycle (see Chapter 5 for more details).

Each uterine horn continues into an oviduct that ends with the infundibulum, which envelops the ovaries. The ovaries are almond-shaped structures about 1.5×1 cm in diameter. The ovarian stroma produces a gray ultrasound image, the size of which depends on reproductive status (Figure 11.7).

Once the ovaries are located, the best image is frozen and the largest section of each structure (follicles ≥ 2 mm and CL) is measured with the built-in calipers. The structures are drawn on ovarian maps (Figure 11.8) and the images are recorded in individual videos for future reference.

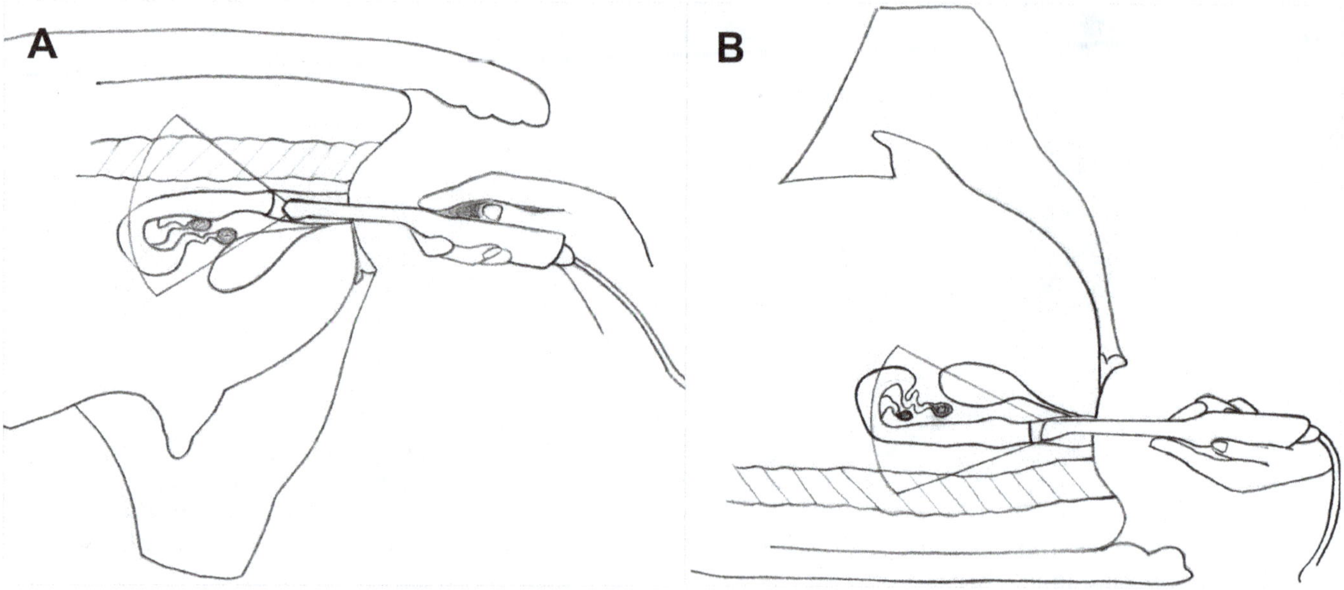

Figure 11.4. Illustration of the transvaginal approach to study the reproductive tract of small ruminants. The transvaginal approach is another option for examining the reproductive tract in detail, and it can be done with the animal in a standing position or in dorsal recumbency. Images are obtained from several different orientations to get the best views of the uterus and ovaries. A: The probe is inserted into the vagina, with the ewe restrained in a crate in a standing position, and gently moved up and down to visualize the ovaries; B: The same technique can be applied with the ewe in dorsal recumbency, as described in Figure 11.3.

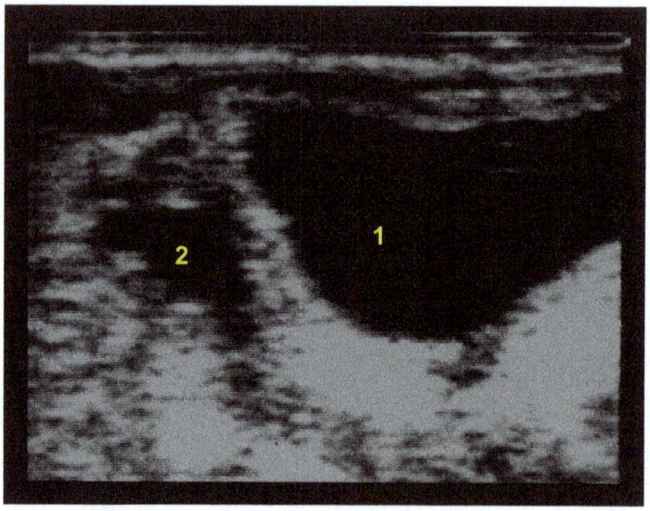

Figure 11.5. Ultrasonographic image of the urinary bladder (5MHz probe; depth 2.5cm). The urinary bladder is the reference structure to locate the reproductive tract. 1: Urinary bladder; 2: Uterus.

It takes 1 to 10 minutes to evaluate all the structures, depending on how easy it is to locate the ovaries (for example, excessive amounts of fat can make the ovaries difficult to find). Using this technique to measure ovulation rate on a farm, an average of 35 ewes per hour can be scanned. To accomplish this, a good setup and labor force are needed to assure a continuous flow of animals into the scanning tent.

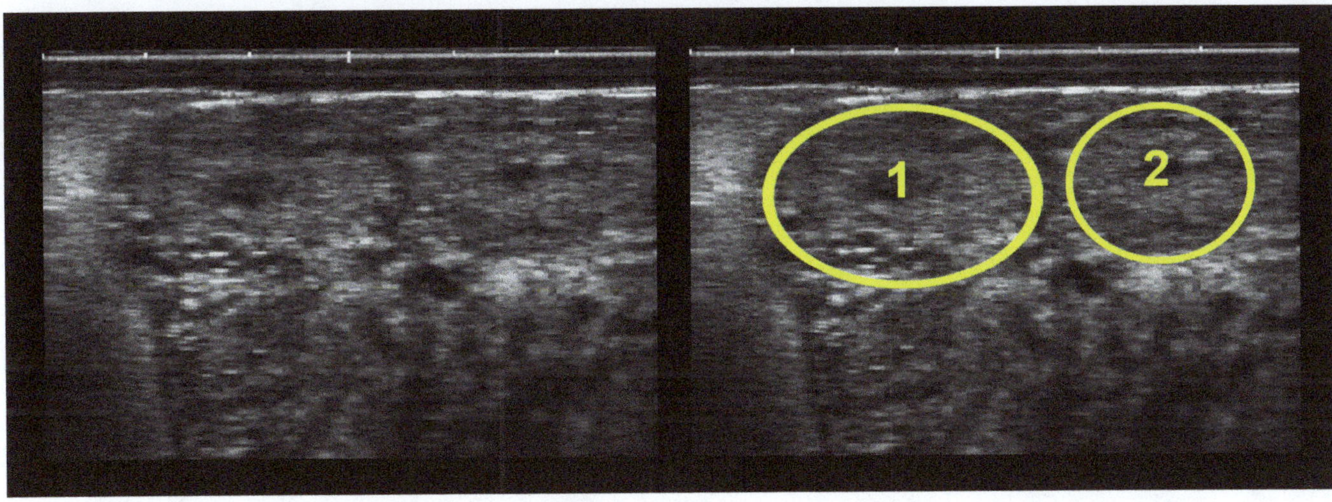

Figure 11.6. Ultrasonographic image of two uterine horn sections in transverse view (8 MHz probe; depth 4 cm). Ewes and does have a bipartite uterus that is divided into the uterine body and uterine horns, but these two structures cannot be differentiated by ultrasonography. The horns turn downward and backward and form two coils. This is important because ultrasound images are cross sections; hence, different images will be generated depending on the direction taken by the ultrasound waves as they pass through the uterus and horns. Typically, an image containing circular and longitudinal shapes is generated. 1 and 2: Uterine horn portions in transverse sections.

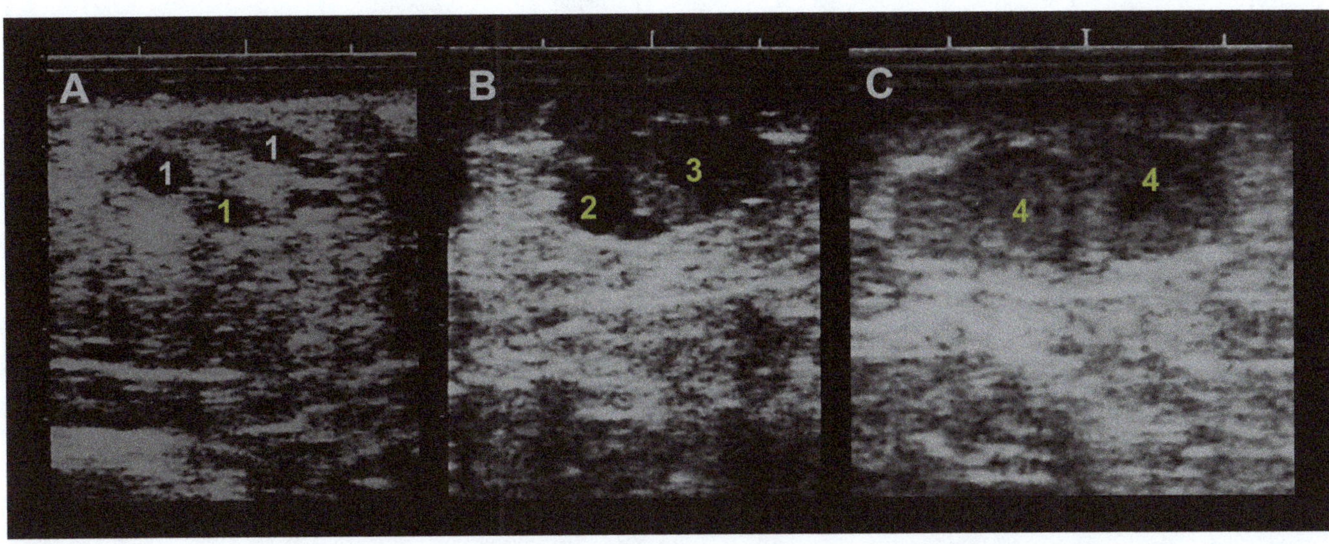

Figure 11.7. Ultrasonographic images of ovaries in anestrous and cyclic females (A to C) (5 MHz probe; depth 4 cm). During anestrus (A) only small follicles are visible in the ovarian tissue. As the ewe or doe begins to cycle, the size of the follicles increases. Prior to ovulation, the preovulatory follicle increases in size giving an anechoic (black) image due to fluid in the antrum (B). Immediately after ovulation, corpora hemorrhagica will also appear as anechoic structures because the antral cavities fill with blood. As the corpora hemorrhagica develop into corpora lutea (CL), they will appear as gray structures, usually solid but often with an anechoic central cavity (C). A: Ovary during anestrus with various small anechoic follicular structures (1) in the ovarian parenchyma; B: In the breeding season with a medium-sized preovulatory follicle (2); disappearance of the large follicle means ovulation has occurred; that day is defined as day 0 of the reproductive cycle; 3: Corpus luteum (CL) visible 3 days after ovulation; C: Double ovulation; 4: CL becomes more echogenic until day 9 after ovulation and remains well defined until after day 12 when the boundaries start to lose definition concurrent with a decline in progesterone concentrations. Note that the right CL has a small central cavity.

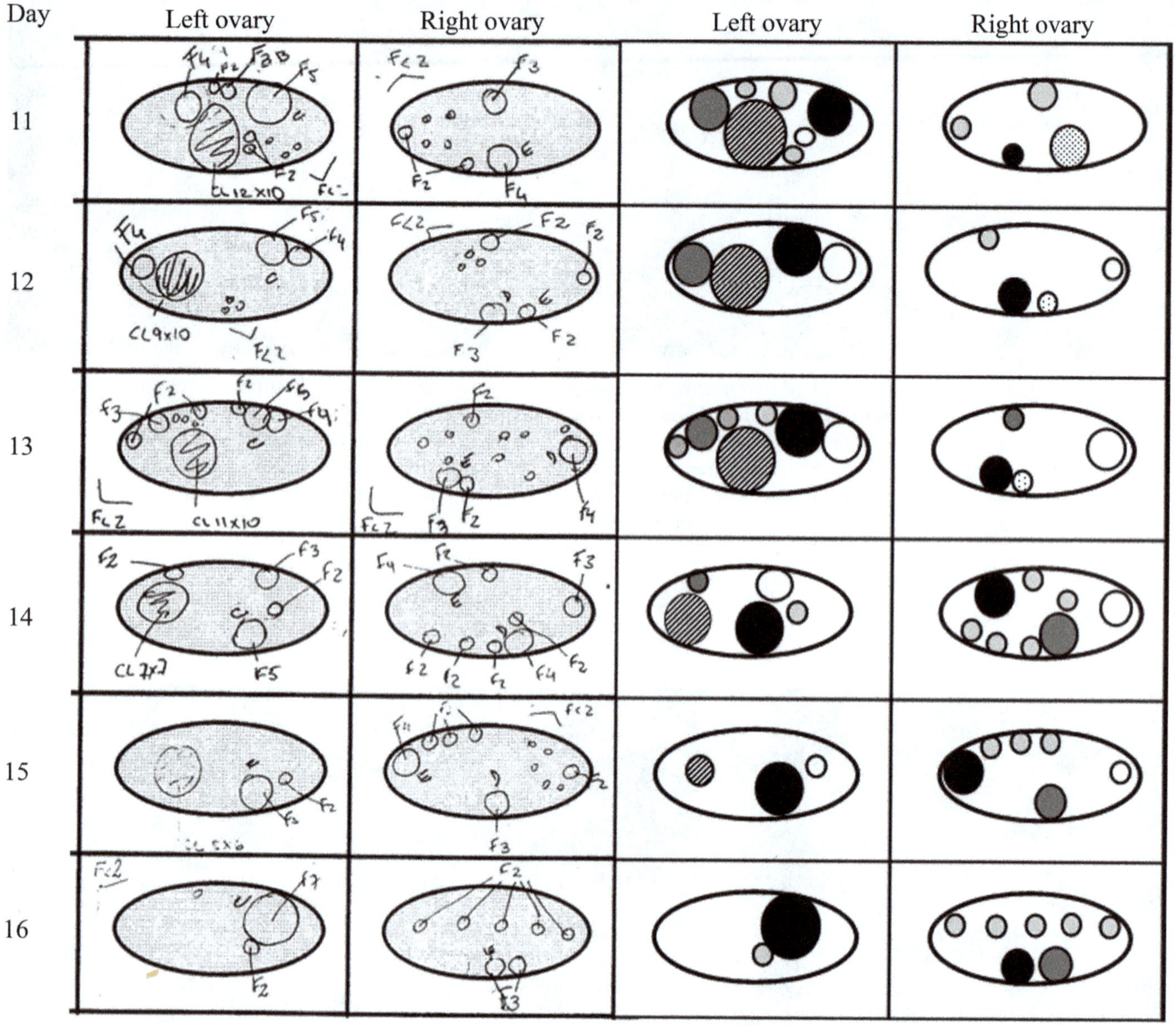

Figure 11.8. Ovarian maps. Daily maps obtained by ultrasound examination of ovarian follicles and CL, presented as raw data (left) and analyzed data (right) for pairs of ovaries. Circles with the same colors in the same ovary represent the development of the same structure between days 11 and 16 of the estrous cycle.

Endocrine and Ovarian Processes that Comprise the Normal Estrous Cycle and Pregnancy

Follicles

The estrous cycle is driven by a sequence of endocrine events regulated by the brain, ovary, and uterus (Figure 11.9).

The crucial role played by FSH in the short-term control of follicular development in does and ewes and was not elucidated until the wavelike pattern of follicular growth was confirmed by ultrasonography[5].

A rise in FSH concentration precedes each follicular wave, from which one follicle (the *dominant follicle*) is selected to continue its growth while all the others regress through atresia (Figure 11.10). When a CL is present, the dominant follicle will also regress, leading to the emergence of a new wave[16]. If the CL regresses, the dominant follicle continues to expand until ovula-

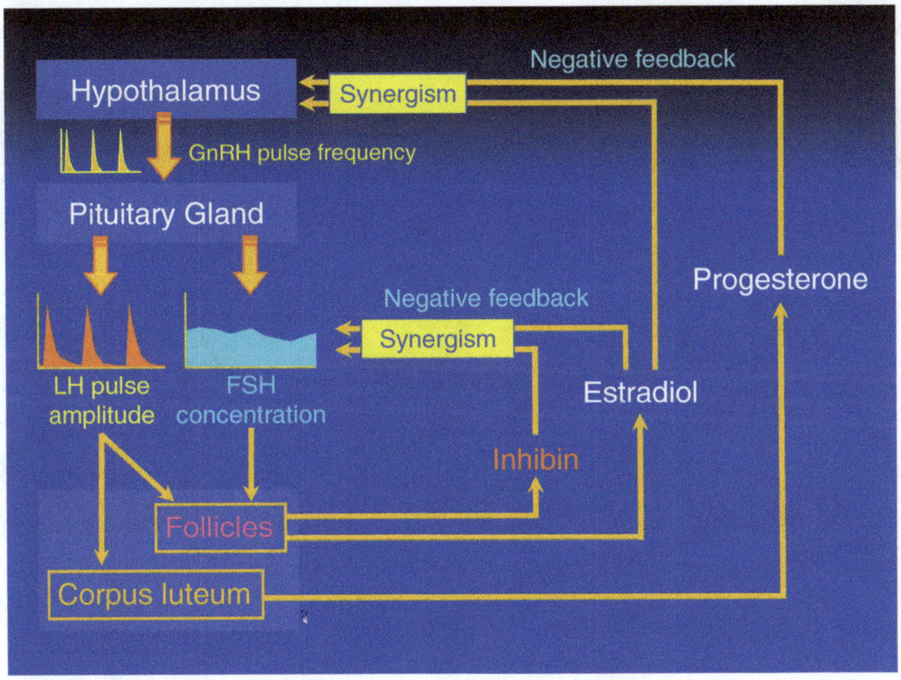

Figure 11.9. Illustration of the endocrine regulation of the estrous cycle. The major endocrine pathways that control ovarian function in the female, illustrating the pituitary control of ovarian production of inhibin and sex steroids, and the roles of these hormones in negative feedback. The secretion of FSH is inhibited by actions primarily at the pituitary level, whereas the frequency of secretion of GnRH (and LH) pulses is reduced by actions on the gonadotrophic centers in the brain. The maintenance of homeostasis involves two synergistic feedback loops, the first involving the follicle(s) and the pituitary gland, and the second involving the follicles, the CL, and the brain. These processes explain the follicular waves that can be documented during the estrous cycle by ultrasound imaging. High progesterone concentrations produced by the corpus luteum at midcycle will inhibit GnRH pulse frequency, leading to reduced estradiol production by the follicles. Low progesterone concentrations during the follicular phase allow an increase in GnRH pulse frequency, so estradiol production by the dominant follicle will increase and elicit estrus, the LH surge, and ovulation. Estradiol and inhibin, both of which are follicular products, will reduce FSH concentrations, thus reducing follicular growth.

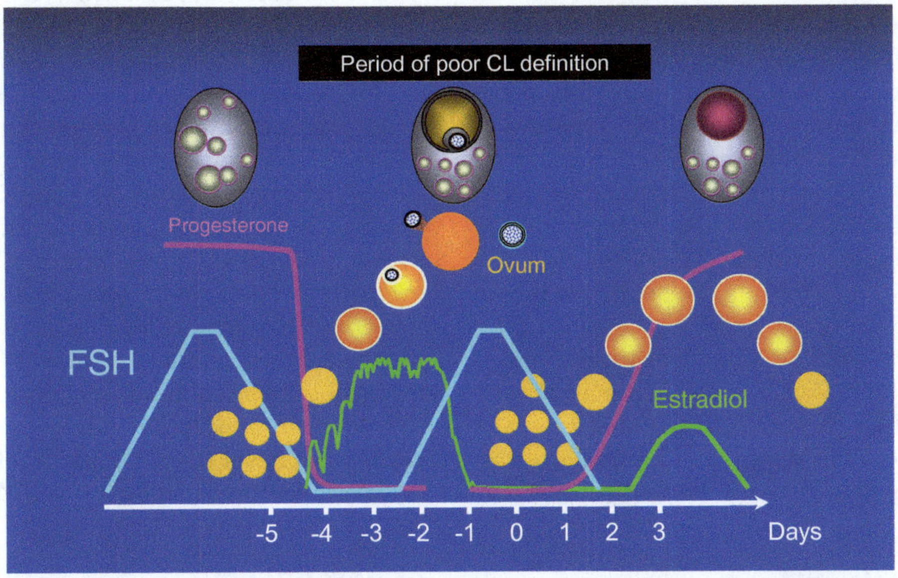

Figure 11.10. Wavelike patterns of follicular growth. Follicular and endocrine events during the late follicular phase, as the final follicular wave becomes an ovulatory wave, and during the early luteal phase as the first follicular wave of the next cycle begins. During the ovulatory wave, a dominant follicle grows, ovulates, and becomes a corpus luteum. Although the whole series of events can be documented with ultrasonography, the CL can be detected most accurately from days 8 to 12 after ovulation.

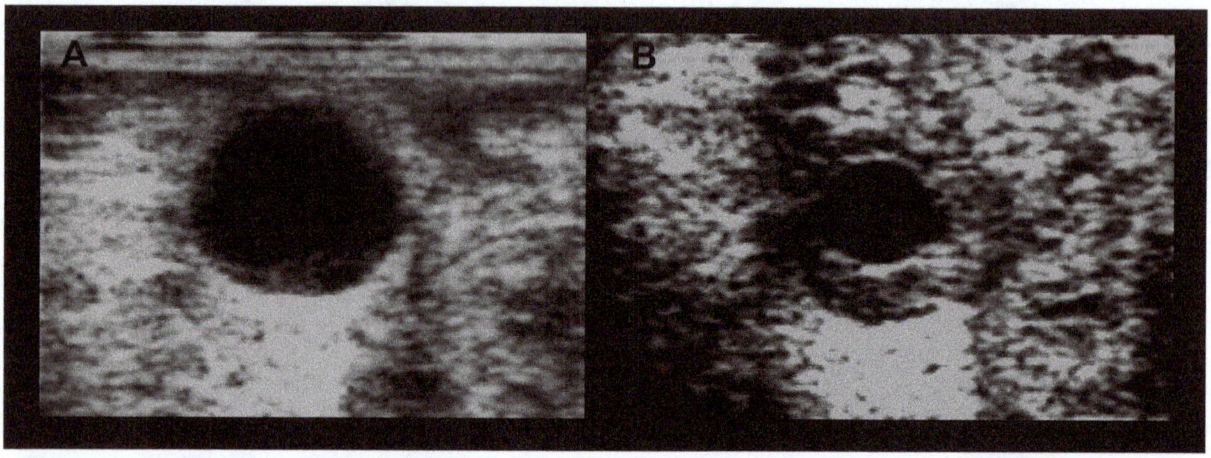

Figure 11.11. Ultrasonographic images of the same corpus luteum with a cavity taken at 3 and 6 days of the estrous cycle. A: Development of a CL with a large cavity 3 days after ovulation; B: Image of the same developing CL 6 days after ovulation. Note that the cavity of the CL (cavitary corpus luteum) has reduced significantly in a 3-day period.

tion takes place. There are two to six waves per estrous cycle, with three waves being most common in ewes and four waves being most common in does.

Corpus luteum (CL)

The CL can be first detected by ultrasonography on day 3 after ovulation, and its patterns of growth are highly correlated with the production of progesterone during the midluteal phase[6]. Ultrasonography is 100% accurate for the detection of a fully functional CL, but less accurate during the growth and regression of a CL and when more than one CL is present[15,16]. Inaccuracies can also occur when CLs develop central cavities[16] (Figure 11.11A). This problem can be avoided by measuring ovulation rate on day 10 of the cycle when most CL cavities will be small[14,16] (Figure 11.11B).

Another source of error occurs when the CL develops a large crown (ovulatory papilla) that may be mistaken for a second CL (Figure 11.12). In these cases, a second examination a few days later may be necessary if the operator is uncertain about the number of CL.

Early pregnancy

The embryo reaches the uterus on day 4 and starts to elongate by day 11 (Figure 11.13).

This is the beginning of implantation, but firm adhesion to the endometrium will not occur until day 16. Around day 20 of pregnancy, the embryonic vesicle (Figures 11.14, 11.15) extends to the contralateral horn of the uterus, creating pockets of fluid within the uterine lumen.

From day 21 of pregnancy, the placentomes can be discerned as small echogenic areas on the surface of the endometrium. The embryo becomes more readily visible between days 25 and 30. At this time the amnion (Figures 11.15, 11.16) can be seen as a hyperechoic line that encircles the embryo at a distance of 1–2 mm[9].

The transrectal technique is the best choice for early diagnosis of pregnancy because the uterus will still be located in the pelvic cavity. Accuracy is low before day 24 (50%), but increases by days 32–34[13] (85–100%). Before day 24, the pregnancy diagnosis is based on the presence of anechoic pockets of fluid that can also originate from causes other than pregnancy. It is important to consider that, after a diagnosis of early pregnancy, some animals may lose their embryos, increasing the number of false positive diagnoses. The difference in conception rate between an early transrectal diagnosis (day 30) and a later transcutaneous diagnosis (day 60) can be up to 16%.

Midpregnancy

At 40 to 60 days, it is possible to see echoic fetuses surrounded by large amounts of hypoechoic fluid. Other structures of pregnancy, such as placentomes and the umbilical cord, also become readily visible

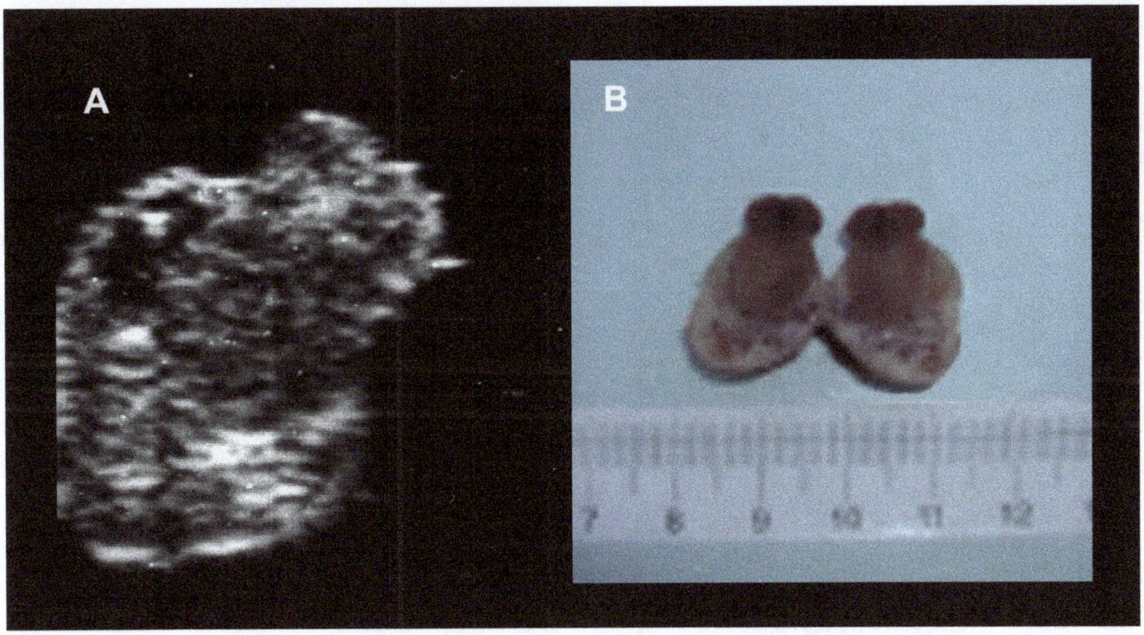

Figure 11.12. Ultrasonographic image of an ovariectomized corpus luteum with a large ovulatory papilla. A: Ultrasound image in vitro after ovariectomy; B: Photograph of the removed ovary (B).

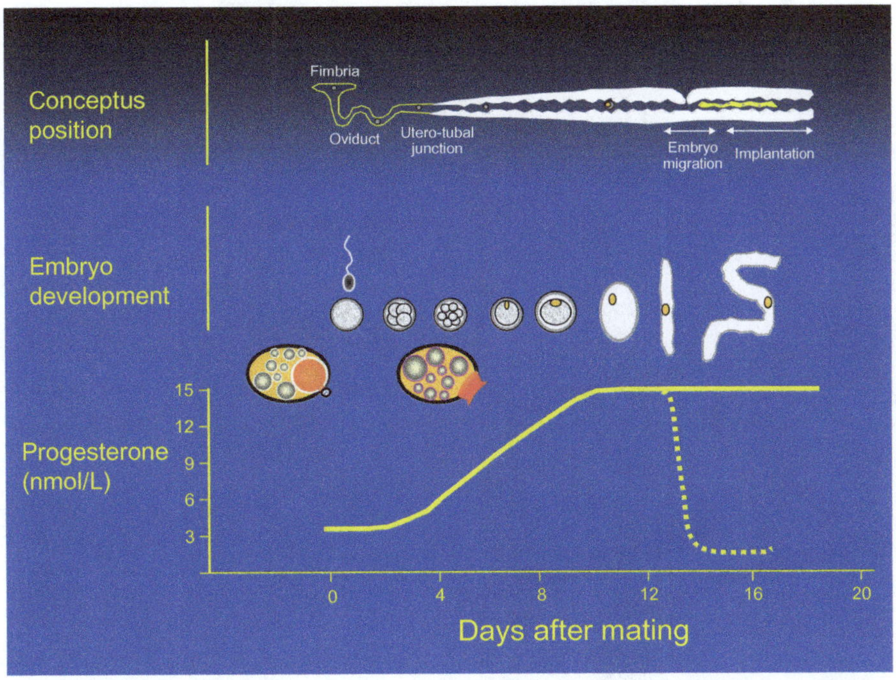

Figure 11.13. The temporal relationships between the development of the embryo, its position in the female tract, and maternal blood concentrations of progesterone during the first 16 days of pregnancy (modified after Thomas E. Spencer). The broken line in the progesterone pattern indicates the time that luteolysis would be expected if conception had failed.

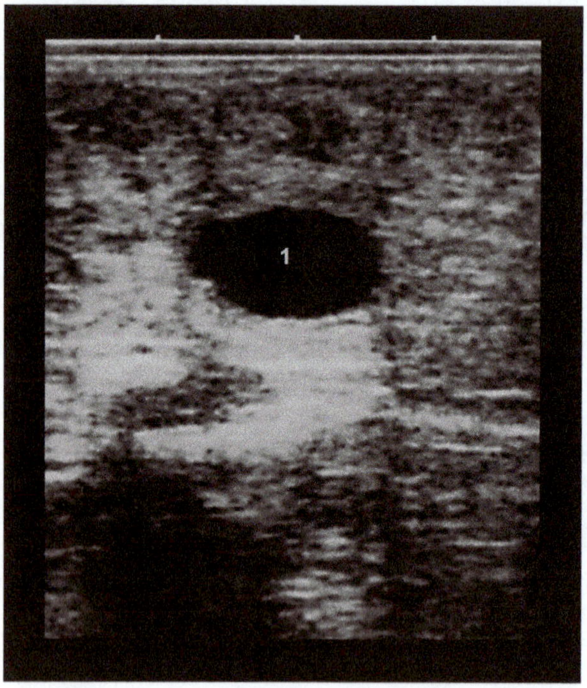

Figure 11.14. Ultrasonographic image of the embryonic vesicle. Image of an embryonic vesicle (1), which becomes visible after day 20 of pregnancy as an anechoic structure inside the uterine lumen.

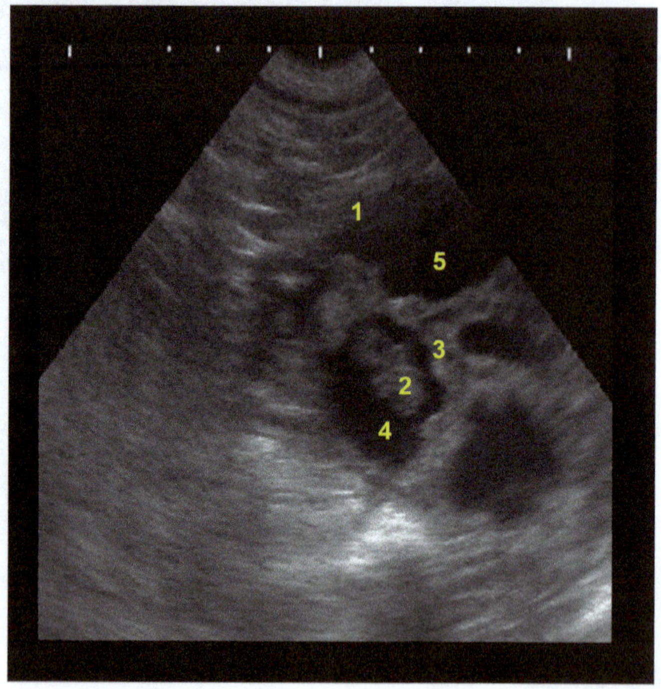

Figure 11.16. A 30-day-old embryo encircled by the amnion, as seen by transabdominal ultrasonography (5 MHz sectorial probe; depth 10 cm). 1: Uterus; 2: Embryo; 3: Amnion; 4: Amniotic fluid; 5: Allantoic fluid.

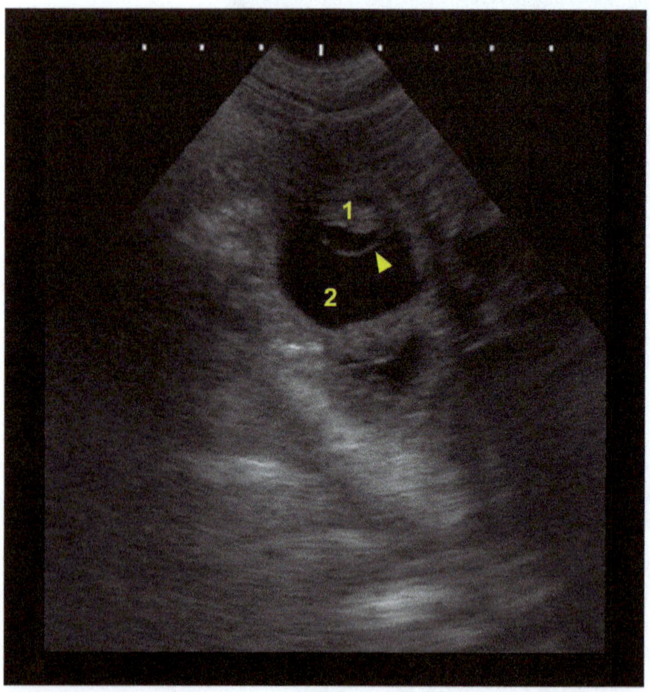

Figure 11.15. Ultrasonographic image of an embryo at 21 days of pregnancy. Notice that at this stage the embryo can be easily confused with a placentome.

(Figure 11.17). At this stage numerous fetal organs such as the heart, liver, digestive tract, and kidneys can be imaged sonographically (Figures 11.17B, 11.18). Due to their intense echogenicity (white), bony parts such as the skull, spinal column, ribs, and extremities can be easily identified.

During midpregnancy, transrectal ultrasonography becomes less accurate and must be replaced by the transabdominal or transcutaneous technique because the uterus descends into the abdominal cavity (Figure 11.19).

Late pregnancy

After day 100 of pregnancy, it is difficult to determine the number of fetuses. Imaging of placentomes is still possible (Figure 11.20), but fetal body parts are only partially visible.

Various approaches can be used for transabdominal diagnosis of pregnancy. The choice of technique and probe depends primarily on the stage of gestation and whether it is important to detect multiple fetuses (Table 11.1). After day 60 (midpregnancy) transcutaneous ultrasonography using a 3.5 MHz sectorial probe is

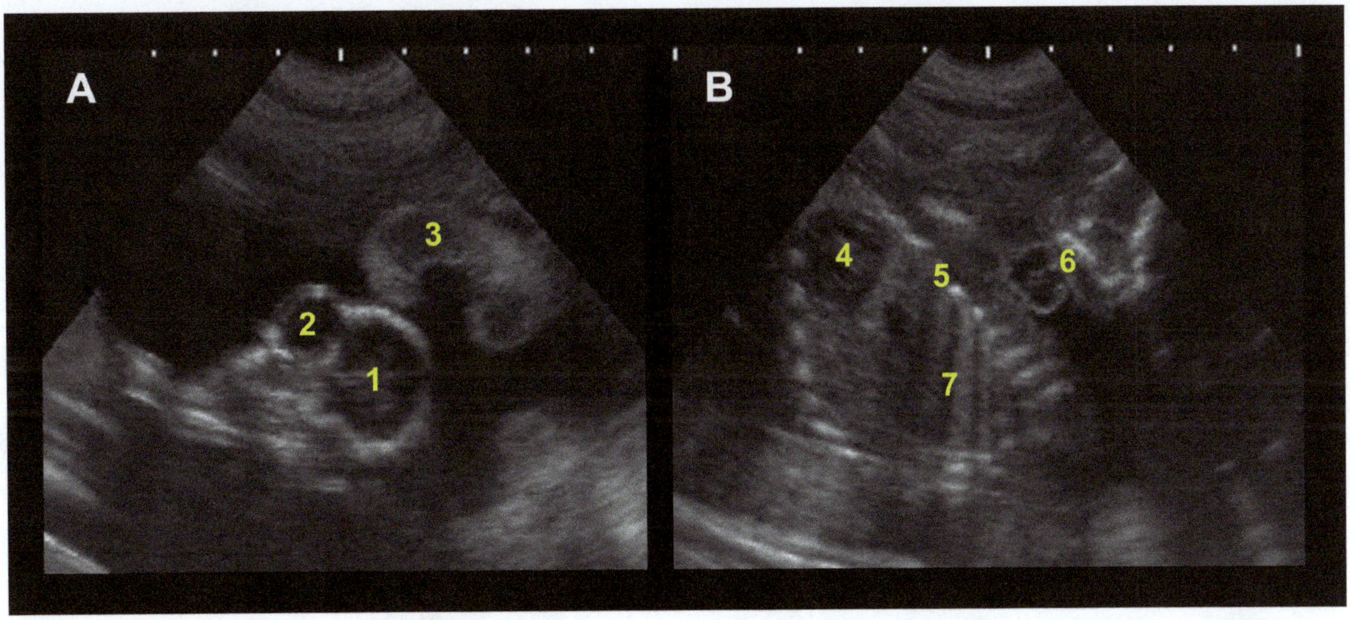

Figure 11.17. Ultrasound images of a 60-day fetus (5 MHz sectorial probe; depth 8 cm). A1: Head appears as a hyperechoic, circular-shaped image; A2: Eye; A3: Placentome; B4: Heart and heart rate can be used as an indicator of fetal viability; B5: Ribs are easily observed due to their hyperechoic characteristics; B6: Umbilical cord; B7: Rumen filled with liquid indicating normal development of this portion of the digestive system.

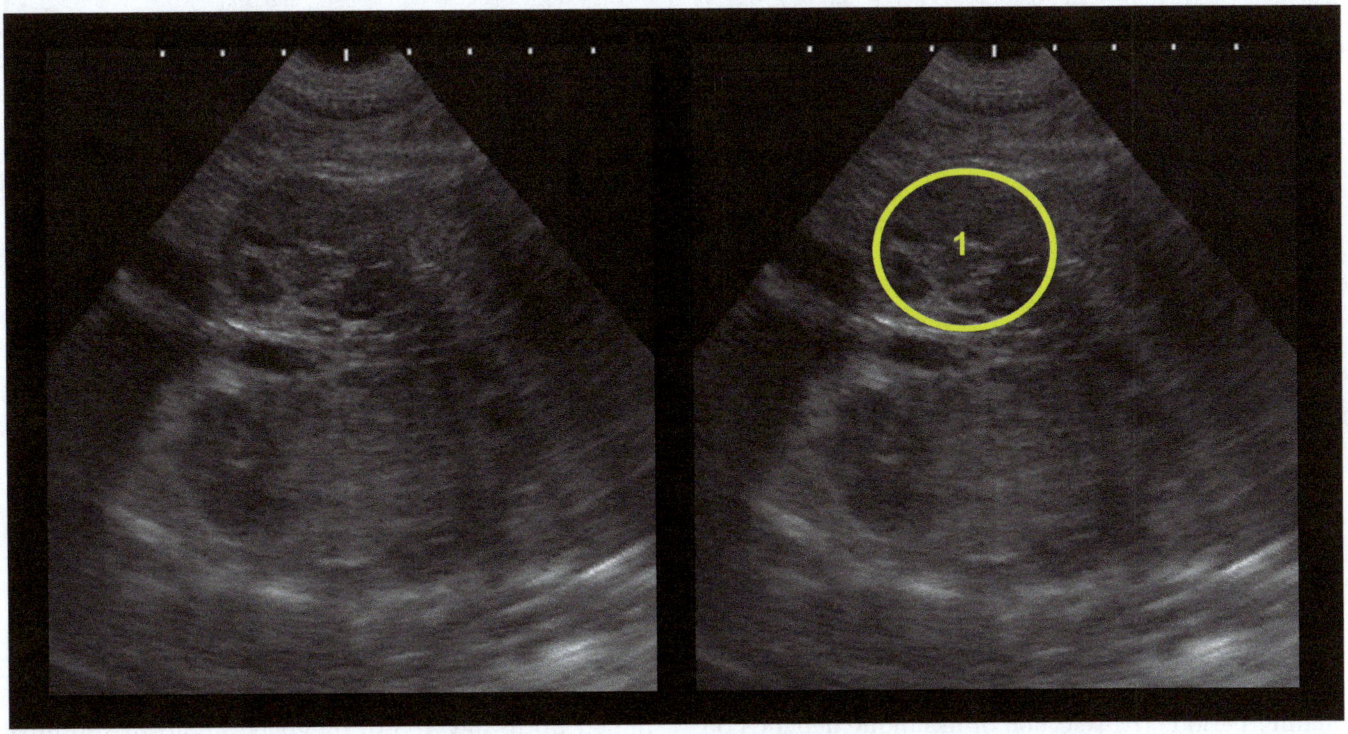

Figure 11.18. Ultrasound image of a 120-day fetus viewed with the transabdominal technique using a 5 MHz sectorial probe (depth 10 cm). 1: The kidney of the fetus can be identified on this sonogram.

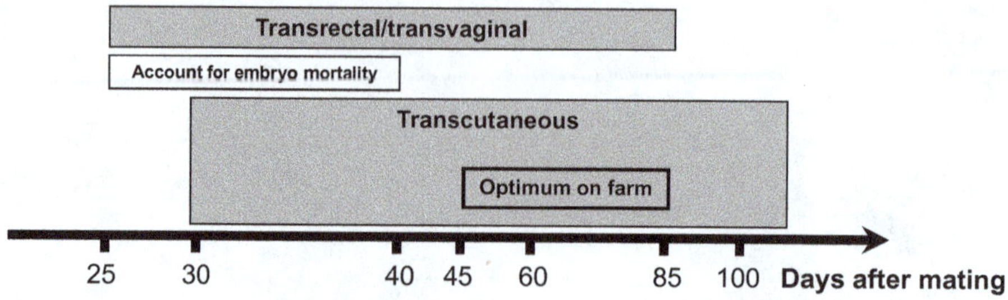

Figure 11.19. Periods during pregnancy when the different ultrasonographic techniques are recommended and when pregnancy scanning on the farm is appropriate. Transrectal and transvaginal ultrasonography for the diagnosis of pregnancy can be done from day 25 to day 85 after mating, but accuracy is not maximized until day 30 and decreases after day 60 after the uterus has descended into the abdominal cavity. Transcutaneous or transabdominal techniques can be used from day 30 until after day 100 but, in the field, the optimum period for accurate diagnosis is between days 45 and 85 after mating. It is important to remember that embryo mortality between days 30 and 40 can lead to a false positive diagnosis of pregnancy.

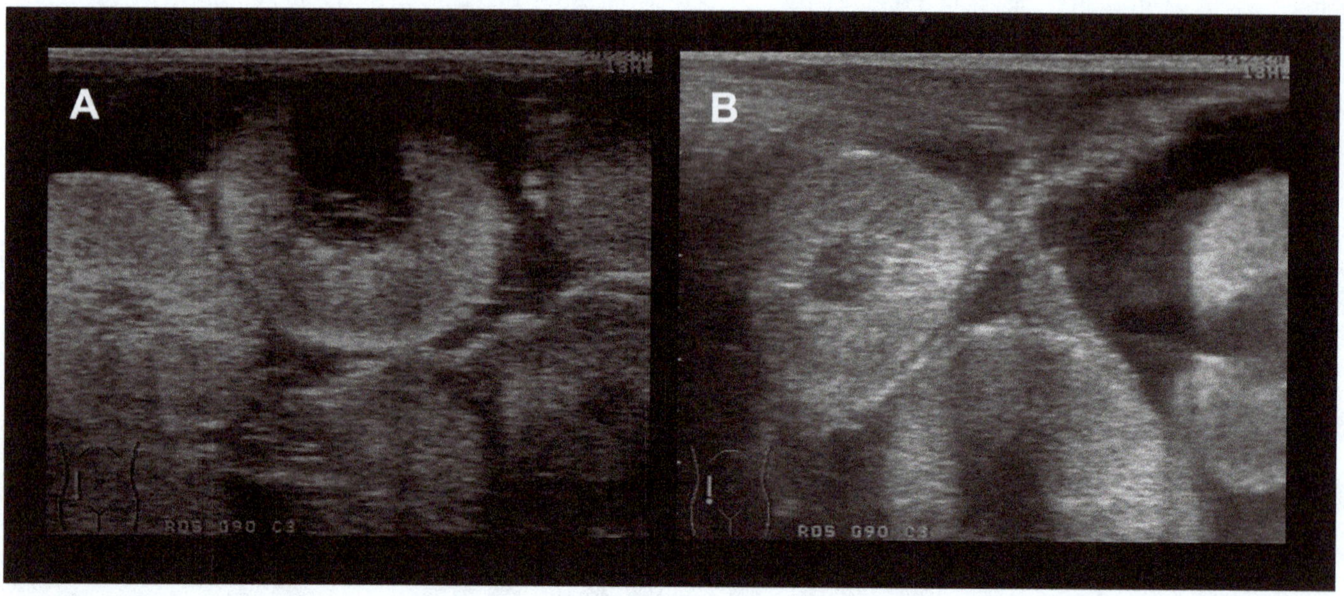

Figure 11.20. Late pregnancy (day 120) ultrasonographic image from a ewe (7.5 MHz linear probe; depth 9 cm). Due to the rapid development of the placenta in the second half of pregnancy the sonographic image is dominated by placentomes that, on cross section, are seen as cup-shaped hyperechogenic structures. They are often the first positive signs of pregnancy during ultrasound examination[9].

best. The accuracy of diagnosis will depend on the range in gestational age at scanning, so it is important to know the dates of the beginning and the end of the mating period. The selection of technique depends on several factors, but a combination of speed and accuracy are important for pregnancy diagnosis in the field. Transcutaneous scanning can be performed under a tent and in a scanning crate with the ewe or doe in a standing (Figure 11.21) or sitting position (Figure 11.22) or with the animals a meter higher than the operator, as is the case in the milking parlor (Figure 11.23).

The number and viability of the fetuses can be determined up to day 100 of pregnancy, with the optimal period being days 45–85[9] (Figure 11.19). To minimize the number of false negatives and positives, the females should be fasted for 12 h and the abdominal wall lifted during the test. With the scanning crate set up appropriately, and three handlers to move animals, it is possible to scan 500 ewes per hour for pregnancy diagnosis

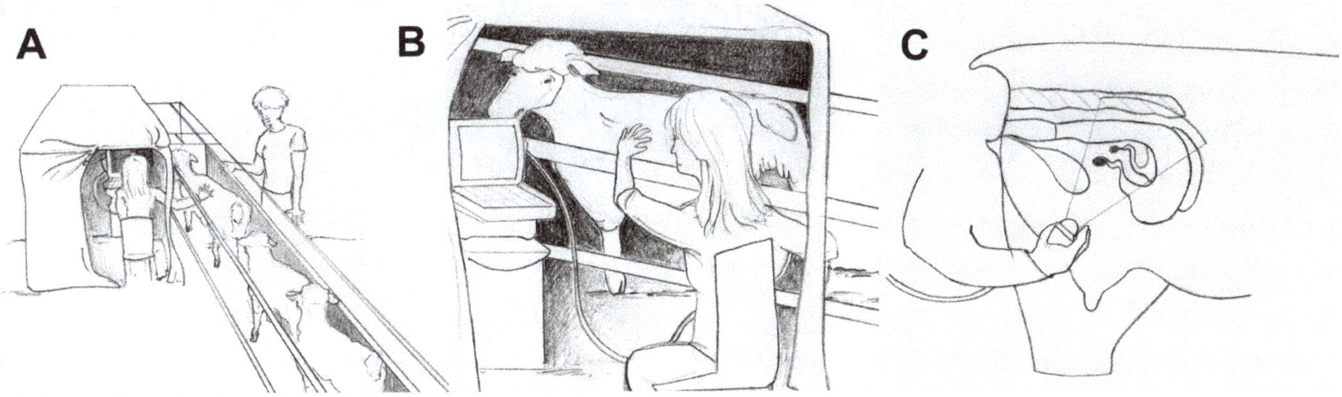

Figure 11.21. Illustration of transcutaneous pregnancy scanning with the female in a standing position. A: The scanning crate will be positioned at the end of the race and a tent is built around the operator to avoid direct light on the screen of the scanner; B: The ewe will enter the crate, which could be elevated 0.5 meter from the floor, and the operator will access the woolless area in front of the udder between the legs of the ewe; C: The sector probe covered with a layer of lubricant will be positioned on the right side of the ewe.

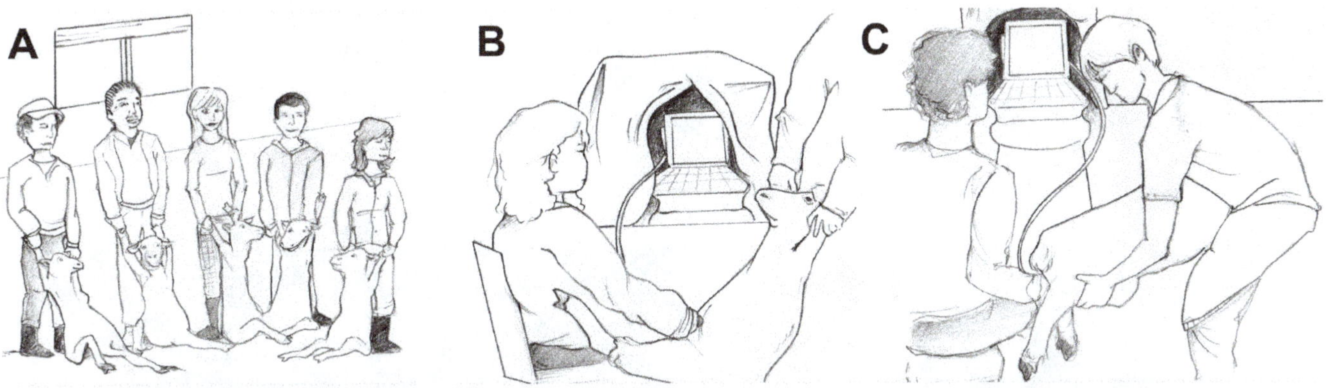

Figure 11.22. Illustration of transcutaneous pregnancy scanning with the female in a sitting position. A: The handlers will catch the ewes from the pen and, while waiting in the queue, another operator will add lubricant in the left and right woolless areas in front of the udder; B: The ewe will be presented to the operator in the sitting position and the sector probe positioned on both sides; C: If the ewe is suspected to be nonpregnant, the handler will reposition her into the standing position for further evaluation.

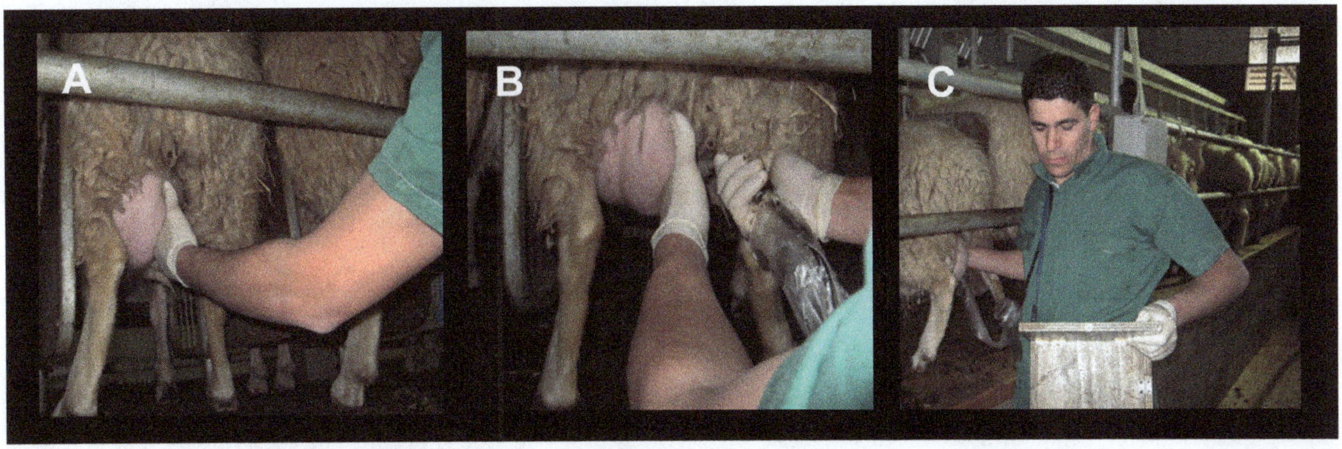

Figure 11.23. Illustration of transcutaneous pregnancy scanning with the female in the milking parlor. A: Using the left hand, the operator will access and clear the area between the udder and the right leg of the ewe; B: Using the right hand, the operator will position the sector 3.5 MHz probe on the right hairless area; C (right): The operator will identify the image on the screen and call out a diagnosis for recording.

and 350 per hour for litter size. By placing the animal in the sitting or standing position, single pregnancies can be detected in about 10 seconds. When twins are suspected, 20–30 seconds are needed to confirm the diagnosis. Nonpregnant ewes require 20–30 seconds for diagnosis. Under commercial conditions, 100–150 ewes can be scanned per hour (1200 per day) if two or three handlers are presenting sheep to the operator and one or two handlers are refilling empty catching pens. The highest daily rate has been 1800 but the quest for speed can lead to loss of accuracy. The sensitivity of ultrasound for detecting pregnancy is 99% and the specificity is 100%. For detecting multiples, the sensitivity is 91% and the specificity 100%, giving a percentage of correct diagnosis of 98%. In the milking parlor, it is possible to detect pregnancies in about 10 to 40 seconds, so it is possible to scan over 90 animals per hour.

Fetal Count, Age, and Sex

Fetal count

It is also possible to determine the stage of pregnancy, the viability of the fetus, the number of fetuses, and their sex. Fetuses can be counted using various approaches. Often the first observation is variation in the volume of uterine fluid, which is greater in animals carrying twins than in animals with a similarly sized single fetus. On some occasions both fetuses are evident although one is in longitudinal section while the other is in cross section. To count the fetuses accurately it is important to identify the same body structure more than once (Figure 11.24A,B).

The expertise of the operator is another factor affecting the accuracy of the diagnosis of multiple fetuses. Newly trained operators are initially not able to scan

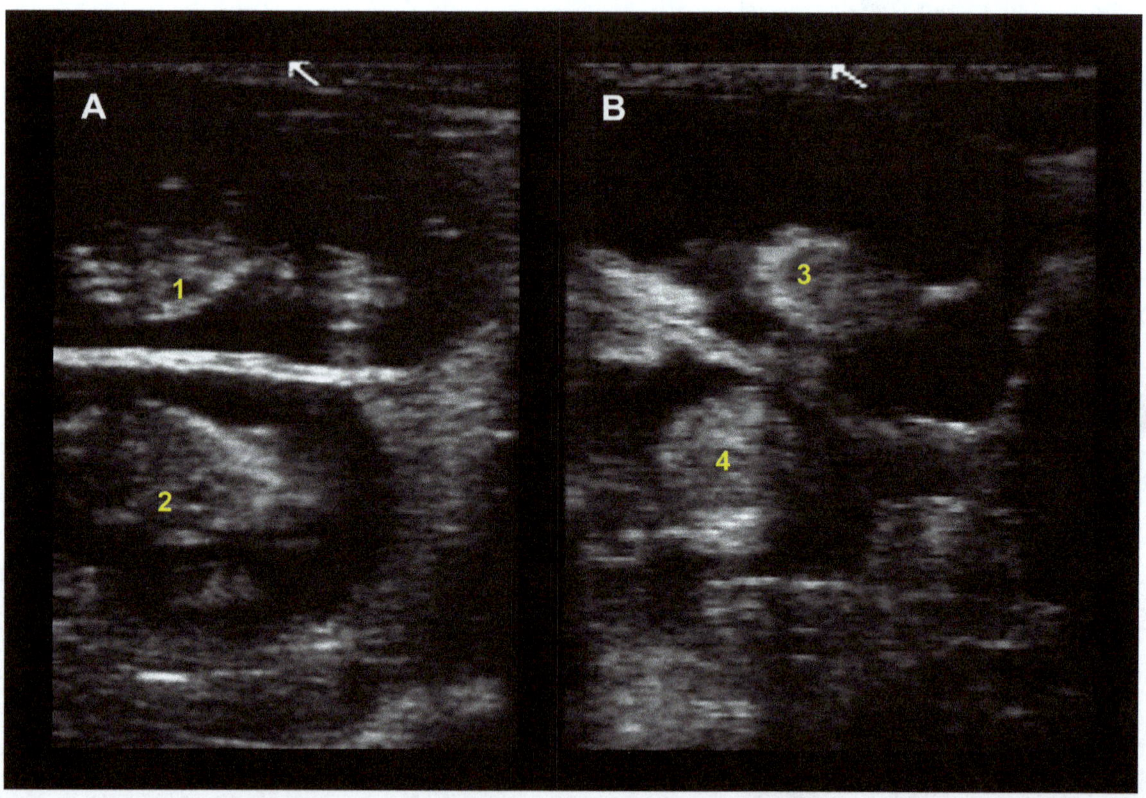

Figure 11.24. Identification of 60-day twins in a doe (3.5 MHz linear probe; depth 12 cm). The ultrasonographer normally looks for the number of trunks or heads (cross or transverse section) or spines (longitudinal section) present in the uterus. The same structures must be identified in both fetuses, in order to avoid errors in fetal counts. The key to accuracy is to always use the same methodology (Figure 11.25) so the same structure is not seen twice. A1: Trunk of fetus #1; A2: Trunk of fetus #2; B3: Head of fetus #1; B4: Head of fetus #2.

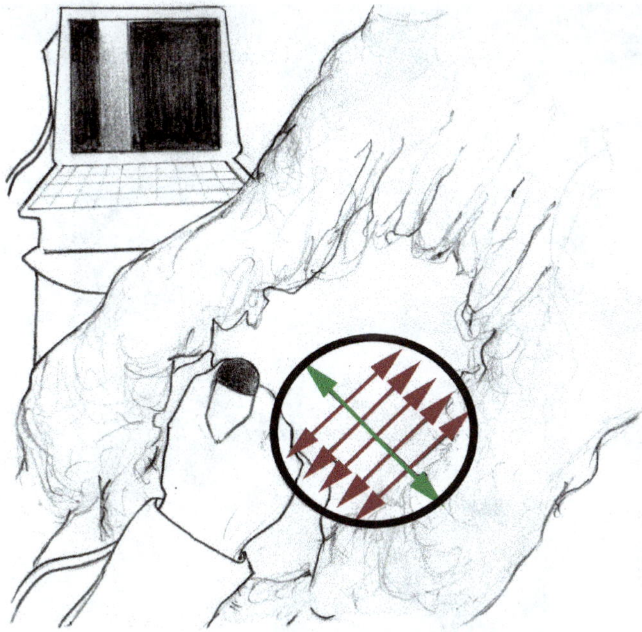

Figure 11.25. Suggested methodology for scanning ewes and does for fetal count in a sitting position. With the probe in the right hand, the operator touches its left surface with the right thumb to confirm that the image is generated on the left side of the screen. The probe is positioned on the skin of the right woolless area of the ewe if she is in standing position and on the left woolless area if the ewe is in the sitting position, as on this drawing (circle). Then the probe is slowly moved right to left at the same level in order to localize the pregnancy and fetal parts (blue arrow). After that, the direction of the scanning movements will be perpendicular to the first set of movements at different levels (red arrows) to cover the complete scanning area systematically, in a way to avoid going back on the same fetus twice.

Table 11.2.
Measurements used to predict the age of the embryo and fetus in sheep

	Embryo/Fetus (Age)				
	24–35 Days	36–40 Days	41–65 Days	66–130 Days	131–147 Days
Embryonic vesicle (cm)	2.0–3.5	3.5–5.0	>5.0		
Crown-rump length (cm)	1.0–2.0	2.0–3.5	>3.5		
Thoracic diameter (cm)	0.5–1.2	1.2–1.5	1.5–3.0	3.0–8.0	>8.0
Biparietal diameter (cm)			1.2–2.5	2.5–5.0	>5.0
Head length (cm)			1.5–3.0	3.0–7.5	>7.5

accurately. Analysis of 0, 1, 2, 3, or 4 fetuses will highlight differences among operators. After training with the technique (500 to 1000 animals) and an appraisal session with an expert, operators will improve their accuracy sufficiently to be of commercial value (Figure 11.25).

Fetal age

Fetal age can be estimated by measuring different parts of the body at different stages of pregnancy (Table 11.2). During the first 3 months, fetal size is not related to litter size[7,13]. For example, the pattern of growth from day 20 to 40, as determined by crown-rump length (CRL) (Figure 11.26), is the same for litters of 1 to 4[13].

Up to day 40, the difference in predicted and actual birth date for sheep, based on the size of the fetus, ranges from −10 to +7 days[13]. Head diameters (Figure 11.27) and lengths provide a good index of fetal development and offer an advantage over other measures because long periods of observation (from 36 to 91 days) are feasible[7].

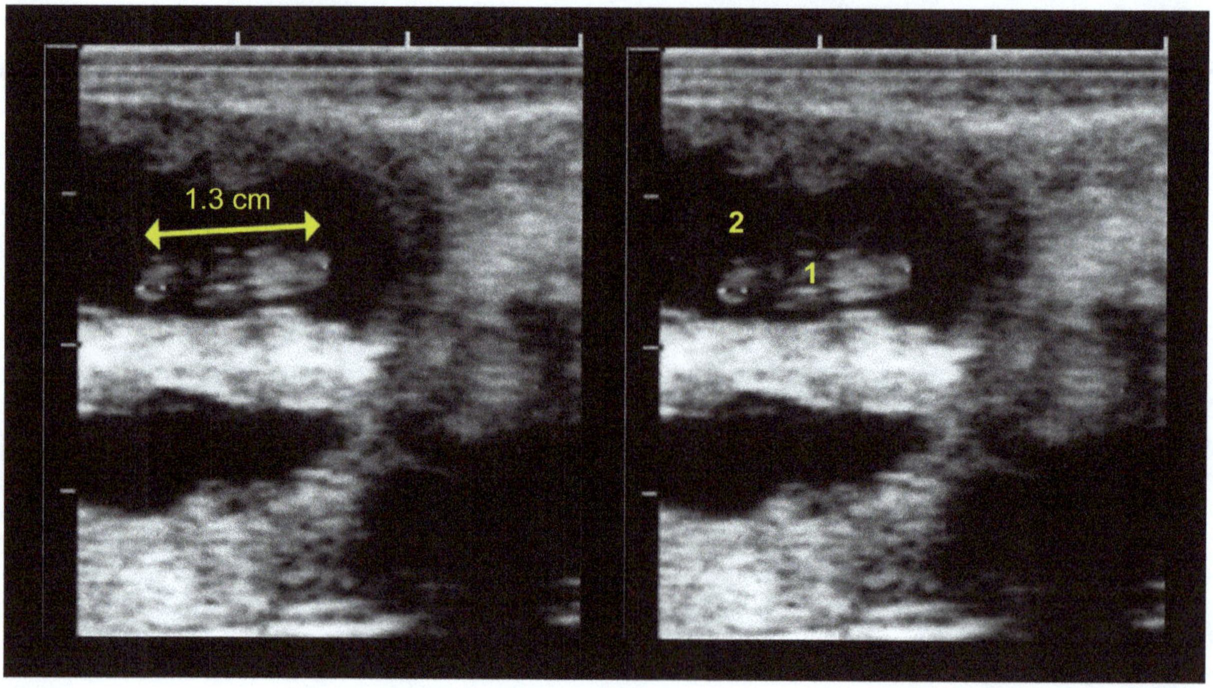

Figure 11.26. Measurement of crown-rump length (CRL), which can be used to estimate fetal age. The length of the fetus from the top of the head (crown) to the end of the buttocks (rump) is called the *crown-rump length (CRL)*. Table 11.2 gives CRL measurements that can be used to predict the age of the embryo and fetus in sheep. On this ultrasound image the 26-day embryo has a CRL of 1.3 cm. 1: Embryo; 2: Amniotic fluid; Yellow arrow: CRL.

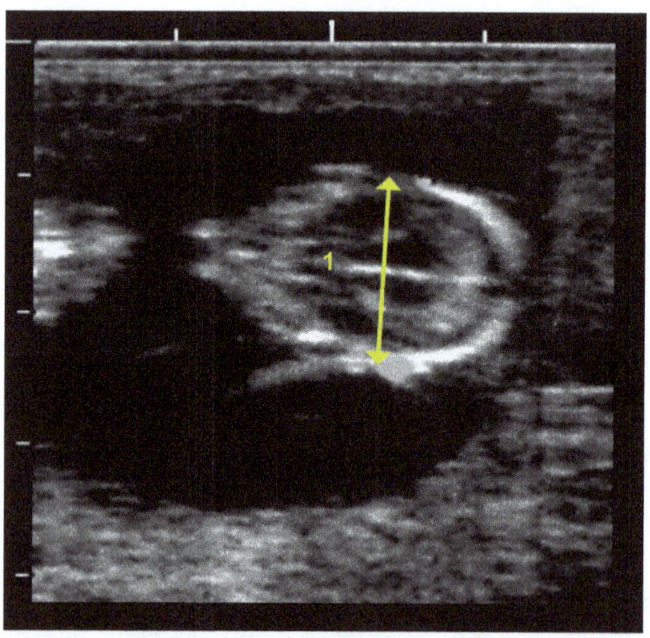

Figure 11.27. Measurements of head diameter, which can be used to estimate fetal age. The biparietal diameter (BD) of the head is strongly correlated with age in fetuses between 40 and 130 days (Table 11.2). On this ultrasound image the 42-day fetus has a BD of 1.3 cm. 1: Head; Yellow arrow: BD.

During the last one-third of pregnancy, estimation of fetal age is affected by the individual characteristics of the fetus, which are determined by genetics, nutrition, and the age of the ewe. Attempts to use the placentomes for the determination of gestational age in ewes and does have been only partially successful because placentomes of different sizes coexist in the same animal throughout gestation.

Fetal sex

For sex determination, it is possible to locate and identify the genital tubercle at 60 to 69 days. With a linear-array 5 MHz transducer applied transcutaneously, the accuracy was 100% for male fetuses but only 76% for females. In this study, fetal sex could not be determined in 7% of the ewes[4]. In goats, the accuracy of fetal sexing is high (100%) for a single fetus, but lower for twins (93%) and triplets (63%)[12].

The ultrasound appearance of the fetal genital tubercle is the same in small ruminants and bovine species. See Chapter 7 for more details.

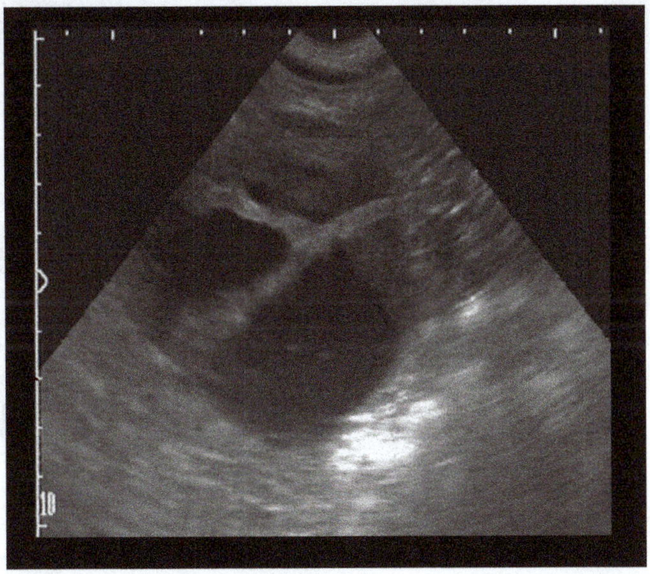

Figure 11.28. Ultrasonographic image of a pseudopregnancy (5 MHz sectorial probe; depth 10 cm). This image shows an enlargement of the uterus due to fluid accumulation that could be easily confused with a normal pregnancy. No fetal structures will be observed nor will other signs of pregnancy, such as placentomes.

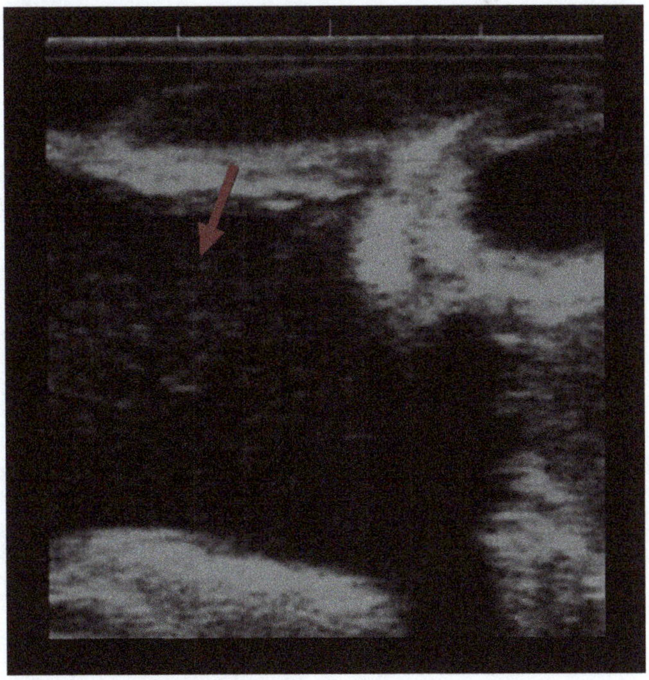

Figure 11.29. Ultrasonographic image of a metrorrhagia. Arrow indicates the accumulation of blood inside the uterus, which may be related to pregnancy, abortion, or other abnormalities of the placenta.

Pathological Conditions in the Female

Ultrasound allows for the determination of abnormal causes of anestrus, such as pseudopregnancy (Figure 11.28) or pathological processes in the uterus (metritis, metrorrhagia) (Figure 11.29) and ovaries (Figure 11.30).

The ultrasonographer can also detect embryonic and fetal abnormalities during the course of pregnancy. Early mortality (Figure 11.31), detected by the absence of the heartbeat, will lead to a late return to estrus; a later mortality may lead to mummification of the uterine contents (Figure 11.32).

It is also possible to see malformations in different parts of the fetal body. Intrapartum uterine torsion in ewes can be diagnosed by transabdominal sonographic

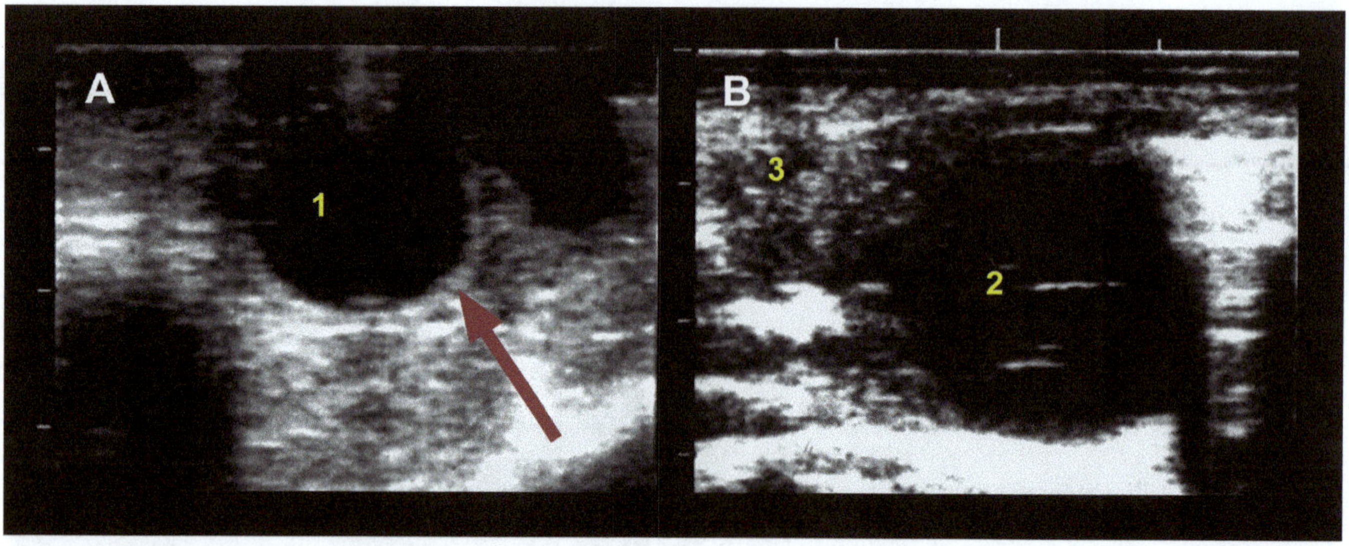

Figure 11.30. Ultrasonographic images of a follicular cyst (A) and a paraovarian cyst (B). A: The follicular cyst is an anechoic structure similar to a follicle but of abnormally large size, located where ovulation did not occur; this condition is one of the most common ovarian pathologies observable by ultrasound in small ruminants; B: This anechoic structure is located alongside the ovary and can be confused with a follicular cyst. To identify these structures correctly, the limits of the ovary and its stroma must be observed. 1: Follicular cyst; 2: Paraovarian cyst; 3: Ovarian stroma.

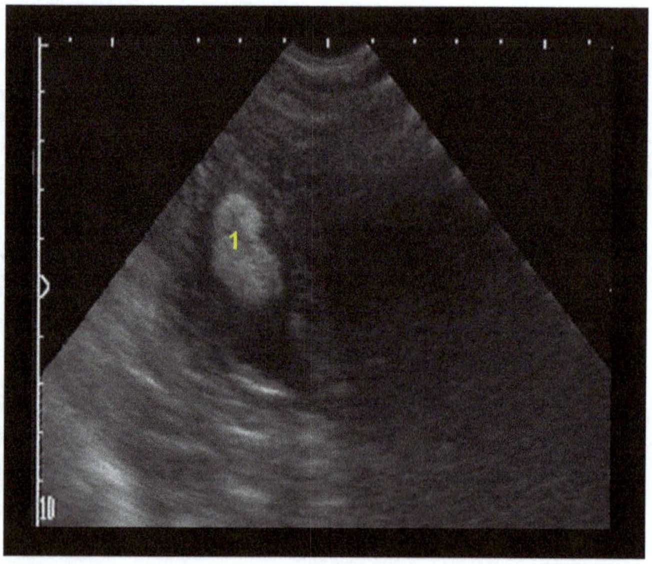

Figure 11.31. Ultrasound image of a dead embryo (5 MHz sectorial probe; depth 10 cm). In this image the dead embryo is more echoic than a normal embryo, with a small amount of amniotic liquid. 1: Dead embryo.

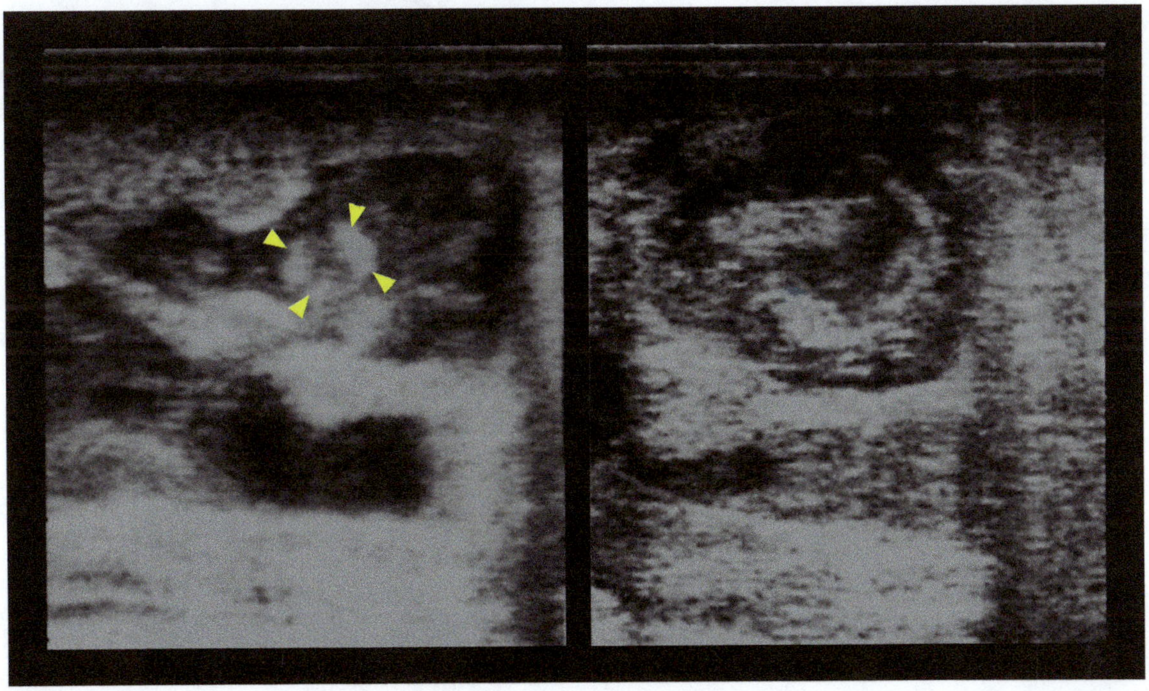

Figure 11.32. Ultrasonographic image of a mummified fetus (5MHz linear probe; depth 4cm). 1: Mummified fetus; Yellow arrows: Placentome.

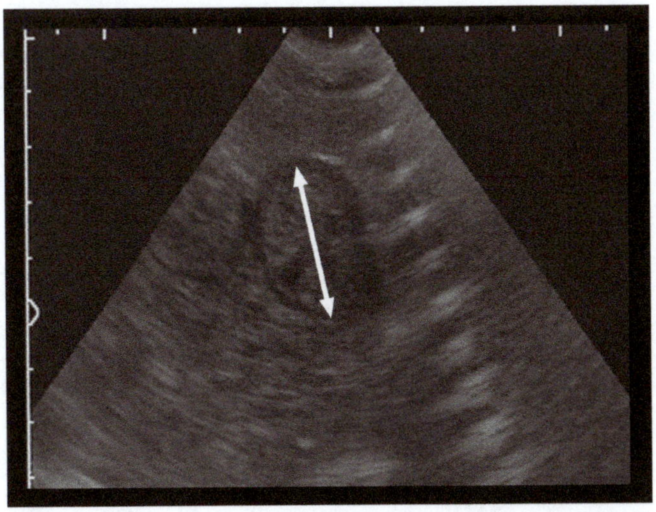

Figure 11.33. Measurement of the uterine horn width to evaluate involution of the uterus postpartum (5MHz sectorial probe; depth 8cm). The arrow indicates the width of the uterus that could be measured in order to identify abnormalities during involution.

measurements of the thickness of the uterine wall[17]. Normal uterine involution postpartum can be followed by measuring the width of each uterine horn by transrectal ultrasonography[8] (Figure 11.33).

Ultrasonographic Evaluation of the Male Genital System

The hormonal control of reproduction in the male is described in Figure 11.34.

Because the formation of sperm takes 49 days, males must be examined at least 2 months before the beginning of the mating season to allow time to treat any pathological process and restore normal fertility. Traditionally, the male genital system is subjected to clinical examination of the penis, testes, and scrotum, followed by macroscopic and microscopic evaluation of the semen[2]. The application of these techniques is the gold standard for diagnosis of the more frequent causes of infertility, but their value as a diagnostic tool

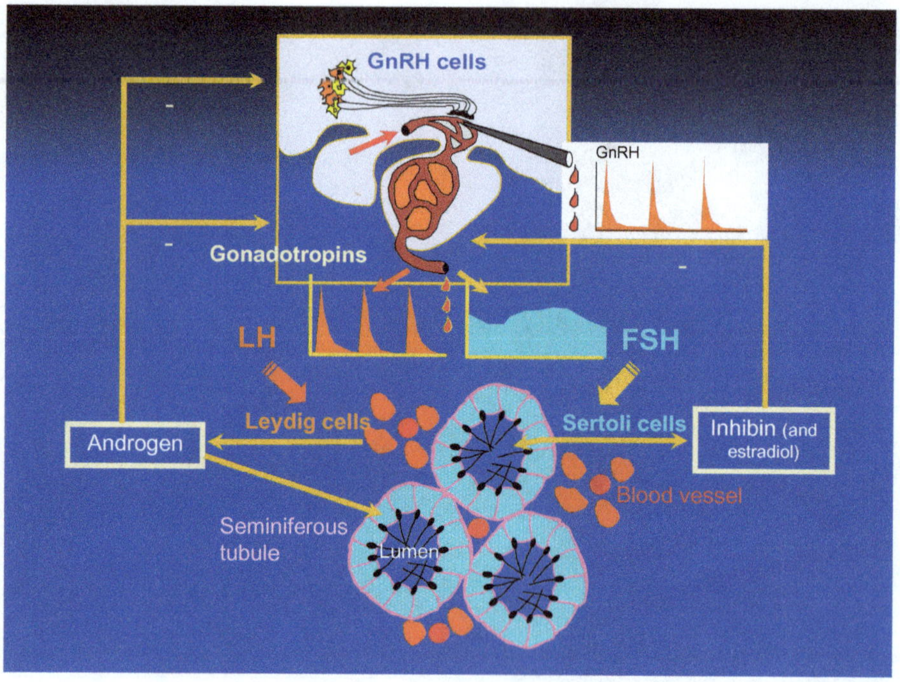

Figure 11.34. Hormonal control of reproduction in the male. Schematic representation of the endocrine control of reproductive function in the male by the hypothalamo-hypophysial-gonadal axis. In brief, GnRH pulses from the hypothalamus induce secretion of the pituitary gonadotropins FSH and LH, which in turn stimulate Sertoli and Leydig cells, respectively. The Sertoli cells secrete inhibin and estradiol; the Leydig cells secrete androgens. All of these hormones exert negative feedback at the pituitary level, but androgens also inhibit hypothalamic GnRH output (probably after conversion to estradiol in brain tissue) while promoting the process of spermatogenesis in the seminiferous tubules.

for the determination of degenerative disease is limited. Ultrasonography offers the possibility of detecting anomalies in the internal accessory glands (e.g., bulbourethral, seminal vesicular glands), all of which are inaccessible by palpation. A combination of all techniques will increase the accuracy of an examination for breeding soundness.

Although ultrasonographic evaluation of the male genital system in small ruminants was first reported 20 years ago[3], private practitioners have not adopted it routinely. The aim of this part of the chapter is to highlight the advantages of using ultrasonography to reach a definitive diagnosis.

Anatomy of the male reproductive tract

Figure 11.35 describes the anatomy of the male reproductive tract. The ultrasonographic pattern of scrotal skin is well defined and echogenic.

The dimensions of the testes in the ram are highly variable, being affected by many factors including age, genotype, photoperiod, and nutrition[1]. The diameter of the testes can be measured by ultrasonography and the values are highly correlated with postmortem measurements[11]. The testes are each suspended in the scrotum by the spermatic cord, which is composed of convoluted testicular arteries, the venous plexus (pampiniform plexus), nerves, and a smooth muscle (the cremaster) (Figure 11.35).

The tunica testis, albuginea, and vaginalis (parietal and vaginal), are composed of fibrous tissue and are seen as two hyperechoic lines between the skin and the testis (Figures 11.35, 11.41).

The testis feeds into the epididymis, which is divided into the head, the body, and the tail (Figure 11.35). The head of the epididymis is a well-defined structure with a more heterogeneous pattern than that of the testis (Figures 11.36, 11.37). The rete testis is seen near the head of the epididymis and is composed of anechoic tubules and hyperechoic interstitial tissue (Figure 11.37).

The body and tail of the epididymis are more difficult to identify due to their smaller size, but they are more easily seen when a pathological process is present

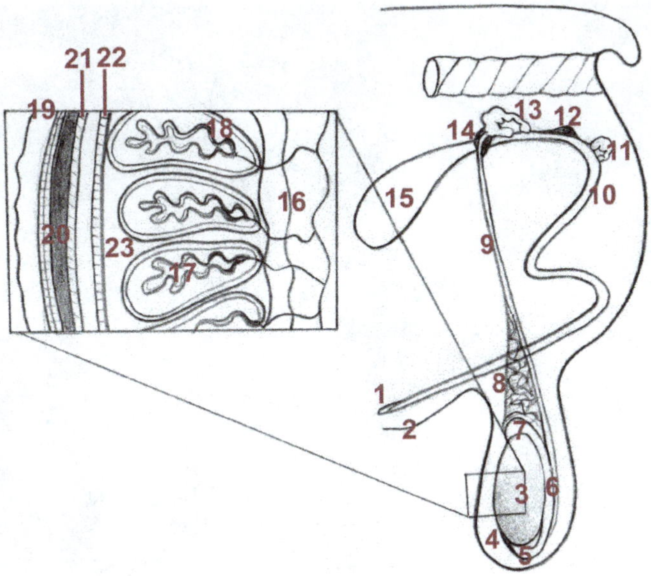

Figure 11.35. Schematic representation of the anatomy of external (testis, epididymis, and penis) and internal (prostate, seminal vesicular glands, bulbourethral glands) components of the male reproductive tract in small ruminants. 1: Penis; 2: Prepuce; 3: Testis; 4: Scrotum; 5: Tail of the epididymis; 6: Body of the epididymis; 7: Head of the epididymis; 8: Blood vessels of the pampiniform plexus; 9: Vas deferens; 10: Urethra; 11: Bulbourethral gland; 12: Prostate; 13: Seminal vesicular glands; 14: Ampulla; 15: Bladder; 16: Mediastinum; 17: Lobule; 18: Seminiferous tubule; 19: Scrotal skin; 20: Scrotal fascia; 21: Parietal tunica vaginalis; 22: Visceral tunica vaginalis; 23: Tunica albuginea.

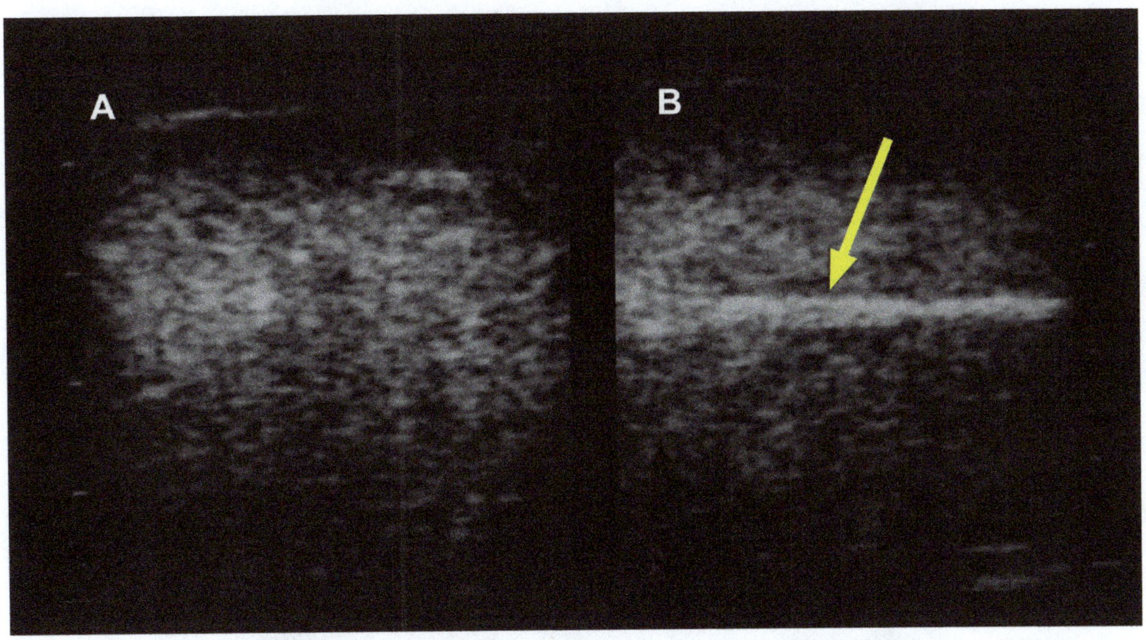

Figure 11.36. Transverse (A) and longitudinal (B) ultrasonographic images of the normal testicular parenchyma and mediastinum. The ultrasonographic appearance of normal parenchyma of the testis is homogeneous, with anechoic areas that correspond to seminiferous tubules and hyperechoic areas that correspond to interstitial connective tissue. The mediastinum is a cord of connective tissue that extends along the long axis of the testis. In longitudinal sections it can be seen as a centrally located hyperechoic line (arrow).

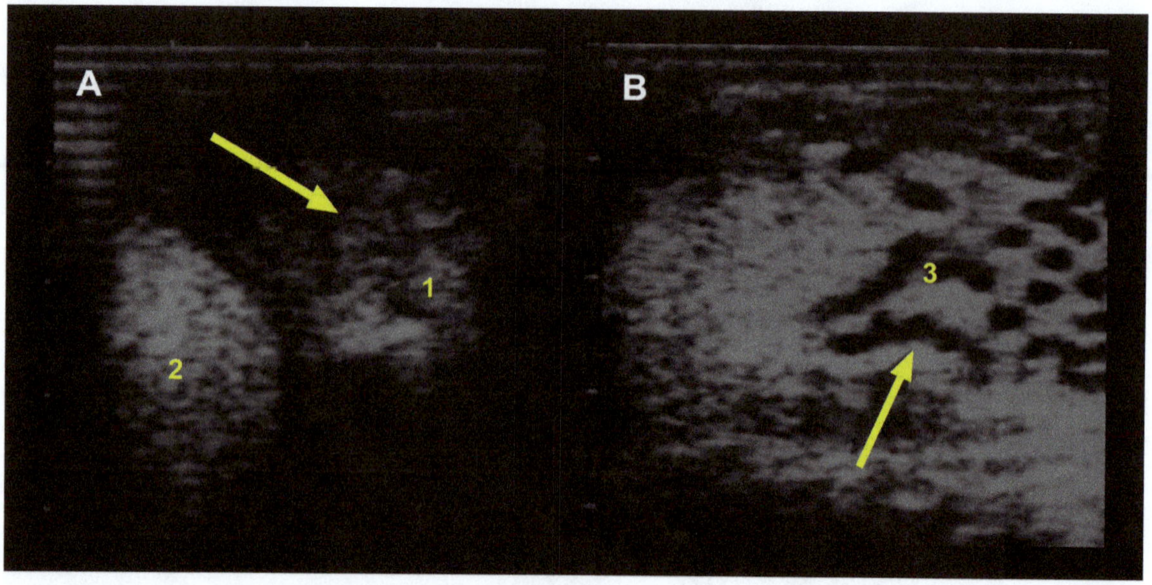

Figure 11.37. Ultrasonographic image of the head of the epididymis (A) and rete testis (B). 1: Head of the epididymis (yellow arrow) with a pattern that is more heterogeneous than the testis seen alongside; 2: Testicular parenchyma; 3: Rete testis (white arrow) composed of anechoic tubules and hyperechoic interstitial tissue.

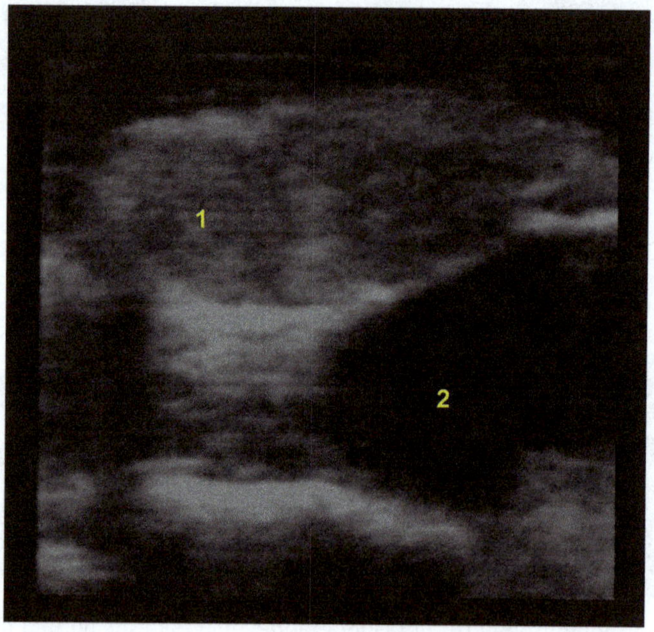

Figure 11.38. Ultrasonographic image of normal seminal vesicular glands. Seminal vesicular glands appear as twin spherical or ovoid structures with an isoechoic central pattern and hyperechoic edges. 1: Vesicular glands; 2: Bladder.

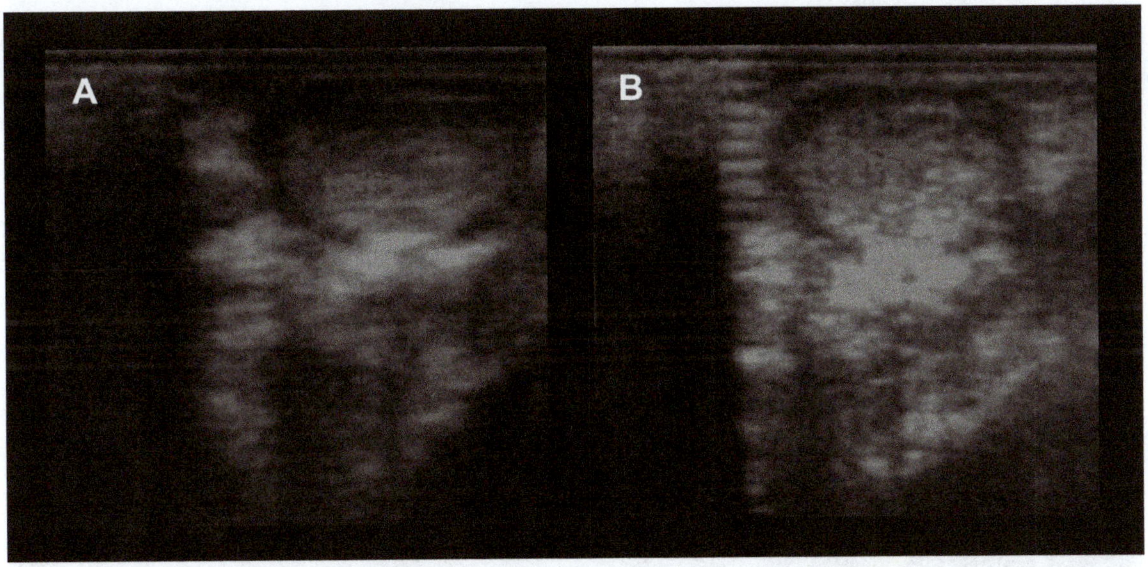

Figure 11.39. Ultrasonographic image of bulbourethral glands. Bulbourethral glands, like normal seminal vesicular glands, appear as twin spherical or ovoid structures with a slightly hyperechoic pattern. A: Left bulbourethral gland; B: Right bulbourethral gland.

(e.g., hydrocele). The tail is continuous with the ductus deferens, which appears as an anechoic tubular structure with hyperechoic walls. The vas deferens emerges from the head of the epididymis and enters the urethra, a common duct for the reproductive and urinary systems.

The accessory glands are located along the pelvic portion of the urethra (Figure 11.35). Ultrasonographic examination of the accessory glands is focused mainly on the vesicular and bulbourethral glands (Figures 11.38, 11.39).

The prostate is too diffuse and irregularly located for ultrasonographic observation. The ultrasonographic pattern of the bulbourethral glands is slightly hyperechoic (Figure 11.39). In sagittal section, the measurement of normal bulbourethral and seminal vesicular glands correlates with direct postmortem measurements after dissection from surrounding fat and connective tissue[11].

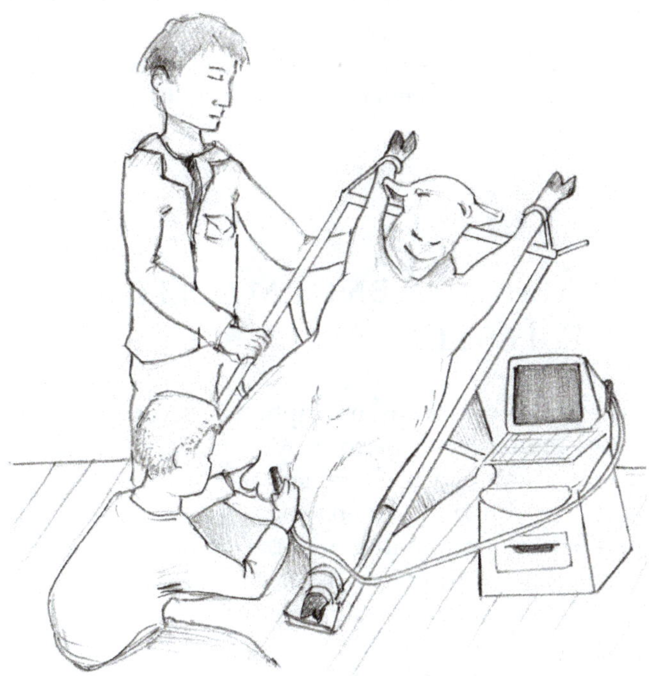

Figure 11.40. To securely perform a transcutaneous ultrasonographic evaluation of the testes of small ruminants, the animal must be restrained in this position.

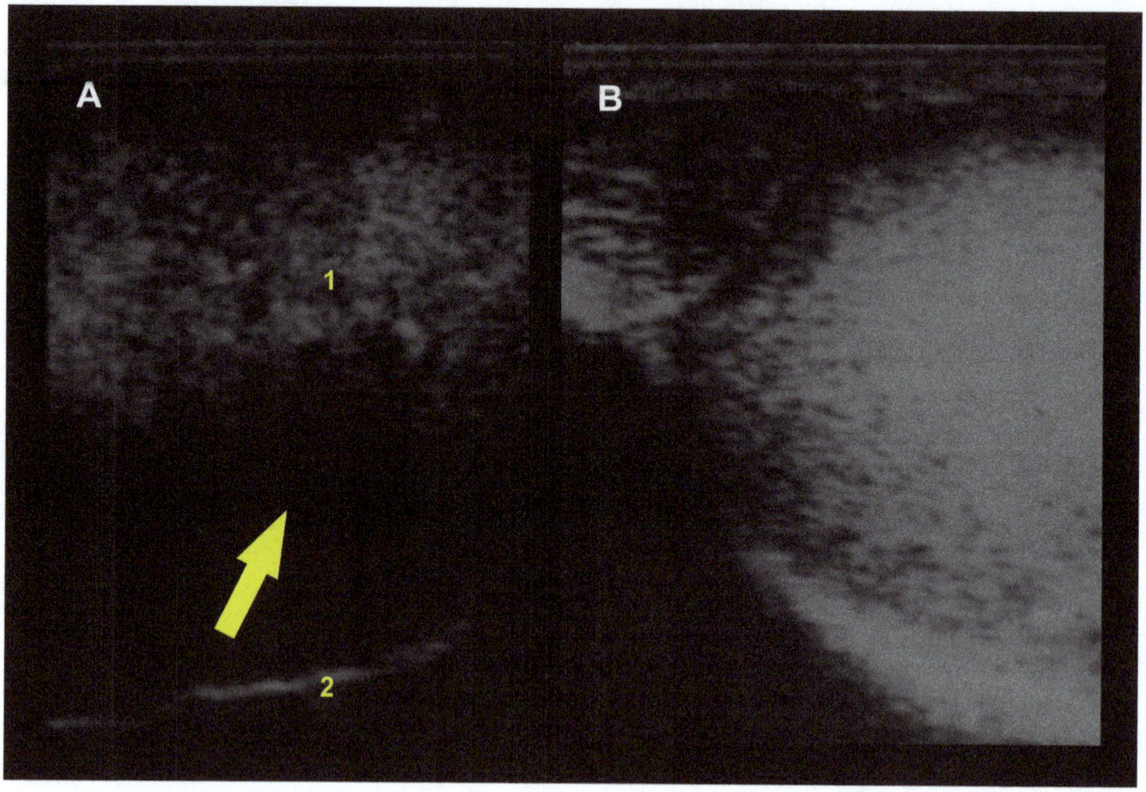

Figure 11.41. Ultrasonographic images of acute orchitis (A) and chronic orchitis (B) in a buck. A: Acute orchitis shows anechoic areas of edema (arrow) between the parenchyma and the membranes of the testis; B: Chronic orchitis is characterized by a hyperechoic pattern throughout the testis; 1: Parenchyma; 2: Membranes of the testis (scrotal fascia, parietal and visceral tunica vaginalis).

Common Abnormalities of the Testis

Transcutaneous ultrasonographic observations of the testes are easier to perform with the male in dorsal recumbency, either restrained in a metallic cradle (Figure 11.40) or on the floor, although it is possible to perform this examination with the animal in a standing position, as with bulls (Chapter 9). Sedation may be required depending on the temperament of the animal. A hydrosoluble contact gel is applied to the area of study. The transducer is firmly pressed against the skin and swept back and forth over the area of interest.

The study of the scrotum, testis, and epididymis is useful for diagnosing causes of infertility or sterility, with or without the presence of deformation, pain, swelling, or trauma. The usual findings are calcifications, cystlike structures (varicocele, hydrocele, cysts, hematoma, abscesses), solid nodular lesions (infarcts, neoplasms), and diffuse lesions (orchitis, hyperplasia). Ultrasound can also be useful for identifying retained testes and testicular torsion.

The most common findings in small ruminants are acute and chronic orchitis and epididymitis. Acute orchitis is characterized by a diffuse hypoechoic pattern, due to edema and fluid collection in the testicular tissues (Figure 11.41A).

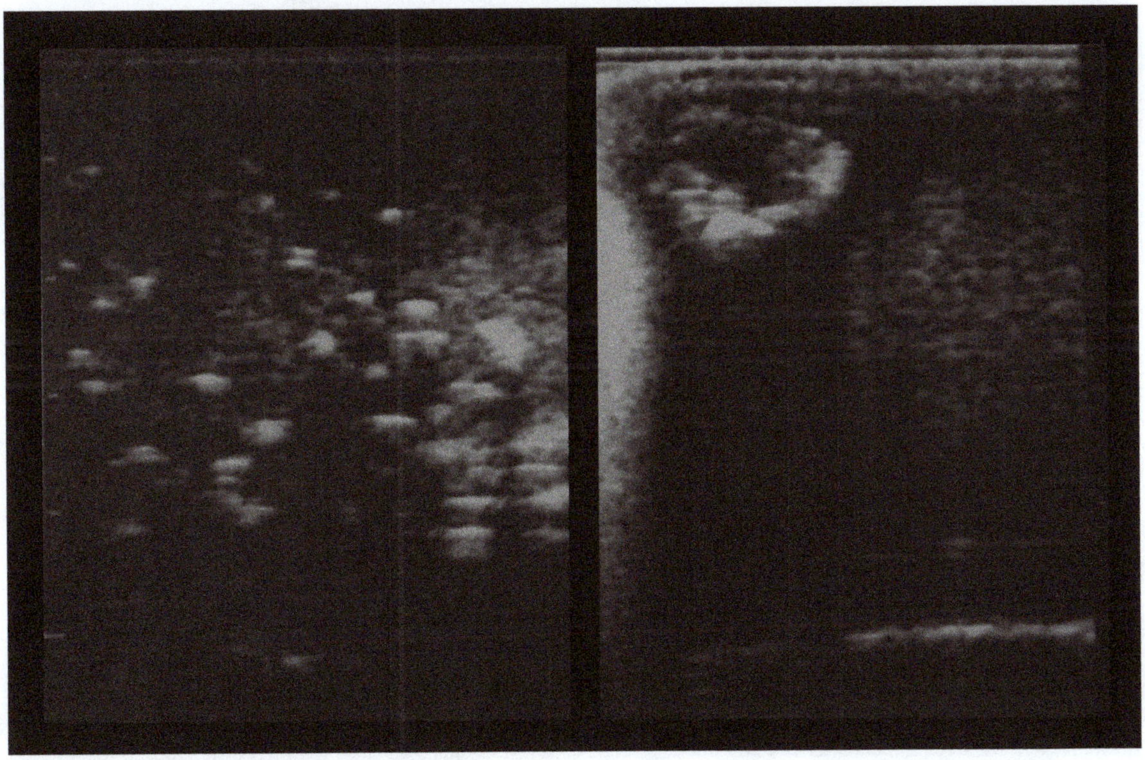

Figure 11.42. Ultrasonographic image of chronic testicular degeneration in a buck. Many areas of calcification can be visualized within the parenchyma of the testis.

It is normal to find anechoic foci in orchitis of infectious origin. Chronic inflammation of the testis is usually accompanied by fibrosis, so the disease is represented by a generalized hyperechoic pattern (Figure 11.41B), with hyperechoic spots signifying testicular degeneration and calcification (Figure 11.42). Finally, advanced degeneration may end in atrophy (Figure 11.43).

Acute epididymitis, as a rule, is hypoechoic whereas chronic epididymitis is hyperechoic (Figure 11.44). Epididymal cysts are rare and difficult to differentiate from spermatocele by ultrasound (Figure 11.45). Thus, aspiration of fluid is necessary to confirm the diagnosis. Clear serous fluid signifies an epididymal cyst, whereas creamy fluid signifies a spermatocele.

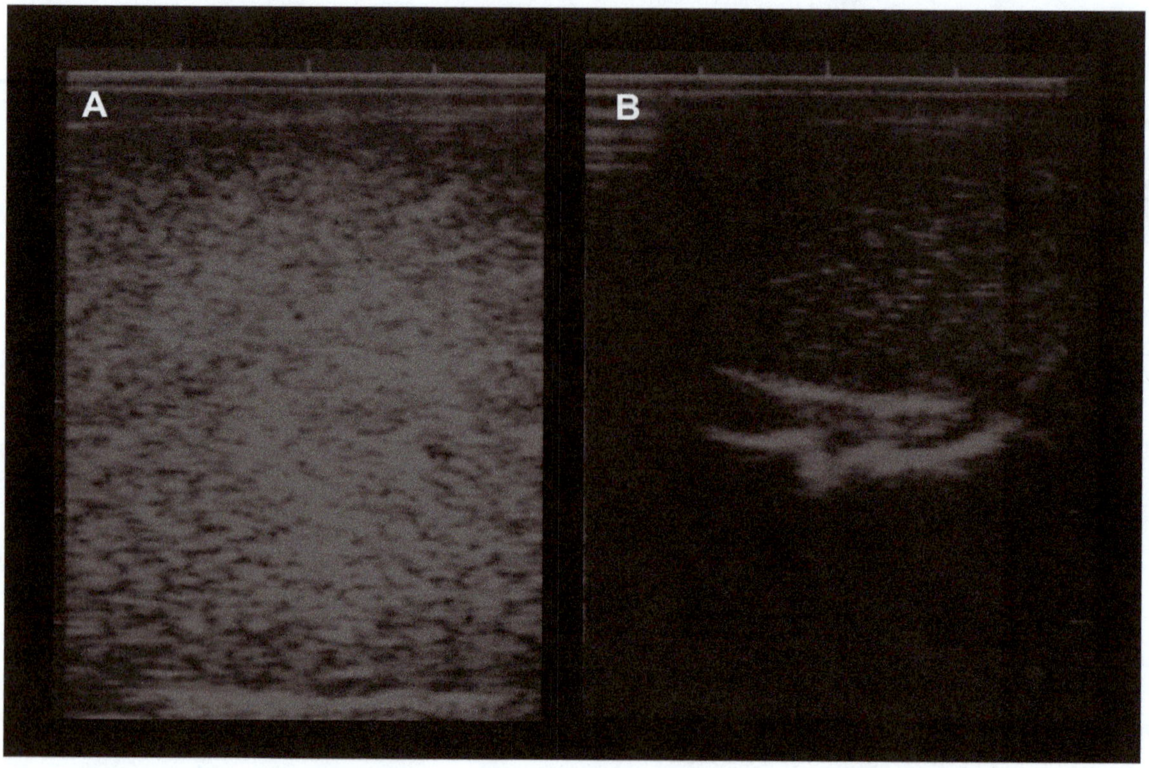

Figure 11.43. Ultrasonographic image of testicular atrophy in a ram. Comparison of ultrasonographic images of a normal testis (A) and an atrophied testis (B) in rams.

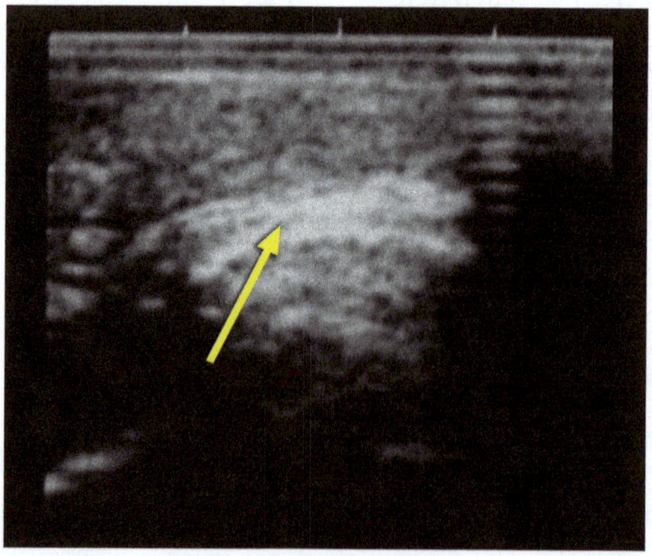

Figure 11.44. Ultrasonographic image of chronic epididymitis. In this ultrasound image, it is possible to differentiate the hyperechogenic pattern of the enlarged epididymis (arrow).

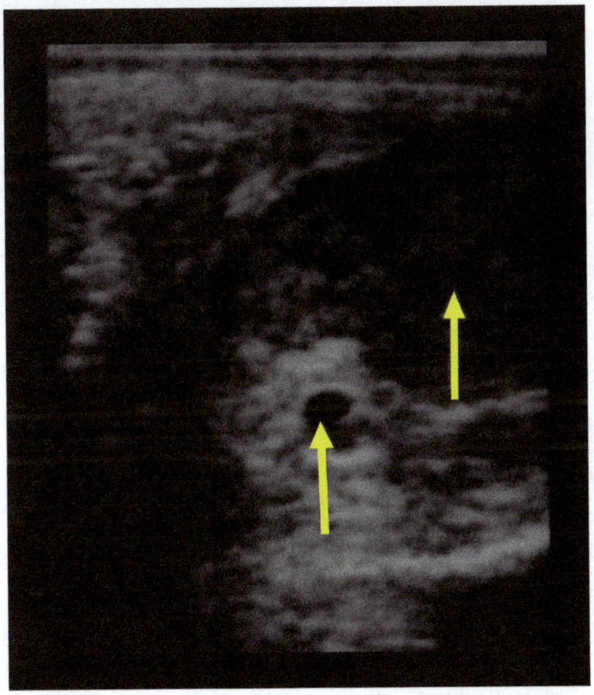

Figure 11.45. Ultrasonographic image of spermatocele in a ram. The fluid accumulation corresponds to spermatoceles in the body of the epididymis (arrows).

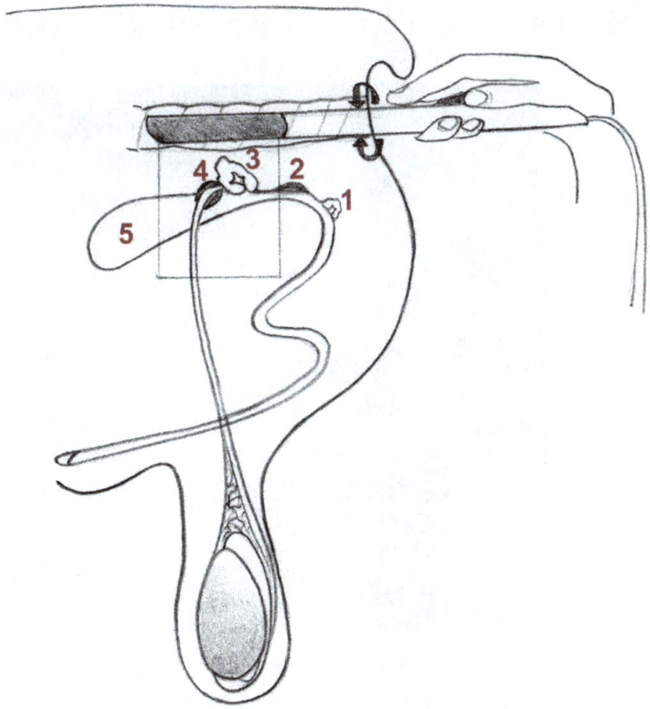

Figure 11.46. Transrectal technique for ultrasonographic evaluation of internal reproductive accessory glands in the male. The probe is inserted into the rectum with the transducer oriented perpendicularly to the abdominal wall. When the urethra is located the probe is slightly rotated laterally to observe the internal glands. 1: Bulbourethral glands; 2: Prostate; 3: Seminal vesicular glands; 4: Ampulla; 5: Bladder.

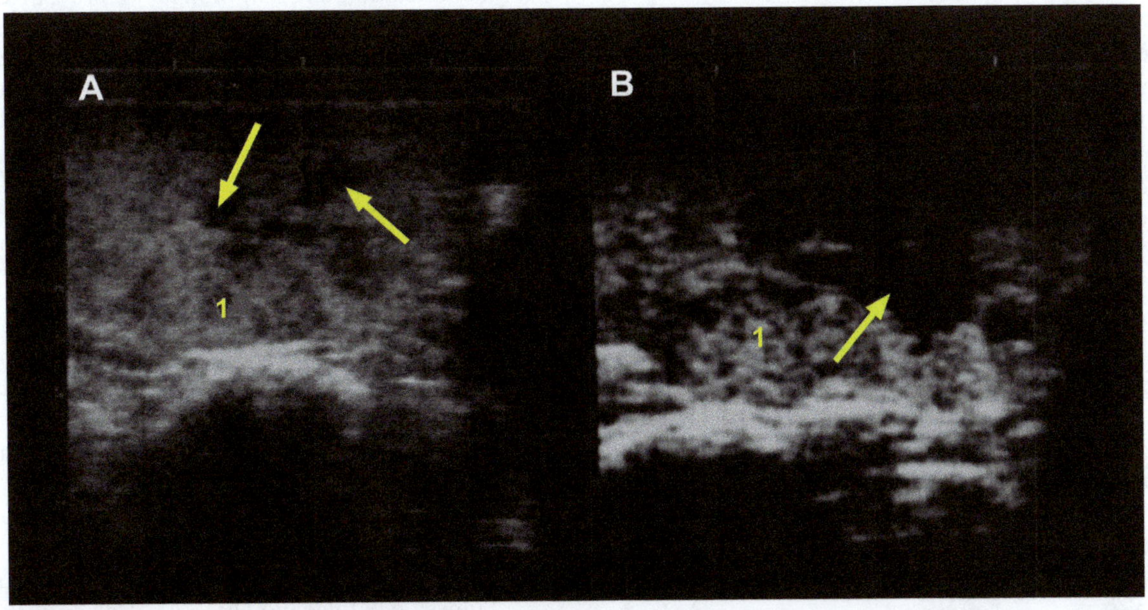

Figure 11.47. Ultrasonographic images of chronic inflammation of the seminal vesicular glands without abscesses (A) and with abscesses (B) in a buck. A: Discrete chronic inflammation and anechoic areas (arrows) in the vesicular gland (1); B: Abscessed seminal vesicular glands showing large areas of pus accumulation (arrow).

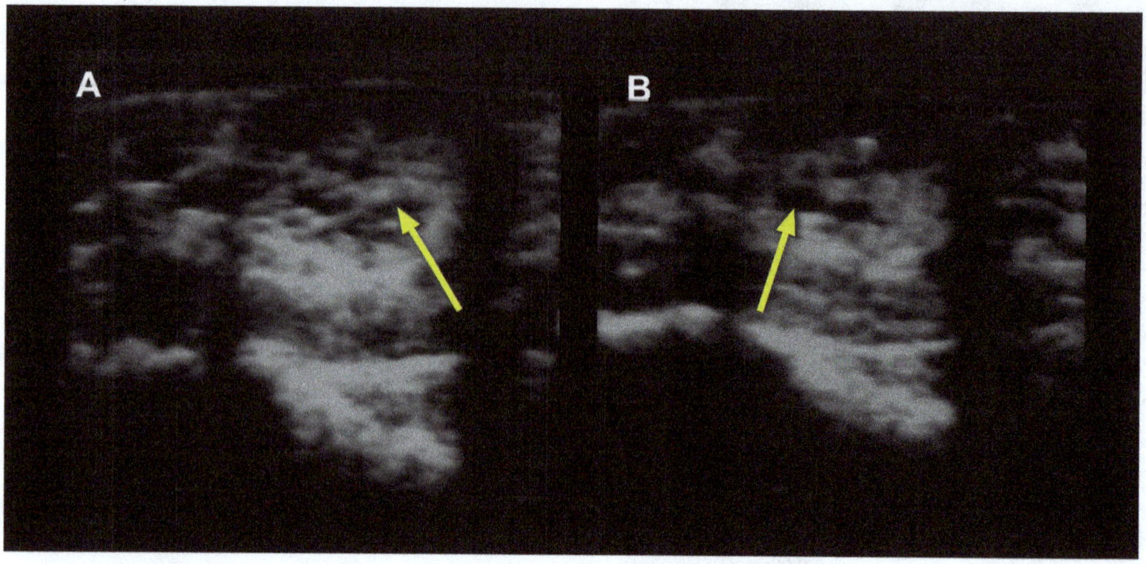

Figure 11.48. Ultrasonographic image of chronic inflammation in the bulbourethral glands of a buck. Chronic inflammation and anechoic areas (arrows) in both bulbourethral glands. A: Left gland; B: Right gland.

Common Abnormalities of the Accessory Glands

Transrectal ultrasonography is also used for evaluation of internal accessory glands (Figure 11.46).

The most common anomalies visualized by ultrasonographic examination in small ruminants are acute and chronic seminal vesicular and bulbourethral gland inflammations, usually associated with orchitis and epididymitis. The most common pattern of inflammation in both bulbourethral and seminal vesicular glands is mixed and heterogeneous, with anechogenic foci indicative of the presence of abscesses (Figures 11.47, 11.48).

References

1. Blache D, Zhang S, Martin GB (2003). Fertility in male sheep: modulators of the acute effects of nutrition on the reproductive axis of male sheep. Reproduction 61 Supplement.
2. Boundy T (1992). Routine ram examination. In Pract 14: 219–228.
3. Buckrell BC (1988). Applications of ultrasonography in reproduction in sheep and goats. Theriogenology 29(1): 71–84.
4. Coubrough CA, Castell MC (1998). Fetal sex determination by ultrasonically locating the genital tubercule in ewes. Theriogenology 50: 263–267.
5. Ginther OJ, Kot K (1994). Follicular dynamics during the ovulatory season in goats. Theriogenology 42: 987–1001.
6. Gonzalez de Bulnes A, Moreno JS, Brunet AG, Lopez-Sebastian A (2000). Relationship between ultrasonographic assessment of the corpus luteum and plasma progesterone concentration during the oestrous cycle in monovulvar ewes. Reproduct Domest Anim 35(2): 65–68.
7. Gonzalez de Bulnes A, Santiago Moreno J, Lopez-Sebastian A (1998). Estimation of fetal development in Manchega dairy ewes by transrectal ultrasonographic measurements. Small Rumin Res 52: 243–250.
8. Hauser B, Bostedt H (2002). Ultrasonographic observations of the uterine regression in the ewe under different obstetrical conditions. J Vet Med 49(10): 511–516.
9. Kähn W (1994). Veterinary Reproductive Ultrasonography. Mosby, Germany.
10. Martin GB, Milton JT, Davidson RH, Banchero Hunzicker GE, Lindsay DR, Blache D (2004). Natural methods for increasing reproductive efficiency in small ruminants. Anim Reprod Sci 82–83: 231–245.
11. Santiago Moreno J, Gomez-Brunet A, Gonzalez de Bulnes A, Toledano-Diaz A, Malpaux B, Lopez-Sebastian A (2005). Differences in reproductive pattern between wild and domestic rams are not associated with inter-specific annual variations in plasma prolactin

and melatonin concentrations. Domest Anim Endocrinol 28: 416–429.
12. Santos M, E.P. M, Bezerra F, Moura R, Paula-Lopes FF, Neves F, Lima JP, Oliveira M (2007). Early fetal sexing of Saanen goats by use of transrectal ultrasonography to identify the genital tubercle and external genitalia. Amer J Vet Res 68(5): 561–564.
13. Schrick FN, Inskeep EK (1993). Determination of early pregnancy in ewes utilizing transrectal ultrasonography. Theriogenology 40: 295–306.
14. Simoes J, Almeida JC, Valentim R, Baril G, Azevedo J, Fontes P, Mascarenhas R (2006). Follicular dynamics in Serrana goats. Anim Reprod Sci 95: 1–2, 16–26.
15. Simoes J, Potes J, Azevedo J, Almeida JC, Fontes P, Baril G, Mascarenhas R (2005). Morphometry of ovarian structures by transrectal ultrasonography in Serrana goats. Anim Reprod Sci 85 (3–4): 263–273.
16. Viñoles C (2003). Effect of nutrition on follicle development and ovulation rate in the ewe. Department of Clinical Chemistry. Uppsala ISSN:1401–6257. ISBN: 91-576-6650-4, Doctor of Philosophy. Swedish University of Agricultural Sciences. PhD: 120.
17. Wehrend A, Bostedt H, Burkhardt E (2002). The use of trans-abdominal B-mode ultrasonography to diagnose intra-partum uterine torsion in the ewe. Vet J 164 (1): 69–70.

Points to Remember

- B-mode ultrasonography has led to major breakthroughs in our understanding of basic reproductive physiology and has had a great impact on the reproductive management of small ruminants in the field.
- Appropriate use of ultrasonography requires thorough knowledge of the anatomy of the reproductive tract and the physiological processes that control reproductive function, because the images change with changes in the reproductive status of the animals.
- Selection of appropriate equipment and technique is critical for producing accurate observations and diagnoses.
- The transrectal technique is the only option for studying the accessory glands in the male, and it is also the best choice for pregnancy diagnosis 30–45 days after conception.
- The transabdominal technique is the best choice for the diagnosis of single or multiple pregnancies between 45 and 85 days after conception because it combines speed and accuracy.
- The expertise of the operator is crucial in the interpretation of the images, so extensive training is required.
- Ultrasonography is a useful tool for the diagnosis of reproductive pathologies in both male and female small ruminants.

Summary Questions

FEMALE

1. Which of the following statements regarding the structures of the urogenital system is true?
   a. The bladder is an irrelevant structure when working with the transrectal ultrasound technique.
   b. The cervix can be easily seen by ultrasound.
   c. Follicles are seen as gray structures and CLs as black structures.
   d. The ovaries are larger and easier to find during the breeding season.

2. When measuring ovulation rate, it is important to remember that
   a. The accuracy for detecting double ovulations is 100% throughout the estrous cycle.
   b. All CL present similar images.
   c. A CL with a large cavity can be mistaken for a large anovulatory follicle.
   d. CLs with cavities are associated with pathological processes.

3. Pregnancy can be diagnosed by
   a. Transrectal ultrasonography from day 20.
   b. Transabdominal ultrasonography from day 45 to 85.
   c. Transvaginal ultrasonography after day 90.
   d. The selection of the technique and times from conception are not relevant to accuracy of the diagnosis.

4. To detect multiple pregnancies it is crucial to
   a. Fast the ewes for 24 hours.
   b. Have an appraisal session with an expert and practice on 50 ewes.
   c. Detect one head and one trunk.
   d. Make sure that the same body structure is seen twice using the appropriate methodology.

MALE

5. Testes and accessory glands of small ruminants may be observed by
   a. Transrectal examination.
   b. Transcutaneous examination.
   c. Both transrectal and transcutaneous examination.
   d. Transcutaneous and transrectal examination, respectively.

6. Which are the most common testicular pathologies that can be observed by transcutaneous ultrasonography in a buck?
   a. Orchitis and spermatocele
   b. Orchitis and epididymal cysts
   c. Orchitis and epididymitis
   d. Orchitis and infarct of the testis

7. In small ruminants which internal accessory glands of the male can be observed by ultrasonography?
   a. Seminal vesicular and bulbourethral glands
   b. Prostate and bulbourethral glands
   c. Prostate and seminal vesicular glands
   d. Seminal vesicular glands and rete testis

Answers

1. d
2. c
3. b
4. d
5. d
6. c
7. a

CHAPTER TWELVE

CAMELIDS

Víctor H. Parraguez, Gregg Adams, Marcelo Ratto, and Luis A. Raggi

USEFULNESS OF ULTRASONOGRAPHY IN CAMELIDS

Real-time B-mode ultrasonic scanning has been demonstrated to be a very useful technique for the evaluation of the reproductive status in female camelids. Currently the main uses of this technique are

- Reproductive tract evaluation
- Pregnancy diagnosis
- Estimation of the fetal age
- Evaluation of fetal growth and fetal viability

There are also other specific, but less frequent, uses of ultrasonography in female camelids:

- Follicular and uterine dynamic evaluation
- Detection of ovulation
- Evaluation of superovulatory treatments
- Follicular aspiration

The introduction of ultrasound scanning for reproductive management has been shown to improve the pregnancy rate from 50–60% up to 85–90% in camelid herds located in their site of origin, the Andean highlands.

EQUIPMENT AND SCANNING TECHNIQUES

Ultrasound equipment

The criteria for selecting a specific scanner are cost, image quality and resolution, external power source, and portability. Based on the experience of one author, there is a direct relationship between the cost and durability of the equipment. Important issues to consider for use under farm conditions is the capability of working with a dual power supply (DC/AC) and the capability of connecting different types of probes to the ultrasound unit. For transrectal use, a slim linear- or convex-array or curvilinear probe with a frequency between 5 and 7.5 MHz is ideal. These characteristics ensure a clear and well-defined image with sufficient depth penetration to examine the entire female reproductive tract.

Restraint and technique

Llamas and alpacas are usually docile and amenable to ultrasonographic examination and other management procedures. Examination of the reproductive tract may be done transrectally or transabdominally, but the transrectal approach is preferable (Figure 12.1). Examination is usually done without sedation, with the animal restrained manually or in a chute, and may be done with the animal in a standing or recumbent position (Figures 12.1, 12.2). The probe may be introduced into the rectum with a gloved hand, as in transrectal palpation, in most adult llamas and many adult alpacas, particularly if multiparous. However, in young or small females, the pelvic space may be too small for intrarectal placement of the hand of the examiner, so the use of a rigid probe extension of the probe is very effective (e.g., PCV pipe ~2.0 to 2.5 cm diameter and 40 cm in length; Figures 12.2, 12.3). With experience, it may become easier and quicker to use an extended probe in all animals. Before the probe is introduced into the rectum, it should be lubricated using ultrasonographic gel or vegetable oil. Although it is not necessary, a plastic sleeve around the probe may provide additional protection against wear and tear (Figure 12.2).

Ultrasound examination of the pregnant female has not been associated with embryo loss or abortion[11].

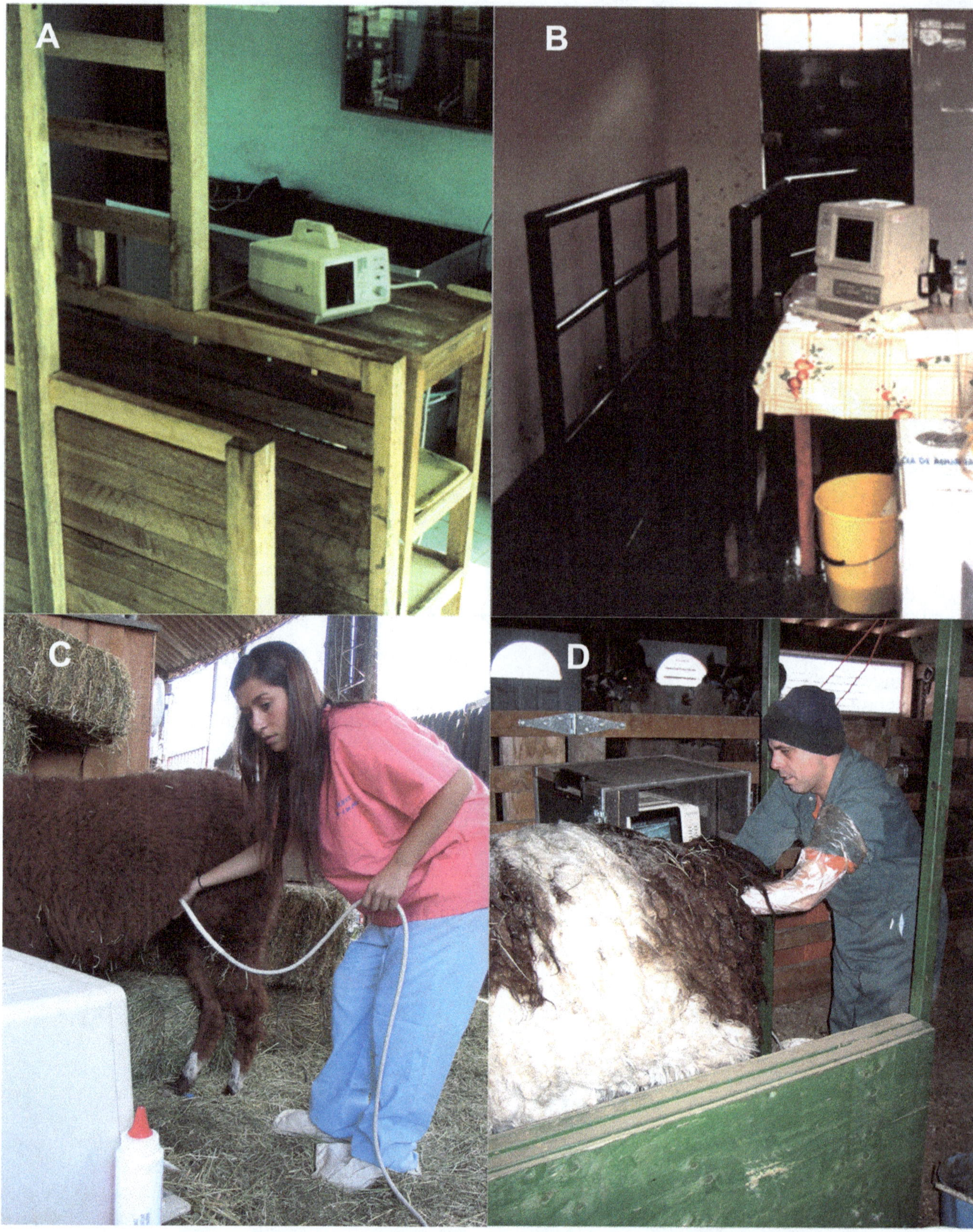

Figure 12.1. Restraint and technique for ultrasonographic examination of the reproductive tract in llamas and alpacas. Examples of restraint chutes are shown in (A) and (B). A transabdominal (C) or transrectal (D) approach may be used to evaluate the reproductive tract of camelids with the use of ultrasound.

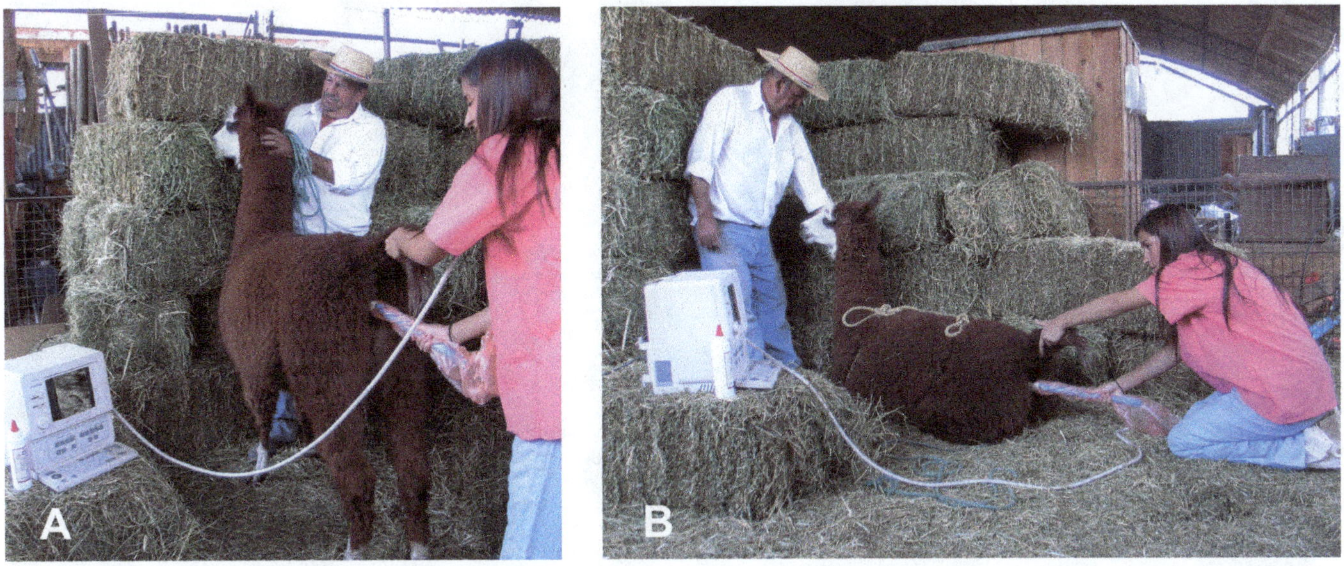

Figure 12.2. Ultrasonographic examination of the reproductive tract of a female alpaca. Note that a rigid probe extension is demonstrated and that the female may remain standing (A) or assume sternal recumbency (B) during examination.

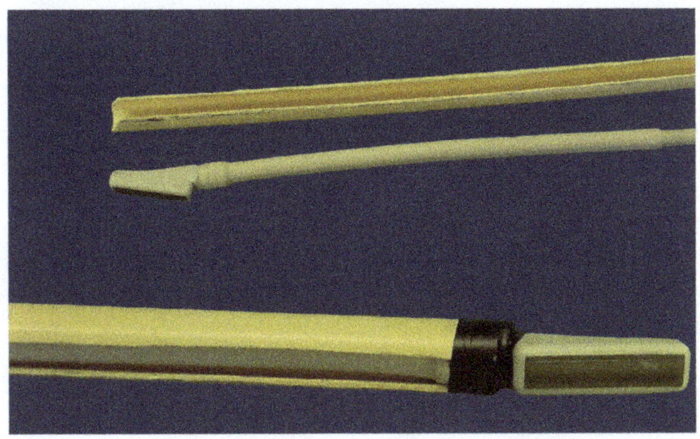

Figure 12.3. Rigid PCV extension of the probe for a linear-array ultrasound transducer designed for intrarectal use in llamas and alpacas.

Ultrasonographic Anatomy

The ultrasonographic appearance of the ovary, uterus, and cervix is illustrated in Figure 12.4. Similar to other domestic species, the uterus of the alpaca and llama is bicornuate, but the left uterine horn is slightly longer than the right (7.9 ± 1.3 cm versus 7.4 ± 0.9 cm), even in nulliparous animals. Llama and alpaca ovaries are round to oval and globular in shape, containing numerous follicles on the surface. Ovarian size depends on the structures present, but in general the average length of the ovaries is 1.8 cm. Several fluid-filled follicles ranging in diameter from 2 to 10 mm, in the presence or absence of a corpus luteum (CL), may be detected in the ovaries at any given time. Follicles are characteristically arranged along the periphery of the ovary and large follicles and the corpus luteum protrude distinctly from the ovarian surface. The preovulatory follicle grows at a mean rate of 0.8 mm/day and the average diameter on the day before ovulation is 10 mm. Ovulation occurs on average 29 hours after mating[13] and may take place at any spot on the surface of the ovary. The mature corpus luteum is 11 to 13 mm in diameter and is characteristically a well-delineated hypoechogenic structure with a white (echogenic) horizontal area in the center (Figures 12.4C, 12.6EF). The echotexture of the uterus and the cervix is darker during follicular dominance than during luteal domi-

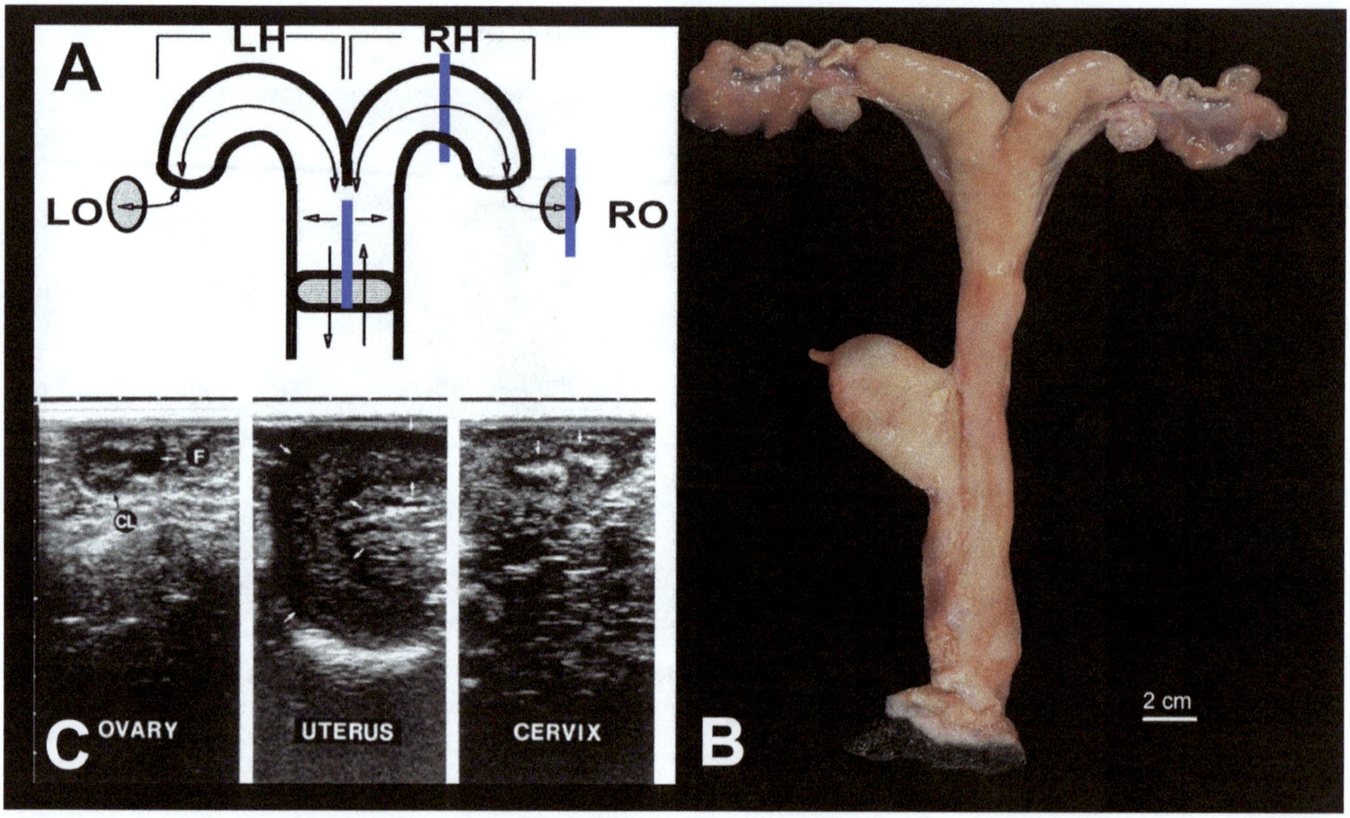

Figure 12.4. Scanning sequence (A) and the gross (B) and ultrasonographic (C) anatomy of the reproductive tract of female llamas and alpacas. Reproduced with permission of Elsevier Limited. Previously published in *Current Therapy in Large Animal Theriogenology* and modified from Sumar J and Adams GP, 2007[15]. B: The oviducts are long and tortuous and end in an open bursa that normally covers the ovary. The tip of the uterine horns is blunt and rounded, unlike other ruminants in which it tapers slowly toward the uterotubal junction. Accordingly, the oviduct of alpacas and llamas opens into the uterine horns via a small, raised papilla, which acts as a well-defined sphincter. The vagina is deceptively long and commonly exceeds 20 cm. C: By ultrasonography, the cervical folds appear as transverse echogenic bands, and they are especially prominent during the luteal phase and pregnancy. Curling of the uterine horns is greater for the left horn than for the right horn and is greater during the luteal phase and pregnancy than during the follicular phase. Profound uterine turgidity occurs during follicular dominance. CL: Corpus luteum; F: Follicle.

Table 12.1.
Morphologic dynamics of the reproductive tract of female llamas and alpacas during the follicular and luteal phases (adapted from Adams et al. 1989)

	Follicular Dominance	Luteal Dominance
Prevailing ovarian hormone	Estrogen	Progesterone
Ovaries	Preovulatory follicle	Corpus luteum
Uterine horn shape	Minimum curl	Maximum curl
Uterine echotexture	Heterogeneous, becoming dark	Homogeneous, gray
Uterine tone	Turgid	Flaccid
Cervical echotexture	Folds indistinct (gray)	Folds distinct (black)

nance, indicative of an increase in intercellular fluid (edema) during follicular dominance.

Changes in appearance of the reproductive tract in accordance to follicular or luteal dominance are shown in Table 12.1.

Ovarian Function and Endocrinology in South American Camelids

Ovarian follicular dynamics

Llamas and alpacas are species in which ovulation depends upon mating—i.e., copulation induces ovulation. Hence, they do not have regular estrous cycles as in other ruminants. Instead they have a continuous follicular phase, during which the female is sexually receptive to the male. This is interrupted by a luteal phase if mating and ovulation occurs, during which the female is nonreceptive. If mating and subsequent ovulation results in pregnancy, the luteal phase persists throughout pregnancy and the female remains nonreceptive. If mating and subsequent ovulation does not result in pregnancy, the luteal phase lasts approximately 10 days, after which the female once again becomes receptive. Ovarian follicular development occurs in a wave pattern during both follicular and luteal phases. As in other ruminants, a wave of follicular development is characterized by synchronous growth of a group of follicles followed by continued growth of a single dominant follicle (selection) and regression of the remaining subordinate follicles[3,16] (Figure 12.5).

The use of ultrasonography has revealed that dominant follicles grow to a maximum diameter of 10 to

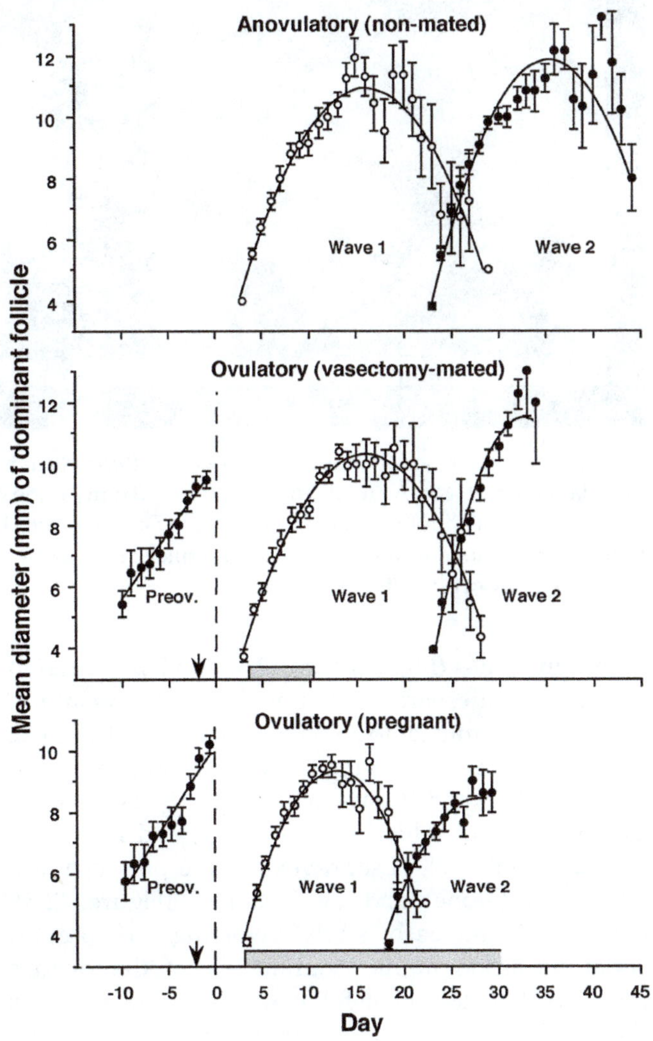

Figure 12.5. Mean (±SEM) diameter of the dominant follicle for anovulatory (top), ovulatory nonpregnant (middle), and ovulatory pregnant (bottom) llamas. Reproduced with permission of BioScientifica, member of the STM Agreement accessible at http://www.stm-assoc.org/stm-permission-guidelines. From Adams et al. 1990[3]. The arrow indicates the day of mating (Day 0 = day of ovulation) and the lightly shaded bars indicate the days of detection of the corpus luteum for the ovulatory groups.

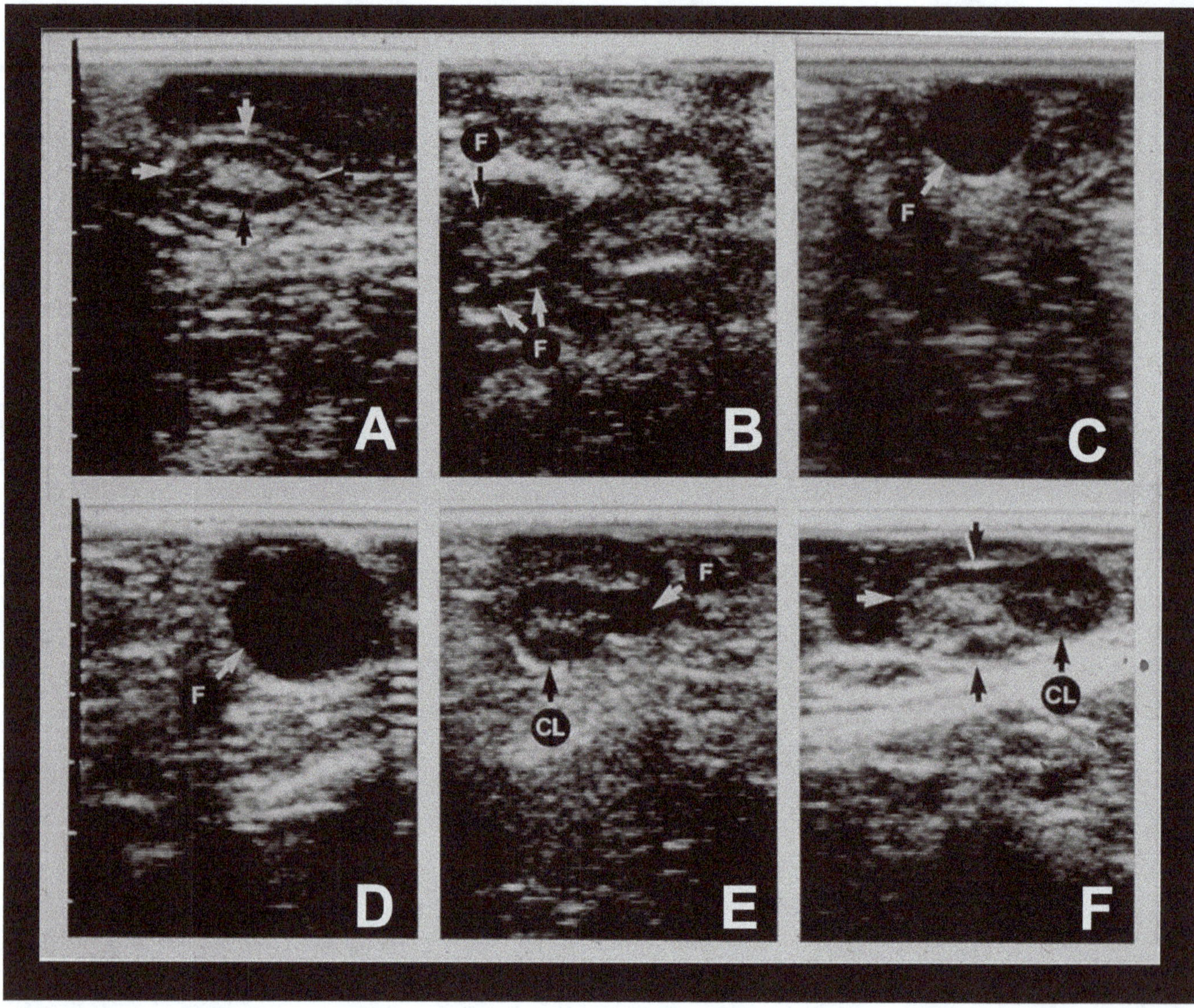

Figure 12.6. Ultrasonograms of llama ovaries. Reproduced with permission from *Biology of Reproduction*, originally published by Adams et al. 1989[2]. A and B: Small follicles (≤3 mm) at the periphery of the ovary. Periphery of ovary is indicated by arrows; C: Ovulatory-sized follicle (14 mm diameter); D: Oversized dominant follicle that failed to ovulate (22 mm); E: Corpus luteum with central echogenic area and adjacent follicle; F: Corpus luteum protruding from ovary. Periphery of ovary is indicated by arrows. CL = Corpus luteum; F = Follicle.

15 mm in llamas (Figures 12.5, 12.6) and 7 to 12 mm in alpacas. The lifespan of the anovulatory dominant follicles ranged from 20 to 25 days in llamas and 15 to 22 days in alpacas with an interwave interval of approximately 20 days and 16 days in the respective species[3,9,16]. The duration of follicular dominance, and hence the interwave interval, is shortened by the presence of a CL (progesterone) and by lactation[3] (Figure 12.5). Contrary to an early study involving laparoscopy, serial ultrasonographic examination of the ovaries revealed that dominant follicles of successive waves are equally as likely to develop in the same as in the opposite ovary—i.e., they do not regularly alternate between ovaries[3].

Reproductive endocrinology in camelids

Studies in which endocrine and ultrasonographic data were collected contemporaneously have validated the relationship of ultrasonographic dynamics of the ovaries with physiologic events. Several studies have reported circulating profiles of reproductive hormones in camelids, and the most consistent data are those of progesterone and estradiol concentrations. Maximum

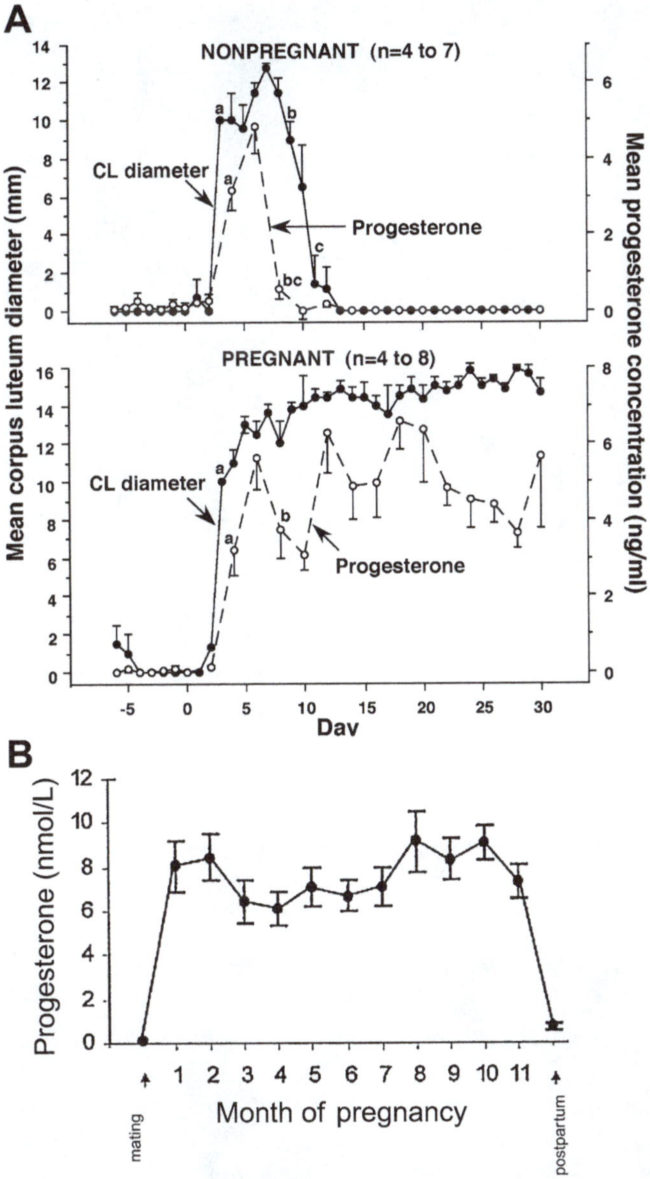

Figure 12.7. Ultrasonographic assessment of the CL and circulating concentrations of progesterone in llamas (A) and pregnant alpacas (B). Reproduced with permission of Animal Reproduction Science (Elsevier Limited) and modified from Adams et al. 1991a[4] and Raggi et al. 1999[12]. CL diameter: Diameter of the corpus luteum in mm; A (top): Chart is for nonpregnant llamas; A (bottom): Chart is for pregnant llamas; B: Chart is for pregnant alpacas.

plasma estradiol concentration (23 to 31 nmol/L) and urine estrone sulphate concentration (20 to 30 ng/mg creatinine) have been correlated with the maximum diameter of the dominant follicle[1,7]. Progesterone profiles (Figure 12.7) have also been well characterized in the nonpregnant luteal phase as well as during pregnancy[1,4,12]. Ultrasonographically detected CL diameter

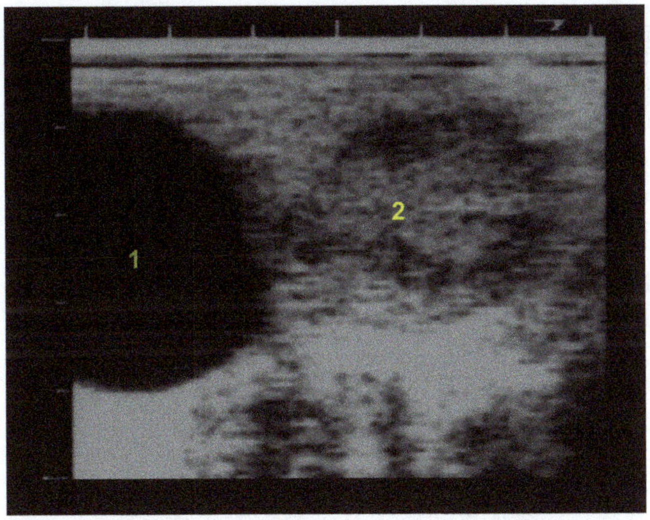

Figure 12.8. Urinary bladder (1) is observed as a well-defined anechoic structure. It is the most obvious landmark to localize the uterus (2) (5 MHz probe; depth 5 cm). The scale along the top of the image is in 1 cm increments.

is highly correlated with plasma progesterone concentration[4,13]. Maximum CL diameter and maximum plasma progesterone concentration were detected 7 to 9 days after mating in llamas, and the first significant decrease in CL diameter and plasma progesterone concentration during luteolysis in nonpregnant females occurred 11 and 10 days after mating, respectively. Regarding gonadotrophins, a significant increase in circulating LH concentration occurs 15–30 minutes after mating with a maximum concentration (4–6 ng/ml) at 2 hours[1,6–8]. Measurement of FSH in llamas and alpacas has provided equivocal data; a reliable assay for camelid FSH has yet to be established.

Pregnancy Diagnosis and Evaluation of Fetal Growth

Early pregnancy diagnosis by ultrasound

Pregnancy diagnosis using ultrasonography involves the recognition of uterine changes associated with the development of a gestational sac and embryo/fetal structures.

The nonpregnant uterine horns in camelids appears, in a transverse plane, as a spherical or ovoid structure with an intermediate echogenic density, located dorsal and cranial to the urinary bladder (Figure 12.8). The lumen of the normal, nongravid uterus (potential

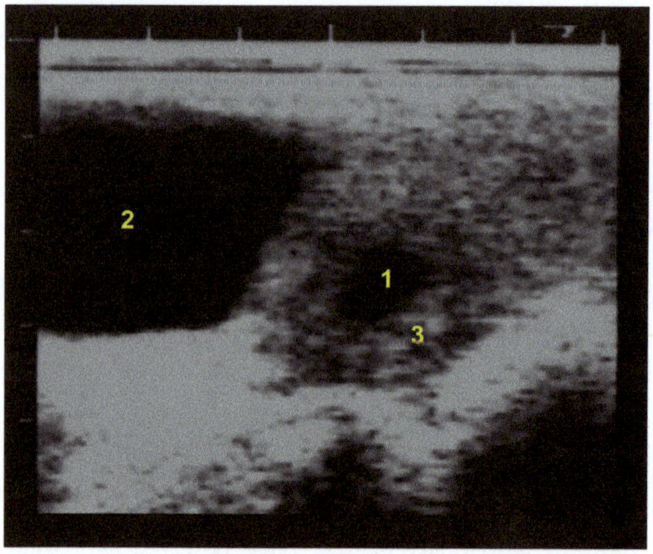

Figure 12.9. Ultrasonographic image of the gestational sac in a camelid pregnancy of 15 days (5 MHz probe; depth 5 cm). The gestational sac (1) is observed as an anechoic sphere in the central zone of the uterus. 1: Gestational sac; 2: Urinary bladder; 3: Uterus. The scale along the top of the image is in 1 cm increments.

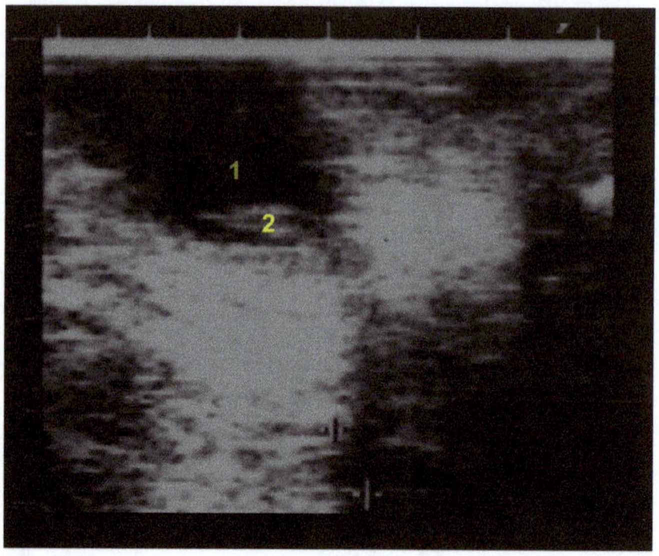

Figure 12.10. Ultrasonogram of a 25-day pregnancy in an alpaca (5 MHz probe; depth 5 cm). 1: Gestational sac (allantoic fluid); 2: Embryo located on the base of gestational sac. The scale along the top of the image is in 1 cm increments.

space) is not clearly distinguished by ultrasonography in these species. The earliest echographic sign of pregnancy is the appearance of a spherical dark structure (anechoic) with well-defined external limits, located at the center (lumen) of the uterus. This structure corresponds to the gestational sac (Figure 12.9). In alpacas and llamas, the gestational sac can be observed from day 10 after mating, with a diameter of 0.5 ± 0.04 and 0.54 ± 0.03 cm, respectively. At day 23 after mating this structure can be observed in 100% of the alpacas, with a diameter of about 1.0 ± 0.14 cm. In more than 90% of llamas, the gestational sac can be observed from day 21 after mating (diameter = 0.9 ± 0.03 cm) and in 100% of animals by day 34.

The daily growth of the gestational sac diameter between days 15 to 30 of pregnancy is about 0.9 mm in alpacas and llamas. By day 25 it is possible to observe the appearance of the embryo in both species. It appears as a small spot of high echogenic density (hyperechoic), usually occupying the basal zone of the gestational sac (Figure 12.10). By day 35 of pregnancy, the embryo may be clearly defined (Figure 12.11) and the appearance of the heartbeat at this gestational age is also an important echographic finding, both in alpacas and llamas[11].

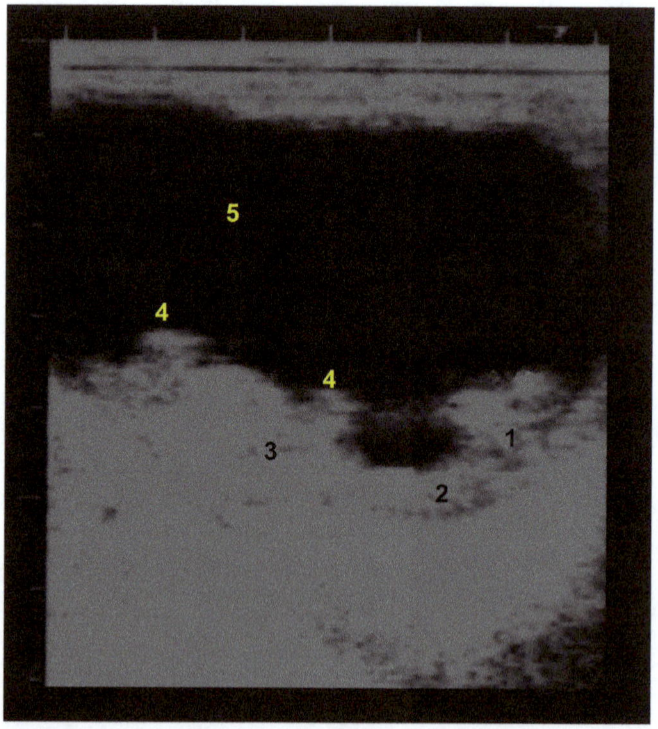

Figure 12.11. Ultrasonogram of a 35-day pregnancy in a llama (5 MHz probe; depth 7 cm). The fetus is clearly observed in the basal zone of the gestational sac. Note that the head, neck, trunk, and legs can be defined. 1: Head; 2: Neck; 3: Trunk; 4: Legs; 5: Allantoic fluid. The scale along the top of the image is in 1 cm increments.

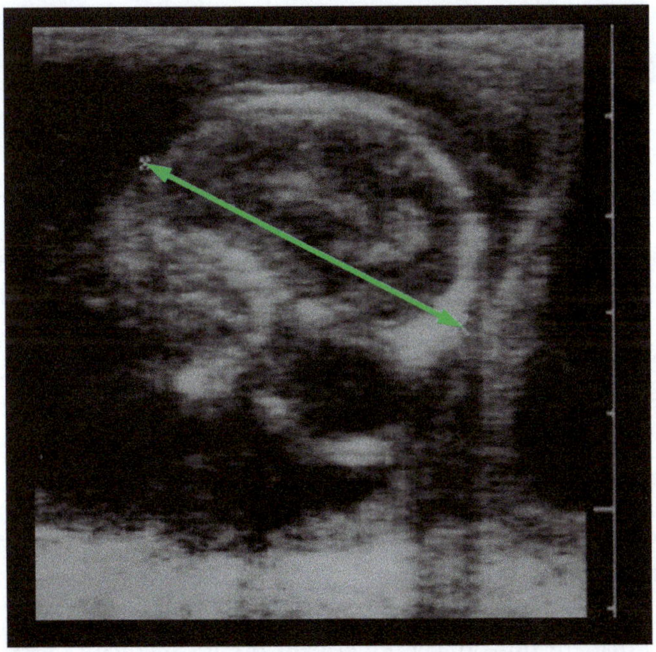

Figure 12.12. Ultrasonographic image of the head of a 165-day pregnancy in an alpaca (5 MHz probe; depth 6 cm). The calipers show the fetal biparietal diameter measurement (BPD = 3.6 cm). Equations for estimation of the gestational age (GA, measured in days) using fetal BPD (measured in centimeters) according to Gazitúa et al. 2001[10]. Alpacas: GA = (BPD-0.11376) 47.23287; $r = 0.98$; $P < 0.001$. Llamas: GA = (BPD-0.002399) 43.02293; $r = 0.98$; $P < 0.001$.

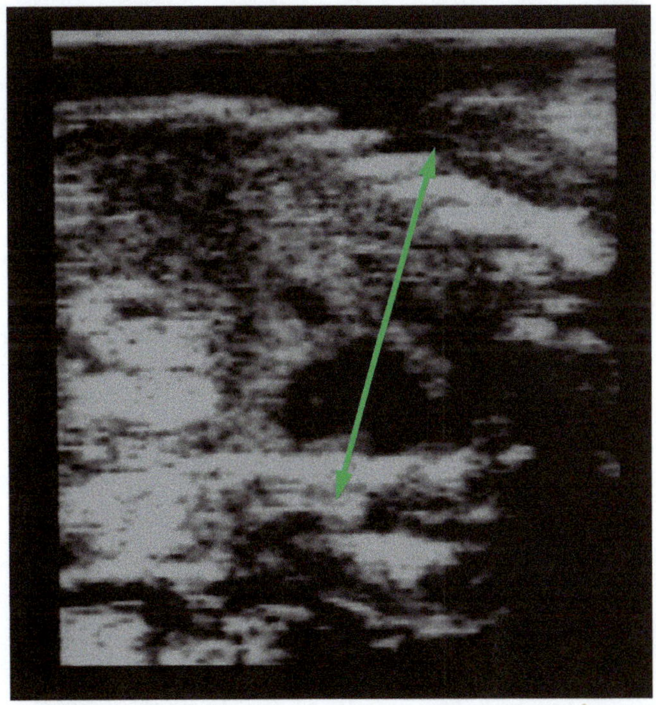

Figure 12.13. Ultrasonographic image of the thorax of a 173-day-old fetus in a llama (5 MHz probe; depth 7 cm). The calipers show the fetal thorax height measurement (TH = 3.8 cm). Note that the line defining the distance between the vertebral column and the sternum should cross the fetal heart. Equations for estimation of the gestational age (GA, measured in days) using the fetal TH (measured in centimeters) according to Gazitúa et al. 2001[10]. Alpacas: GA = (TH-0.36436) 52.87663; $r = 0.96$; $P < 0.001$. Llamas: GA = (TH-0.07137) 46.94485; $r = 0.95$; $P < 0.001$.

Ultrasound fetal growth evaluation

The ultrasound examination of the pregnant uterus allows discrimination among different anatomical structures of the fetus after the first month of pregnancy. It has been demonstrated in different species, including the domestic South American camelids, that the growth of some fetal biometric characteristics is well correlated with gestational age. The ultrasound measurements of these characteristics allow evaluation of fetal growth dynamics when the date of mating is known, or estimation of gestational age when the date of mating is unknown. Among the fetal biometrics characteristics observed by ultrasound are biparietal diameter (BPD) and thorax height (TH). BPD should be measured as the distance between the external edges of the temporoparietal bones, in a transversal plane to the occipitofrontal axis, selecting the largest and clearest image (Figure 12.12). TH should be measured as the distance between the external edges of the sternum and vertebral column, following the sagittal plane and crossing the middle of the heart (Figure 12.13). It has been found that BPD and TH show consistent correlation with fetal development at any gestational age in both alpacas and llamas. Although we have found a significant correlation between each attribute and gestational age (see legends for Figures 12.12, 12.13), the BPD is considered the best fetal biometric trait to estimate fetal growth or to determine gestational age in both species[10].

Uterine and Ovarian Abnormalities

In general, 15–20% of females exhibit some reproductive abnormality, either congenital or acquired[14].

Congenital uterine and ovarian abnormalities

Ovarian hypoplasia

This is the most common ovarian anomaly recorded in camelids[14]. It has been found in 16.8% of the infertile females and in 6.0% of females without reproductive history[14]. Hypoplastic ovaries are small (1 × 1.5 cm) and follicular development is suppressed or completely absent. During ultrasound examination it can be observed as a small ovary with scarce or no follicular development. This abnormality may be observed in one or both ovaries. When it is present in both ovaries, it is usually concomitant with uterine/vaginal hypoplasia and females are infertile.

Uterine/vaginal hypoplasia

This is the most common congenital anomaly of the reproductive tract of South American camelids. It is characterized by a significant reduction in diameter and length of the uterine body and horns. In normal herds it can be observed with a frequency less than 1%[14]. During ultrasound examination it can be detected by the small uterine horn diameter and dark (hypoechogenic) homogeneous uterine echotexture.

Uterus unicornis (one-horned uterus), segmental aplasia, and uterus didelphys

These anomalies have been described as incidental postmortem findings, with very low frequency[14]. These abnormalities may be readily apparent during routine ultrasound examinations or transrectal palpation.

Acquired uterine and ovarian abnormalities

Endometritis

Inflammation of the uterus is a common condition in llamas and alpacas[14]. Ultrasonographic signs of endometritis may include slight thickening of the uterine wall, small accumulations of anechoic intraluminal fluid, and irregular echotexture of the endometrium.

Pyometra

This condition is uncommon in llamas and alpacas, but data on the incidence and pathogenesis of the condition have not been reported. The condition may be predisposed by endometritis, but the authors have seen some cases that appeared to result from a cervical tear and subsequent closure. Ultrasonographically, the uterine lumen is distended to varying degrees by purulent fluid that may appear homogeneously black or contain a mixture of echogenic debris within otherwise nonechogenic (black) fluid. The echogenicity of the fluid is not necessarily indicative of the visual opacity or thickness of the purulent fluid.

Ovarian follicular cyst

The existence of an ovarian follicular cystic condition, as a clinical entity, remains equivocal in camelids.

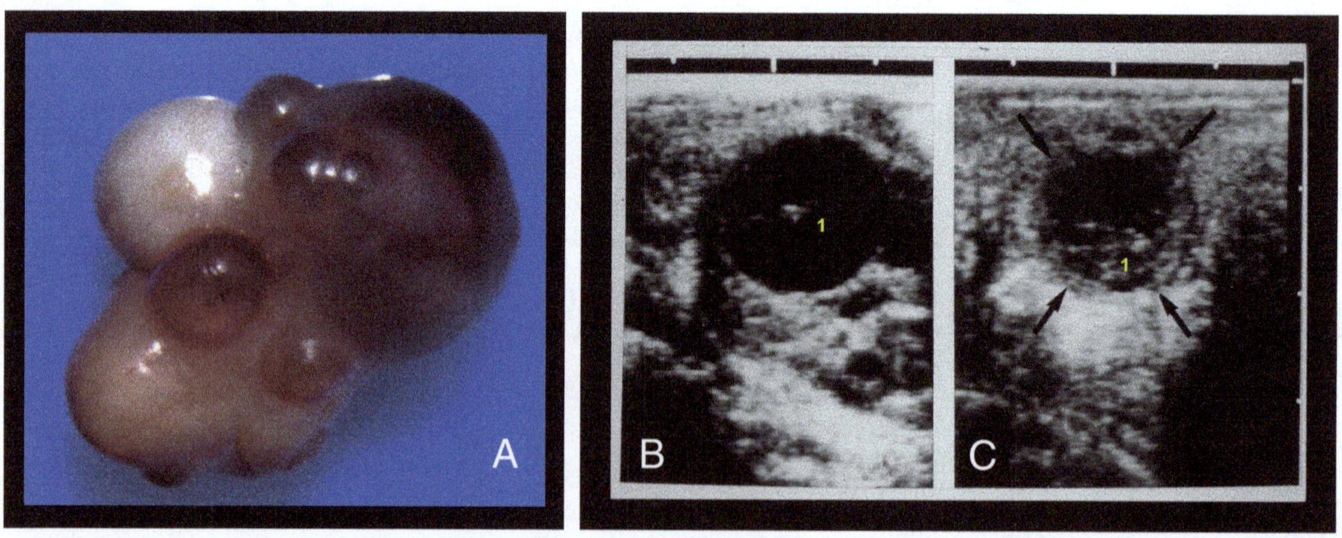

Figure 12.14. Gross (A) and ultrasonic appearance (B and C) of hemorrhagic follicles in llamas. Reproduced with permission of Theriogenology (Elsevier Limited) and modified from Adams et al. (1991b)[5]. B: Echogenic lines (1) in follicular antrum indicate fibrinous bands of a forming blood clot; C: Note the prominence of echogenic debris in the antrum (1) and thickened (apparently luteinized) follicle wall; arrows delineate outer follicle wall.

Based on older literature, follicles >12 mm in diameter were considered "cystic" and therefore subject to hormone treatment to correct the condition. However, based on later ultrasound studies, it appears that "cystic" follicles in llamas may have been overdiagnosed and overtreated in the past. The normal range in follicle diameter extended to 16 mm, and the mean (± SEM) maximum diameter of the dominant follicle was 12.1 ± 0.4 mm^3.

The readers are invited to consult Chapters 4 and 5 to visualize ultrasonographic images of acquired uterine and ovarian abnormalities.

Hemorrhagic follicles

Oversized (≥25 mm in diameter) hemorrhagic follicles are common in females that are not exposed to a male (16% of nonovulatory follicles; Figure 12.14). These oversized follicles contain bloody fluid and appear to be the result of a vascular accident as the dominant anovulatory follicle nears the end of the growing phase, resulting in leakage of blood into the antrum causing it to balloon to an oversized state. Ultrasonographically, the condition is characterized by scattered free-floating echogenic spots within the follicular antrum, which swirl upon ballottement. The antral contents may become organized and swirling may no longer occur. Hemorrhagic follicles become very large (up to 35 mm) and persist for a prolonged period (weeks); however, they resolve spontaneously and they do not disrupt ovarian function or fertility.

REFERENCES

1. Aba MA, Forsberg M, Kindhal H, Sumar J, Edqvist L (1995). Endocrine changes after mating in pregnant and non pregnant llamas and alpacas. Acta Vet Scand 36: 489–498.
2. Adams GP, Griffin PG, Ginther OJ (1989). In situ morphologic dynamics of ovaries, uterus and cervix in llamas. Biol Reprod 41: 551–558.
3. Adams GP, Sumar J, Ginther OJ (1990). Effects of lactational and reproductive status on ovarian follicular waves in llamas (*Lama glama*). J Reprod Fertil 90: 535–545.
4. Adams GP, Sumar J, Ginther OJ (1991a). Form and function of the corpus luteum in llamas. Anim Reprod Sci 24: 127–138.
5. Adams GP, Sumar J, Ginther OJ (1991b). Hemorrhagic ovarian follicles in llamas. Theriogenology 35: 557–568.
6. Adams GP, Ratto MH, Huanca W, Singh J (2005). Ovulation-inducing factor in the seminal plasma of alpacas and llamas. Biol Reprod 73: 452–457.
7. Bravo PW, Fowler ME, Stabenfeldt GH, Lasley BL (1990a). Ovarian follicular dynamics in the llama. Biol Reprod 43: 579–585.
8. Bravo PW, Fowler ME, Stabenfeldt GH (1990b). Endocrine response in the llama to copulation. Theriogenology 33: 891–899.
9. Chavez MG, Aba MA, Aguero A, Egey J, Berestin V, Rutter B (2002). Ovarian follicular wave pattern and the effect of exogenous progesterone on follicular activity in non-mated llamas. Anim Reprod Sci 69: 37–46.
10. Gazitúa FJ, Corradini P, Ferrando G, Raggi LA, Parraguez VH (2001). Prediction of gestational age by ultrasonic fetometry in llamas (*Lama glama*) and alpacas (*Lama Pacos*). Anim Reprod Sci 66: 81–92.
11. Parraguez VH, Cortéz S, Gazitúa FJ, Ferrando G, MacNiven V, Raggi LA (1997). Early pregnancy diagnosis in alpaca (*Lama pacos*) and llama (*Lama glama*) by ultrasound. Anim Reprod Sci 47: 113–121.
12. Raggi LA, Ferrando G, Parraguez VH, MacNiven V, Urquieta B (1999). Plasma progesterone in alpaca (*Lama pacos*) during pregnancy, parturition and early postpartum. Anim Reprod Sci 54: 245–249.
13. Ratto MH, Huanca W, Singh J, Adams GP (2006). Comparison of the effect of natural mating, LH, and GnRH on interval to ovulation and luteal function in llamas. Anim Reprod Sci 91: 299–306.
14. Sumar J (1989). Defectos congénitos y hereditarios en la alpaca. Teratología. Centro de Investigación IVITA. Gráfica Bellido, Lima, Perú.
15. Sumar J, Adams GP (2007). Reproductive anatomy and life cycle of the male and female llama and alpaca. In: Youngquist RS, Threlfall WR (Eds.), Current Therapy in Large Animal Theriogenology, 2nd Edition. Saunders Elsevier, St Louis MO, pp. 855–865.
16. Vaughan J, Macmillan KL, D'Occhio MJ (2004). Ovarian follicular wave characteristics in alpacas. Anim Reprod Sci 80: 353–361.

Points to Remember

- Real-time B-mode ultrasonic scanning is a very useful technique for reproductive status evaluation in female camelids, improving reproductive management and fertility rate. No pregnancy losses have been associated with ultrasound procedures.
- Camelids are usually docile, so ultrasonographic examination of the reproductive tract may be done with the animal restrained manually or in a chute, with the animal in a standing or recumbent position. The transrectal exam using of a rigid probe extension is easier and very effective.
- The ultrasound echotexture of the female reproductive tract changes with the follicular (estrogenic) or luteal (progestational) phases, being less echogenic and heterogeneous during the follicular phase. Follicles can be observed as dark spots at the periphery of the ovary. The corpus luteum is a well-delineated hypoechogenic structure with a white (echogenic) horizontal area in the center.
- Female camelids are induced ovulators, without regular estrous cycles. They have a continuous follicular phase (sexually receptive to the male), which is interrupted by a luteal phase if mating and ovulation occurs. Follicular development occurs in waves during both follicular and luteal phases. The dominant follicles grow to a maximum diameter of 10–15 mm in llamas and 7–12 mm in alpacas. The lifespan of anovulatory dominant follicles ranges from 20 to 25 days in llamas and 15 to 22 days in alpacas.
- Maximum diameter of the dominant follicle is correlated with maximum plasma estradiol concentration and urine estrone sulphate concentration. Maximum CL diameter and maximum plasma progesterone concentration are present at 7 to 9 days after mating in llamas. A significant decrease in CL diameter and plasma progesterone concentration during luteolysis in nonpregnant females occurs 11 and 10 days after mating, respectively.
- The earliest echographic sign of pregnancy (gestational sac) can be observed at day 23 after mating in 100% of alpacas and at day 21 in more than 90% of the llamas. The earliest image of the embryo can be observed at day 25 in both species. By day 35 of pregnancy the embryo may be well defined, and the appearance of the heartbeat is also an important echographic finding.
- Ultrasound is also a powerful tool for evaluating intrauterine fetal growth and well-being. Ultrasonographic measurement of embryo-fetal biometric characteristics may also allow estimation of gestational age or probable date of parturition.

Summary Questions

1. Beginning at which age is it possible to recognize the fetal camelid head, trunk, and legs using ultrasound?
   a. 15 days
   b. 25 days
   c. 35 days
   d. 45 days

2. Identify the fetal structure observed in the center of the following image:
   a. Head
   b. Thorax
   c. Abdomen
   d. Neck

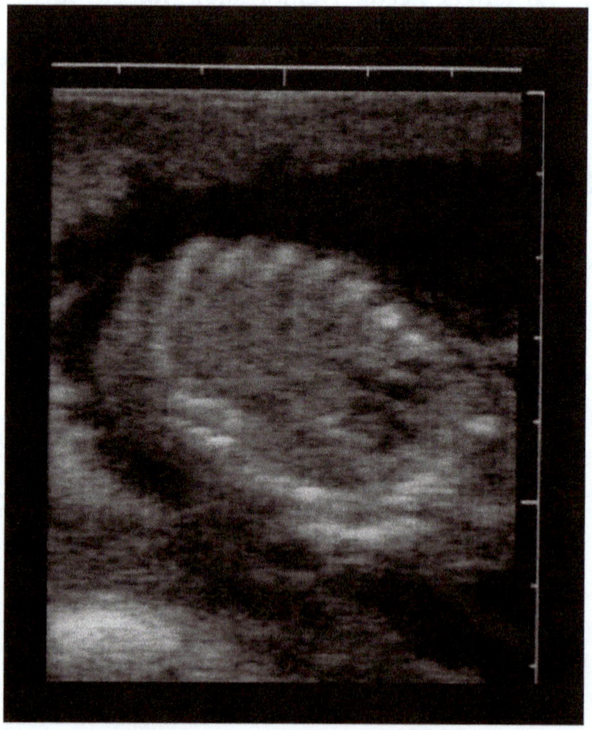

3. According to the appearance of the alpaca gestational sac shown in this image, what is the gestational age?
   a. Less than 10 days
   b. Between 10 and 24 days
   c. Between 25 and 34 days
   d. a, b, and c are false because the image does not show a gestational sac.

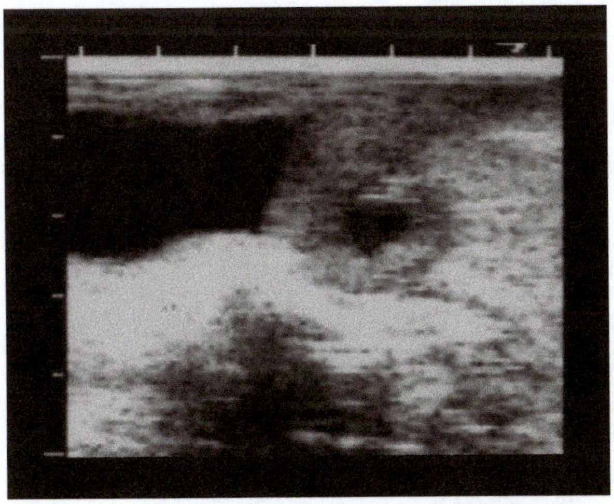

4. By using fetal biparietal diameter (BPD = 3.5 cm), give an estimation of gestational age in this image obtained from a pregnant llama.
   a. 50 days
   b. 75 days
   c. 125 days
   d. 150 days

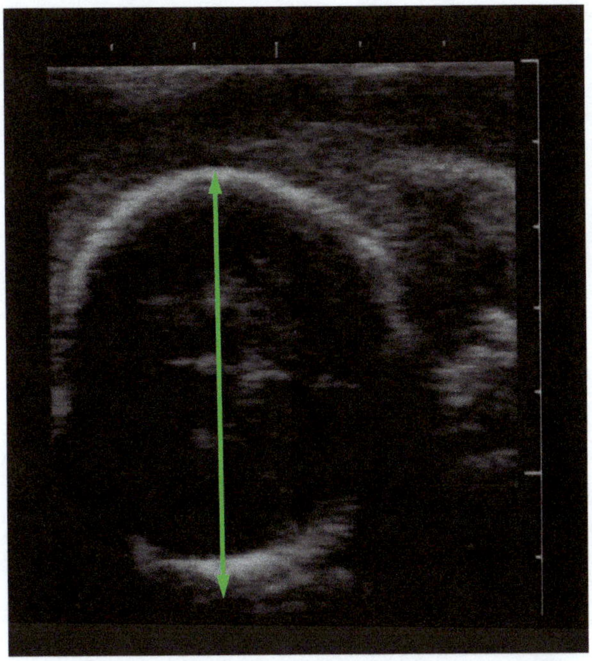

5. How long does the luteal phase in nonpregnant llamas last?
   a. 10 days
   b. 15 days
   c. 20 days
   d. None of the above

6. The interwave interval in alpacas is
   a. Longer than llamas
   b. Shorter than llamas
   c. Similar to llamas
   d. None of above

7. Luteolysis in the nonpregnant llama female occurs
   a. On day 8 after mating
   b. On day 10 after mating
   c. On day 12 after mating
   d. On day 14 after mating

Answers

1. c
2. b
3. b
4. d
5. a
6. b
7. c

INDEX

Printed in the USA/Agawam, MA
August 20, 2026

909404.003